The Pediatric Eye Exam Quick Reference Guide:

Office and Emergency Room Procedures

Lily Zhu-Tam
Citywide Eye Care Optometry, USA

Ida Chung
College of Optometry, Western University of Health Sciences, USA

A volume in the Advances in Medical Diagnosis, Treatment, and Care (AMDTC) Book Series

IGI Global
PUBLISHER of TIMELY KNOWLEDGE

Published in the United States of America by
IGI Global
Medical Information Science Reference (an imprint of IGI Global)
701 E. Chocolate Avenue
Hershey PA, USA 17033
Tel: 717-533-8845
Fax: 717-533-8661
E-mail: cust@igi-global.com
Web site: http://www.igi-global.com

Library of Congress Cataloging-in-Publication Data

Names: Zhu-Tam, Lily, 1978- editor. | Chung, Ida, 1967- editor.
Title: The pediatric eye exam quick reference guide : office and emergency room procedures / [edited] by Lily Zhu-Tam and Ida Chung.
Description: Hershey, PA : Medical Information Science Reference, [2022] | Includes bibliographical references and index. | Summary: "This reference book is a clinical procedure book that provides step-by-step pediatric eye care examination techniques and will serve as a great learning and teaching tool for all eye care professionals"-- Provided by publisher.
Identifiers: LCCN 2021061137 (print) | LCCN 2021061138 (ebook) | ISBN 9781799880448 (hardcover) | ISBN 9781799880455 (ebook)
Subjects: MESH: Eye Diseases--diagnosis | Child | Infant | Adolescent | Diagnostic Techniques, Ophthalmological | Handbook
Classification: LCC RE48.2.C5 (print) | LCC RE48.2.C5 (ebook) | NLM WW 39 | DDC 618.92/0977--dc23/eng/20211227
LC record available at https://lccn.loc.gov/2021061137
LC ebook record available at https://lccn.loc.gov/2021061138

This book is published in the IGI Global book series Advances in Medical Diagnosis, Treatment, and Care (AMDTC) (ISSN: 2475-6628; eISSN: 2475-6636)

British Cataloguing in Publication Data
A Cataloguing in Publication record for this book is available from the British Library.

Advances in Medical Diagnosis, Treatment, and Care (AMDTC) Book Series

ISSN:2475-6628
EISSN:2475-6636

Mission

Advancements in medicine have prolonged the life expectancy of individuals all over the world. Once life-threatening conditions have become significantly easier to treat and even cure in many cases. Continued research in the medical field will further improve the quality of life, longevity, and wellbeing of individuals.

The **Advances in Medical Diagnosis, Treatment, and Care (AMDTC)** book series seeks to highlight publications on innovative treatment methodologies, diagnosis tools and techniques, and best practices for patient care. Comprised of comprehensive resources aimed to assist professionals in the medical field apply the latest innovations in the identification and management of medical conditions as well as patient care and interaction, the books within the AMDTC series are relevant to the research and practical needs of medical practitioners, researchers, students, and hospital administrators.

Coverage

- Experimental Medicine
- Disease Management
- Emergency Medicine
- Medical Procedures
- Internal Medicine
- Medical Testing
- Diagnostic Medicine
- Patient Interaction
- Critical Care
- Disease Prevention

IGI Global is currently accepting manuscripts for publication within this series. To submit a proposal for a volume in this series, please contact our Acquisition Editors at Acquisitions@igi-global.com or visit: http://www.igi-global.com/publish/.

The Advances in Medical Diagnosis, Treatment, and Care (AMDTC) Book Series (ISSN 2475-6628) is published by IGI Global, 701 E. Chocolate Avenue, Hershey, PA 17033-1240, USA, www.igi-global.com. This series is composed of titles available for purchase individually; each title is edited to be contextually exclusive from any other title within the series. For pricing and ordering information please visit http://www.igi-global.com/book-series/advances-medical-diagnosis-treatment-care/129618. Postmaster: Send all address changes to above address.

Titles in this Series

For a list of additional titles in this series, please visit: www.igi-global.com/book-series

Medical Atlas of Cornea and External Diseases in Middle Eastern Populations
Anna Hovakimyan (Malayan Ophthalmologic Centre, Armenia)
Medical Information Science Reference • © 2022 • 507pp • H/C (ISBN: 9781799869375) • US $265.00

Using Narrative Writing to Enhance Healing During and After Global Health Crises
Jennifer Lynne Bird (Oxbridge Academy, USA)
Medical Information Science Reference • © 2022 • 241pp • H/C (ISBN: 9781799890515) • US $295.00

Handbook of Research on Pathophysiology and Strategies for the Management of COVID-19
Omar El Hiba (Chouaib Doukkali University, Morocco) Jayakumar Radhakrishnan (Veterans Affairs Medical Center, USA) Tiziano Balzano (University Hospital HM Puerta del Sur, Spain) and Faical Isbaine (Emory University, USA)
Medical Information Science Reference • © 2022 • 352pp • H/C (ISBN: 9781799882251) • US $425.00

Strategies to Overcome Superbug Invasions Emerging Research and Opportunities
Dimple Sethi Chopra (Punjabi University, India) and Ankur Kaul (Institute of Nuclear Medicine and Allied Sciences, India)
Medical Information Science Reference • © 2021 • 319pp • H/C (ISBN: 9781799803072) • US $225.00

Integrated Care and Fall Prevention in Active and Healthy Aging
Patrik Eklund (Umea University, Sweden)
Medical Information Science Reference • © 2021 • 348pp • H/C (ISBN: 9781799844112) • US $345.00

Cases on Applied and Therapeutic Humor
Michael K. Cundall Jr. (North Carolina A&T State University, USA) and Stephanie Kelly (North Carolina A&T State University, USA)
Medical Information Science Reference • © 2021 • 267pp • H/C (ISBN: 9781799845287) • US $255.00

Artificial Intelligence for Accurate Analysis and Detection of Autism Spectrum Disorder
Sandeep Kautish (Lord Buddha Education Foundation, Nepal & Asia Pacific University of Technology & Innovation, Malaysia) and Gaurav Dhiman (Government Bikram College of Commerce, India)
Medical Information Science Reference • © 2021 • 224pp • H/C (ISBN: 9781799874607) • US $295.00

Diagnostic and Treatment Methods for Ulcerative Colitis and Colitis-Associated Cancer
Ashok Kumar Pandurangan (B. S. Abdur Rahman Crescent Institute of Science and Technology, India)
Medical Information Science Reference • © 2021 • 309pp • H/C (ISBN: 9781799835806) • US $295.00

IGI Global
PUBLISHER of TIMELY KNOWLEDGE

701 East Chocolate Avenue, Hershey, PA 17033, USA
Tel: 717-533-8845 x100 • Fax: 717-533-8661
E-Mail: cust@igi-global.com • www.igi-global.com

This book is dedicated to my family for their unconditional love and support. I could not have done it without their understanding.
Lily Zhu-Tam

I dedicate this book project to my students, mentors, and other pediatric eye doctors who have changed the lives of countless children and who will continue to do so every day.
Ida Chung

Table of Contents

Detailed Table of Contents

Section 1
History

A pediatric case history is essential before proceeding with an examination. This section will focus on birth, developmental, educational, and social histories, as well as active listening skills and flexibility of the clinician for an effective start to the examination. Clinical pearls are provided within the chapter for a more efficient and effective eye exam, including a section on assisting children with special needs.

The art of taking a patient's case history is essential for a solid understanding of pertinent details before proceeding with an examination. While establishing rapport with the patient, the clinician should ask questions about birth history, developmental history, educational and social history. Active listening skills and flexibility of the provider are useful tools for an effective start to the examination. This chapter reviews categories of questions needed for optimization of case history for the pediatric patient. This includes questions focused on specific age categories, including infants and toddlers, preschoolers, elementary-aged children, and adolescents. The chapter author provides clinical pearls for a more efficient and effective exam, including a section on assisting children with special needs.

Section 2
Examination

A pediatric comprehensive eye examination consists of several components, ranging from visual acuity, stereopsis, and binocularity to ocular health. The following chapters will cover in detail the examination of color vision, stereopsis, visual acuity, visual field, pupil, ocular motility, refraction, binocularity, accommodation, anterior segment, and posterior segment. Additionally, this book includes sections specifically on the use of diagnostic agents, slit lamp examination, direct ophthalmoscopy, and indirect ophthalmoscopy with special emphasis in children. A focus on the special needs of premature infants, management of ocular emergencies, and children with myopia are also covered. Clinical pearls are provided within each chapter for a more efficient and effective exam, including modifications to enable a successful eye exam in children of all ages and cognitive abilities.

It is important to screen for acquired or hereditary color vision defects as early as possible. Color vision is a critical part of the early learning experience, and children who have color deficiencies may have difficulties compared to their peers if there is color-based schoolwork. It becomes important for career interests/goals for older children as some jobs may require normal color vision. Hereditary red-green deficiencies are X-linked and therefore affect approximately 8% of males and less than 1% of females. Acquired color vision defects and blue-yellow defects are rare in the pediatric population; therefore, these conditions will be discussed minimally in this chapter. Infants are able to discern color by 2-3 months of age, but accurate color naming may not develop until 4-6 years of age. Screening tests are sensitive, fast, and easy to administer. If a deficiency is suspected through screening, further testing must be evaluated in order to determine the type and severity of the color vision defect. Color vision is typically tested starting at age 3 years and up.

Stereopsis develops very early in life and is thought to be present in a normally developing child by six months of age. In order to develop stereopsis, multiple components of visual development must be intact including visual acuity and bifoveal fixation. Stereopsis is the most sensitive way to assess sensory fusion but can be unreliable in very young age groups due to difficulty understanding the test or instructions. It is best to choose an option with global stereopsis (high level cortical stereo), as local stereopsis may overestimate ability due to available monocular cues. Global is created using random dot stereograms (RDS) – computer-generated patterns to create a stereoscopic form, while local contains line stereograms which create horizontal retinal image disparity giving the perception of depth. Stereopsis can be affected by strabismus, amblyopia, and other binocular vision dysfunctions that interfere with visual efficiency (especially in school-age children). The chapter discusses the most commonly used clinical tests of global and local stereopsis.

Visual acuity measurement is an essential component of any eye exam. In adults and older children, letter-based acuity (i.e., recognition acuity) is commonly used to measure vision. However, in infants and toddlers, performing traditional visual acuity testing is nearly impossible. Instead, modified optotypes such as gratings and pictures are shown to observe the young child's visual behavior. Additionally, there are objective visual acuity methods that negate the need for observing visual behavior. For the practicing clinician, the choices are many and can be confusing. With new commercial products coming into the market every day, it is nearly impossible to comprehensively cover each one of them. Instead, in this chapter, commonly used and/or studied visual acuity tests are covered. For each test, the set-up, procedure, documentation, and scientific evidence supporting or negating its use are discussed.

Visual fields in the pediatric population are an essential part of the eye exam that remain challenging to even the most experienced clinicians. Becoming educated in the multiple ways a child's visual field can be tested regardless of age and cognitive and physical abilities will allow the clinician to gain better insight into the child's function and in some cases, allow the clinician to identify pathological or neurological anomalies in the visual pathway. Gross visual field or functional visual field extent can be estimated by tests such as confrontation visual field testing, finger counting field testing, and white sphere kinetic perimetry. For threshold measurements of a child's visual fields, the Goldmann perimeter, or the more advanced computerized tests such as the Humphrey perimeter, Octopus perimeter, or frequency doubling technology perimeter can be used. Modifications can be made to certain tests to better suit the child's cognitive and physical abilities. The chapter covers different methods of visual field testing specific for the pediatric population.

Pupillary evaluation is a crucial part of every pediatric eye exam. It provides information about the structure of the eye as well as the afferent and efferent function of the eyes. It remains a quick and efficient test in the ocular evaluation. This chapter reviews the relevant neuroanatomy and the different components of the pupillary exam. The light-reflex and swinging flashlight tests are reviewed, as well as how a reverse afferent pupillary defect is detected. Clinical examples and pearls are provided to help the reader better understand the different aspects of the exam.

The purpose of this chapter is to provide the main indications, background, and procedures when assessing eye movement function in the pediatric patient. The assessment of extraocular motility function includes version and ductions using the H pattern test in order to determine the presence of underaction or overactions of the extraocular muscles (EOM). EOM testing detects abnormalities in the structural and neurological integrity caused by an acquired or congenital disease of the central nervous system. Deficits in eye movement function can also contribute to poor academic performance which requires a developmental approach to the assessment of saccadic and pursuit eye movements to determine if a referral for optometric vision therapy is indicated. For the older child who is reading to learn, an assessment of reading eye movements using objective tests, such as the Visagraph and/or the ReadAlyzer, will guide the direction of the management plan.

Accurate determination of refractive error is one of the most critical components of a pediatric eye examination. According to the National Eye Institute, refractive errors are the most common causes of correctable reduced vision in children. Children with uncorrected refractive error are more likely to have developmental delays, visual-related academic problems, and poor social skills or interactions. In addition to difficulty seeing, uncorrected refractive errors can contribute to developmental deficits of accommodation, binocular vision, and certain forms of strabismus, amblyopia, and perceptual function. The author provides the clinician an in-depth guide on how to determine the refractive error in pediatric patients. The chapter focuses on the specific techniques, advantages and disadvantages, equipment required, and step-by-step procedures for performing retinoscopy, objective refraction, and subjective refraction on children.

This chapter introduces the reader to tests commonly performed in a binocular vision examination to determine a child's binocular status. The testings introduced in this chapter are all chairside techniques that do not involve a significant amount of extra equipment or time. The binocular examination consists of determining the ocular position and then accommodation, vergence, and ocular motor statuses. The ocular position consists of determining where the eyes point in space and if they are correctly aligned. Evaluation of ocular alignment and the ability to move the eyes with coordination can be determined with various techniques, including Hirschberg, Krimsky, cover test, as well as Modified Thorington, motor testing, and vergence ranges. This chapter will familiarize the clinician with the basics of binocular vision testing and improve the reader's comfort with the various elements of the binocular vision examination.

Accommodation disorders are associated with a host of etiologies. Children with accommodative disorders can present with various symptoms including blur, fluctuating vision, eye pain, burning sensation, tired eyes, asthenopia, headaches, fatigue with near work, and excessive rubbing, blinking, or tearing. This chapter provides an overview of accommodation testing on pediatric patients in the clinical setting. The author describes the indications for accommodation testing and provides clinical pearls for testing accommodative function in children. The chapter covers the specific tests, equipment required, and step-by-step procedures for testing accommodative amplitude, accommodative response, and accommodative facility.

Foreword

Vision. It is said that next to life itself, vision is the greatest gift. As eye doctors, we have the privilege of protecting, preserving, enhancing, and rehabilitating vision. What an incredible privilege and opportunity!

Vision is a learned skill. The ability to assess a child's visual development and institute needed treatment and therapy is essential to overall health. A child's best vision enhances and facilitates the developmental process. Children may not complain when they are unable to see properly if they have always seen that way. They often assume that however they see is normal. It is therefore critically important to assess vision in all children to ensure normal learning and development. Vision impacts all areas of development. As John W. Streff, OD, said "when vision is working well, it guides and leads; when not, it interferes".

My father, the late Dr. Edwin C. Thau, OD, FAAO, imparted to me the importance of examining children. From start to finish it takes creativity, flexibility and talent. The examination sequence is different from a normal examination for an adult. You must identify the child's visual strengths and challenges while ensuring that their visual abilities can meet or exceed their current visual demands. In addition, you are also beginning a new partnership with the child's family at a new phase in their life.

Although eye doctors understand that a complete eye examination assesses both vision and eye health, there is very little public awareness of this important distinction. During a children's eye examination, we have an opportunity to not only be a steward of a child's vision, but also to reinforce the value of lifelong care for the child's and family's eye health as well as their overall health and well-being.

As an engaged member and volunteer leader of the American Optometric Association (AOA), I, along with thousands of my colleagues, have aided in advocating for increased access to comprehensive eye examinations for children in many ways including helping to create and promote AOA's InfantSEE® national public health program. Through InfantSEE®, doctors of optometry across the country have provided more than 150,000 no-cost eye and vision assessments for infants, identifying more than 18,000 eye and vision conditions. Additionally, through my work for the American Public Health Association, we have authored public health policies related to children's vision. However, in order to implement these policies and effectuate change, we need to strengthen our delivery of comprehensive eye care to children.

In addition to enjoying examining children, I loved teaching optometry students how to examine them. Examining a child is uniquely challenging. It takes clinical skill combined with art and science to gather the needed health data from each child to obtain a timely diagnosis. Although I taught for over three decades, I was limited by the number of students whom I could teach. Furthermore, there was no reference guide with clinical tips and clinical pearls that the students could refer to; their only option was to learn them from their clinical professors.

This, first of its kind, book, *The Pediatric Eye Exam Quick Reference Guide: Office and Emergency Room Procedures*, edited by Lily Zhu-Tam OD, FAAO and Ida Chung, OD, MSHE, FCOVD, FAAO, is a must-have for all eye doctors. Drs. Zhu-Tam and Chung are extraordinary pediatric clinicians and educators whose compilation of chapters written by doctors of optometry and pediatric ophthalmologists across the country has resulted in an extraordinarily rich resource. Those who are novices at examining children will find the advice from a myriad of experienced eye doctors across the country to be critically useful. It helps you choose the right test and adapt to each child's unique needs. Experienced clinicians will find tips and tricks that they may not have previously considered. With advisement aligned with the AOA's Evidence-Based Clinical Practice Guidelines for comprehensive pediatric eye and vision examination, experienced clinicians will find tips and tricks that they may not have previously considered. It will be incredibly useful as a training tool for students to reference and faculty to refer their students to.

It excites me to read the fantastic clinical pearls that are included in every chapter of this book. This book will enable every optometry student and doctor of optometry to learn the hidden secrets that the best clinicians utilize. For example, one of my father's clinical pearls was that the case history was the most important test and, if conducted properly, you will have created a list of differential diagnoses by the end of the case history and spend the remainder of the examination time confirming the diagnosis. This is precisely the clinical pearl shared in the chapter on case history in this book.

This book is a step-by-step guide to the successful examination of children and is an important addition to the library of every doctor of optometry and pediatric ophthalmologist. It is my hope that all who read this book will derive the expertise needed to increase the number of children they examine thereby ensuring that every child has the opportunity to have vision that leads.

Andrea P. Thau, O.D., F.A.A.O., F.C.O.V.D.
Past President, American Optometric Association, USA
Diplomate, American Board of Optometry, USA
Associate Clinical Professor Emerita, SUNY Optometry, USA
Distinguished Practitioner, National Academies of Practice, USA

Preface

Picture this: An infant staring at you and she is not quite sure what she is looking at yet she seems intrigued as if she wanted to ask you questions but she can't. Then you put on a trial lens of +6.00 D OU and all of sudden this tiny little face starts to smile, and she is now looking around the room and reaching out her hands to feel and touch things. How satisfying is that? You as the doctor are now smiling just as much as this happy baby who is now seeing the world clearly for the very first time in her life. It's moments like this that makes it all worthwhile.

Optometry today is more than just providing general eye care. Many of us choose to specialize in our area of interest and express our passion by being a pediatric eye care provider. Some may choose to specialize in vision therapy or myopia control, while others may choose to specialize in ocular disease, glaucoma or even neuro-optometry. The beauty is that we can choose whatever specialty we have the passion for.

As the role of eye care providers expand, there is an even more urgent need for an organized and comprehensive clinical procedures literature. The purpose of this book is to provide step by step practical and clinical testing procedures for the pediatric population. We want to share the joy of taking care of the pediatric population and we want more doctors to feel comfortable examining and treating young children. According to the American Academy of Pediatrics, the American Academy of Pediatric Ophthalmology, and the American Optometric Association, children should obtain an eye exam by 6 months old, at 2-3 years old and then yearly after they enter school. We want to catch visual problems in children as early as possible so we can provide the proper treatment as soon as possible. Many state legislatures are enacting laws mandating eye exams prior to entering school, which means there will be a higher demand for pediatric eye care providers, and we need to be ready to examine these young children in clinical settings and in private practices. This book can help prepare students, residents, novel and seasoned clinicians to provide comprehensive eye care to children of all ages, and to make sure our future generations of children are seeing well.

During our decades long journey as a clinical professor training students and residents in schools and colleges of optometry and hospitals, we could not find a book that really focused on clinical eye care procedures for the pediatric population. Children are not simply small adults. As a clinician examining small children, we must move quickly, prioritize the most important procedures, and get those done before the child loses their focus. A good clinician is always flexible and the sequence of testing for a pediatric eye exam should be based on prioritizing the test results. A good case history from the start guides your exam, assists you in prioritizing the order of tests, and provides differential diagnoses.

It was the book *Atlas of Primary Eye Care Procedures* by Dr. Linda Casser that motivated and inspired us to create a similar book for the pediatric eye care practitioner. So, the story begins and we searched for top notch pediatric specialists to join our team. We gathered a team of pediatric optometrist, behavioral optometrist, pediatric ophthalmologist, and retinal/ROP specialist from national schools and hospitals such as SUNY College of Optometry, New England College of Optometry, Berkeley School of Optometry, Western University of Health Sciences College of Optometry, Boston Children's Hospital Center, and private practices. After a few years of work with over a dozen specialists, *The Pediatric Eye Exam Quick References Guide: Office and Emergency Room Procedures* book was born.

The Pediatric Eye Exam Quick References Guide: Office and Emergency Room Procedures is a one of a kind clinical procedures book that provides step-by-step eye care examination techniques specifically with the young patient in mind. The chapters are written by leading pediatric optometrists and ophthalmologists in the field. Years of academic and clinical experiences from schools of optometry, hospital-based eye care, and private practice are all presented in a user-friendly format with clinical pearls and insights that will help any clinician perform a pediatric eye exam easily and efficiently. Covering a range of critical topics such as, case history, visual acuity, stereopsis testing, color vision testing, pupil examination, visual field testing, ocular motility testing, refraction, binocular examination, accommodation, diagnostic agents, anterior and posterior segment examination, ROP screening, ocular emergencies and myopia management, this book is ideal for all students, residents, academicians, trainers, and novel and seasoned clinicians who are interested in learning how to examine a pediatric patient and staying on top of the latest pediatric eye care procedures.

This book will be an important addition to the field of eye care. This reference guide will serve as a great learning and teaching tool for all eye care professionals.

We have been so fortunate to meet and work with diverse professional colleagues in eye care throughout our careers. It isn't every day an optometrist has the privilege to enter the NICU (neonatal intensive care unit) with an ROP specialist to perform ROP (retinopathy of prematurity) screenings on infants in a hospital setting. We are thrilled to have this opportunity to compile such a comprehensive yet to the point, a step-by-step clinical procedures reference book that will benefit anyone who is interested in providing pediatric eye care. We are even more grateful to have such an insightful and dedicated group of colleagues to work collaboratively on a project of this magnitude. We are proud to be able to share this finished product with our profession.

ORGANIZATION OF THE BOOK

The book is organized into 16 chapters. Each chapter includes clinical pearls and author wisdoms to provide a more efficient and effective eye examination in the pediatric population. A brief description of each of the chapters follows:

Chapter 1 describes the art of taking a pediatric patient's history. The author stresses the importance of establishing rapport with the child and trying to obtain pertinent information to help lead and guide the pediatric eye examination. An effective case history enables the clinician to prioritize the exam, establish differential diagnosis and formulate the proper treatment plan for a child. The chapter focuses on the different aspects of a comprehensive case history based on specific age categories including a section for children with special needs. The author includes helpful tips for wording history questions, reviews developmental milestones, and provides age-specific history questions.

Chapter 2 presents the various ways to conduct color vision testing in children. It's important to identify children with color vision deficiency as this may affect academic performance when there is color dependent, school related activities. Color vision deficiency affects career choices later in life, so the earlier the detection, the earlier one can prepare for the future. This chapter covers Ishihara plates, Color Vision Test Made Easy, Hardy Rand Rittler book, Farnsworth Panel D 15, Farnsworth Munsell 100 hue, anomalscope and digital color vision tests.

Chapter 3 discusses the purpose and different types of stereopsis testing. It presents child-friendly diagnostic tools such as the Random Dot E test, the Preschool Assessment of Stereopsis with a Smile (PASS), Randot Preschool Stereoacuity Test, Lang stereo test, Titmus fly or butterfly test, Randot with Global stereo shapes, and the Frisby stereotest.

Chapter 4 reviews one of the most important elements of a pediatric eye exam which is visual acuity testing. The most common visual acuity charts used to effectively test children is presented. The chapter includes a discussion on visual acuity testing in infants and toddlers, preferential looking tests, Teller acuity cards, Lea gratings, Patti stripes, Cardiff acuity cards, visual evoked potential, optokinetic drum, Lea symbols, Allen pictures, HOTV, Broken wheel test, and ETDRS visual acuity charts.

Chapter 5 presents different methods of visual field testing in the pediatric population. This chapter includes a discussion on confrontation visual field, Goldmann perimetry, frequency doubling technology perimetry, Humphrey field analyzer perimetry, and white sphere kinetic perimetry.

Chapter 6 reviews the neuroanatomy and the associated pupillary pathways relevant to the visual system. The author covers the clinical usage and the importance of the light reflex, swinging flashlight test, near reflex test, and reverse relative afferent pupillary testing.

Chapter 7 is divided into two parts, structural and neurological status, and visual function and developmental status. Special attention is given to practical clinical procedures to assess ocular motility function in the pediatric population. This chapter includes a discussion on versions, ductions, Bielschowsky head tilt test, three-step test, pursuits, saccades, developmental eye movement test, Visagraph and Readalyzer.

Chapter 8 presents one of the most pertinent components of a pediatric eye exam which is determining the child's refractive status. Refractive errors are the most common causes of correctable vision loss in children. Using proper techniques to objectively assess and obtain the accurate refractive findings is of utmost importance in a pediatric eye examination. This chapter discusses the principles and methodology of retinoscopy, dry retinoscopy with phoropter and in free space, Mohindra retinoscopy, cycloplegic retinoscopy, and subjective and objective refraction in children. The chapter also covers autorefraction with Retinomax, Welch Allyn Sure Sight and Welch Allyn Spot instruments.

Chapter 9 discusses the various ways to assess ocular alignment and perform a binocular vision examination. The author covers objective and subjective tests such as Hirschberg, Krimsky, Bruckner test, cover test, Modified Thorington, Risley prisms in phoropter and prism bars in free space. NPC, FCC, NRA, PRA, positive fusional vergence, negative fusional vergence and vergence facility are also discussed.

Chapter 10 discusses the effect of accommodation on the visual system, the various accommodative disorders and provides step-by-step clinical testing procedures to properly assess the active accommodative system in a child. The author presents how to test accommodative amplitude, accommodative responses, and accommodative facility in this chapter. Clinical pearls are provided throughout the chapter.

Chapter 11 presents the most common topical ophthalmic drops for diagnostic use in a pediatric exam. Topical local anesthetics, mydriatic and cycloplegic agents and their uses based on specific age categories are discussed. A section on how to create your own combination drops and use of spray caps for easy pediatric instillation is included.

Chapter 12 describes in detail how to perform an ocular health examination in the pediatric population with traditional methods, and with other more pediatric friendly techniques. Biomicroscopy, +20 D lens with transilluminator, portable slit lamp, Van Herick, shadow test angle estimation, digital intraocular pressure, Tonopen and Icare rebound tonometer are some of the topics discussed by the author in this chapter.

Chapter 13 presents the examination of the posterior pole using direct ophthalmoscopy. The author discusses and compares the use of the traditional direct ophthalmoscope compared to the panoptic ophthalmoscope.

Chapter 14 reviews the use of binocular indirect ophthalmoscopy and scleral indentation. The important landmarks of the retina and classification system of ROP (retinopathy of prematurity) is presented. The authors also provide detailed techniques on how to perform a ROP examination in a premature infant.

Chapter 15 focuses on ocular emergency care. The authors discuss bedside and chairside examination techniques, the use of an eyelid speculum, management of eye lid laceration, foreign body removal, pressure patching, bandage contact lens, checking for seidel sign, corneal and conjunctival culturing, chemical burns and pH testing and irrigation, forced duction testing, neurological screening, and ordering laboratory testing. Ocular imaging such as B-scan ultrasound, CT scan, MRI, MRA, MRV from an ocular standpoint are also discussed in this chapter.

Chapter 16 is the final chapter of the book and focuses on one of today's hottest topics which is myopia management. The author presents clinical studies on risk factors of myopia onset and progression, evidence-based clinical management of myopia, and various treatment options available. Overnight orthokeratology, the first FDA-approved day time daily disposable MiSight contact lens, and atropine treatment are presented in this chapter with all the latest evidence- based clinical study results.

The Pediatric Eye Exam Quick References Guide: Office and Emergency Room Procedures is an organized and comprehensive pediatric clinical procedure book. It is our sincere hope that this book encourages, facilitates, and prepares those doctors who are interested in caring and improving vision for the youngest of patients.

Lily Zhu-Tam
Citywide Eye Care, USA

Ida Chung
College of Optometry, Western University of Health Sciences, USA

Acknowledgment

The editors wish to acknowledge the help of all the people involved in this project and, more specifically, to the authors and reviewers that took part in the review process. Without their support, this book would not have become a reality.

First, the editors would like to thank each one of the authors for their contributions. Our sincere gratitude goes to the chapter's authors who contributed their time and expertise to this book.

Second, the editors wish to acknowledge the valuable contributions of the reviewers for their improvements of quality, coherence, and content presentation of each chapter. Most of the authors also served as referees; we highly appreciate their double duty.

Illustration Contributor

Tak-Man Kimberly Fung, OD, DiploABO

New England College of Optomtery, USA

Peer Reviewers

Linda Bellomy, OD

Western University of Health Sciences College of Optometry, USA

Joshua Cameron, PhD

Western University of Health Sciences College of Optometry, USA

Pinakin Davey, OD, PhD

Western University of Health Sciences College of Optometry, USA

Tiffenie Harris, OD

Western University of Health Sciences College of Optometry, USA

Naida Jakirlic, OD

Western University of Health Sciences College of Optometry, USA

Philip Kwok, OD

Western University of Health Sciences College of Optometry, USA

Rochelle Mozlin, OD

SUNY College of Optometry, USA

Christine Pham, OD

Western University of Health Sciences College of Optometry, USA

Scott Ritcher, OD

Northwell Health, Staten Island University Hospital, USA

Frank Spors, PhD

Western University of Health Sciences College of Optometry, USA

John Tassinari OD

Western University of Health Sciences College of Optometry, USA

An Vo, OD

Western University of Health Sciences College of Optometry, USA

Kimberly Walker, OD

Western University of Health Sciences College of Optometry, USA

Naveen Yadav, PhD

Western University of Health Sciences College of Optometry, USA

Xiaoying Zhu OD, PHD

SUNY College of Optometry, USA

Lily Zhu-Tam
Citywide Eye Care, USA

Ida Chung
College of Optometry, Western University of Health Sciences, USA

Section 1
History

A pediatric case history is essential before proceeding with an examination. This section will focus on birth, developmental, educational, and social histories, as well as active listening skills and flexibility of the clinician for an effective start to the examination. Clinical pearls are provided within the chapter for a more efficient and effective eye exam, including a section on assisting children with special needs.

Chapter 1
Case History for the Pediatric Eye Examination

Amy Moy
New England College of Optometry, USA & Martha Eliot Health Center of Boston Children's Hospital, USA

ABSTRACT

The art of taking a patient's case history is essential for a solid understanding of pertinent details before proceeding with an examination. While establishing rapport with the patient, the clinician should ask questions about birth history, developmental history, educational and social history. Active listening skills and flexibility of the provider are useful tools for an effective start to the examination. This chapter reviews categories of questions needed for optimization of case history for the pediatric patient. This includes questions focused on specific age categories, including infants and toddlers, preschoolers, elementary-aged children, and adolescents. The chapter author provides clinical pearls for a more efficient and effective exam, including a section on assisting children with special needs.

INTRODUCTION

A patient's case history plays an essential role in setting the direction of the eye examination and identifying differential diagnoses. An effective case history enables a clinician to prioritize and plan out the course of the appointment, which can require special creativity with pediatric patients. At times, obtaining a detailed history from the pediatric patient and/or caregiver can be challenging. While parents tend to be very good observers, they are not always accurate in their observations. This dichotomy is especially challenging as pediatric patients and caregivers may not be able to verbalize and express their symptoms. For example, a parent may report that there is an eye turn but when asked which eye, the parent is uncertain.

This chapter aims to describe the main areas of patient history that should be asked by eye care providers, and indicates specific questions by age group. While the list provided in this chapter is not exhaustive, it provides a framework to assist the clinician in eliciting potential areas that will need further questioning. By asking effective questions and setting the goals of the exam, a more successful visit for

DOI: 10.4018/978-1-7998-8044-8.ch001

both the clinician and the patient can be achieved. A case history is also an opportunity to establish rapport with the adult caregiver(s) present and the child to facilitate the examination and communication of the exam results and treatment plan.

BACKGROUND

The case history, or medical interview, is an examination step that is universal to all healthcare professionals. While there are many technological advances and tools such as online or tablet-based case histories, the importance of interpersonal communication and connection cannot be replaced (Keifenheim et al., 2015). An effective clinician must be able to read both verbal and non-verbal cues, as well as be skilled to ask questions that can elicit quality information from the patient and caregiver (Keifenheim et al., 2015). Peterson and Holbrook (1992) studied 80 outpatients and the doctors who examined them and found that 76% of the doctors' differential diagnoses after their history-taking led to the final diagnosis. In comparison, the physical examination led to 12% of the final diagnoses, and laboratory testing led to 11% of the final diagnoses (Peterson et al., 1992).

The definition of history-taking is a "way of eliciting relevant personal, psychosocial and symptom information from a patient with the aim of obtaining information useful in formulating a diagnosis and providing medical care to the patient" (Keifenheim et al., 2015). While it may be necessary for technicians or other assistants to take a preliminary case history, the clinician should be the main interviewer to assess if further detail is necessary.

For complex medical and developmental histories, some eye care practices may prefer to have a questionnaire sent to their patients before the appointment, so that the bulk of the allotted time can be spent on examination and patient education. Alternatively, a complex case history form may be completed by the adult caregiver in the office while the clinician begins testing the child. This strategy is particularly helpful when the complexity of the child or case type is not known at the time of the appointment. The clinician may select the appropriate case history form after the chief complaint and meeting the child, if the child is able to sit independently in the exam chair.

Efficiency is key with a pediatric exam. At the same time, the clinician should maintain a positive, relaxed, and fun environment, especially for young children. Be fun and flexible! Young children typically have a short attention span and can be uncooperative with the examination. The clinician must prioritize the sequence of exams to maximize the amount of pertinent information obtained. Therefore, having a detailed history helps the clinician to formulate a differential diagnosis and a sequential list of exams to be performed. Each patient is unique and responds differently, so it is up to the clinician to strategically perform all the needed tests to formulate the correct assessment and management. Taking case history with a child differs from that of a typical adult exam due to factors such as the source of the information (caregiver versus the child), details sought by the clinician for the purpose of the examination, and how communication occurs between the clinician and the patient.

Clinical Pearl: *A successful clinician is creative and flexible. The sequence of a pediatric exam should be based on the priority of the test result since the child may not be cooperative.*

CASE HISTORY INTAKE

Equipment

1. Electronic health record or paper charting system
2. Chair/stool to enable sitting at child's height, or enough space to squat at child's level for initial conversation
3. Toys to maintain child's attention as appropriate

Before beginning the case history, the clinician should be positioned in such a way that eye contact can be made and is able to begin observation of the child. If the child can contribute to the case history, the clinician should stay at the child's eye level and avoid towering over the child when speaking. This helps to establish rapport.

When initial questioning is focused on the caregiver, three strategies can be used, depending on the disposition of the child at the time:

1. Child is calm/cooperative and does not need the caregiver's full attention

All questions are directed to the caregiver if the child is very young (usually 4 years old or under). An assistant can begin objective and noninvasive testing of the child with the parent near the child and answering questions.

2. Child is apprehensive / uncooperative

The child can be held or positioned behind the caregiver during the history. The exchange with the caregiver should be friendly and warm so that trust is built as the child observes the interaction. An assistant can give toys to the child to decrease any apprehension.

a. A mildly uncooperative child (not just apprehensive) may need some toys or other distractions to help focus attention. Making a game out of the tests, such as using stickers for general fixation, or waving stimulating light/sound toys are useful tools.
b. A significantly uncooperative child may require a "time out" conversation with the caregiver to discuss if some of the goals for the exam can be achieved, or whether it would be best to find another time that the child is less sleepy, less stressed, etc. The clinician should assess the situation and decide whether it would be better to complete the exam on a different day or time, or to continue with the exam with the firm but loving restraint by the caregiver, and despite the likelihood of the child crying, and the potential for needing a follow-up visit if the child is unable to complete all necessary testing.

3. Child is young/immature such that the parent must hold the child

The caregiver may not be able to answer a lengthy set of questions because the child needs the caregiver's attention. In this case, the clinician should conduct an abbreviated case history to obtain the most vital details, and immediately begin the exam to maximize the time the clinician has available to spend examining the child.

As much as possible, the clinician should avoid typing while conducting the case history, except to record highly complex information. Taking quick notes to remember later can be helpful, whether on paper or on the computer/tablet. For young children, having interesting objects or toys ready to keep attention allows the clinician additional time for making observations while speaking with their caregiver. Positioning of the clinician should be such that eye contact can be made with both the child and the parent. If it is difficult to see both the child and parent in the same view, then the clinician should rearrange herself/himself in a triangular position with the child in the exam chair and the parent in a different chair.

If working with a technician who takes a preliminary history, the clinician should take note of important points related to the chief complaint. This enables the clinician to summarize what has already been said so that further questioning can concentrate on additional details.

The use of electronic health record templates can be a help *and* a hindrance. While an electronic template may contain certain fields that serve as prompts for questioning, the most effective case history is not formulaic, but rather a directed sequenced of targeted and appropriate follow up questions based on the chief complaint.

The clinician will tailor their case history depending on the type of visit. A comprehensive eye exam will involve all portions of the history elements (described below in Elements of Case History) as appropriate to age and situation. For problem-specific visits, the clinician should ask about the chief complaint and probe in detail, asking pertinent medical history, while confirming no changes in medications and allergies or other relevant details. For a follow-up visit, it is not necessary to review all details of the history reviewed at the initial comprehensive exam, but any changes in prior history should be confirmed, documented, and dated. Documenting "No changes in vision or medical history since last visit, MM/DD/YY" is a recommended practice.

Observation During Case History

While taking history, the clinician should take mental notes while making observations of the child, gathering as much of this observational information before starting the actual examination. Some signs to intentionally look for include obvious eye turn, squinting, head tilt, type and quality of communication between caregiver and child, the behavior of the child, and general wellness of the child.

In addition, the quality of the history information from the caregiver should be assessed by the clinician. Throughout the history-taking, the clinician should pay attention to the caregiver's reliability as a historian, any distractions during case history (such as other children in the room, phone calls, and sleeping), and the quality of the interactions and relationship between the child and the caregiver.

Create Rapport

While the question "What brings you in today?" is valid and effective, the pediatric exam especially benefits from learning the child's social history. Starting with social history questions can help establish rapport with the child and caregiver, such that further history-taking is much more effective (Figure 1). Some examples of social history questions directed to the parent and/or child include:

- "What kind of toys does your child like to play with?" Answers to this question may indicate developmental milestones or lead to further discussion about visual development.

- "What's your favorite subject in school? Answers to this question can be indicators of school performance or lead to other important details about vision.
- "What's your favorite thing to do on the weekends?" Answers to this question can lead to details about the amount of screen time and the number of hours spent outdoors, especially in cases of dry eye or myopia progression.
- "What's your favorite sport? I love basketball too! Did you see the game yesterday?"
- "What's your favorite song? I love that song! Do you want to sing it together?"

Ending social history with laughing about something the clinician has in common with the child or complimenting the child on something well done, can help ensure a smooth transition to additional history questions. The clinician can say something like, "That's really great to hear. I'd like to ask you some more questions to help me be able to help you with your eyes" as a transition statement.

Figure 1. Smiling child in exam chair

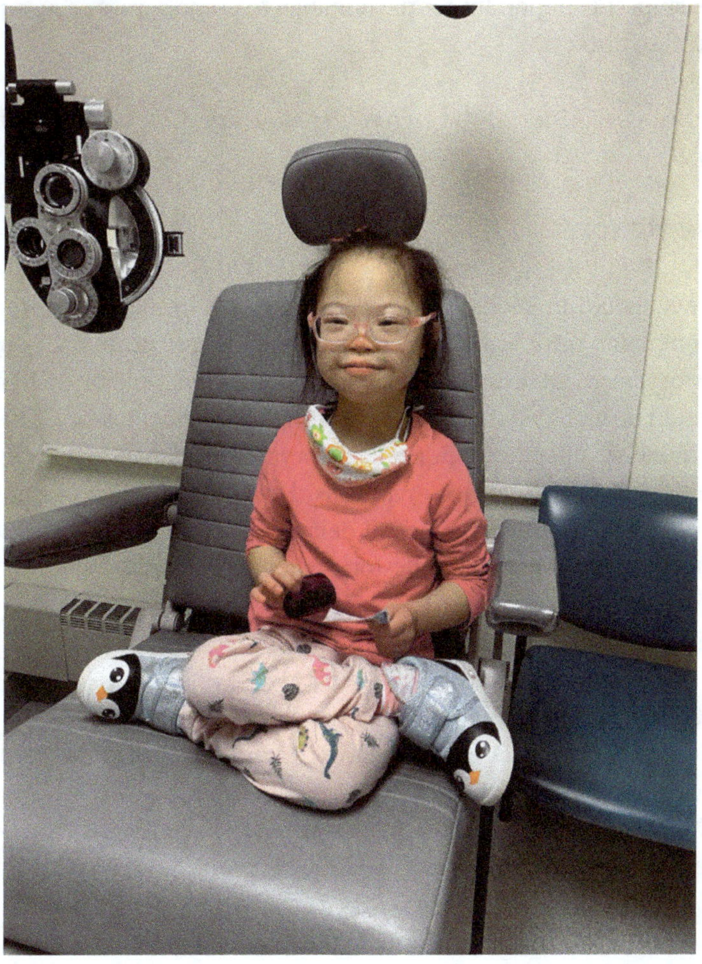

Active Listening

As the listener, the effective clinician will follow the child's or caregiver's leads, ask for their opinions and concerns, and practice attentive listening and open-ended questioning. It has been shown that patients who feel like they were more directed than listened to will leave the encounter with negative emotions (Rosenberg, 1997). Showing the patient and caregiver that they are heard, by summarizing their concerns and setting expectations, allows them to feel an interpersonal connection and reassurance in their care. Taking the time to establish rapport, especially with the adolescent and elementary school-age patient, helps the clinician to perform a more effective exam and management plan. The clinician's tone should be friendly and calm, and able to adapt to a need for higher energy or a quieter environment for a sensory-sensitive child. Smiling is an essential part of providing care for pediatric patients.

Caregiver emotions can play into the quality of the case history. A caregiver may be defensive, appear guilty, or seem overly sensitive. Therefore, open-ended questions are a helpful tool for the clinician, especially when asking potentially sensitive questions. When listening actively to the caregiver or child's history, be sure to use affirmative body language and encourage responses to reinforce a beneficial doctor-patient relationship. It is important for the clinician to come across as non-judgmental and reassuring throughout the case history.

Clinical Pearl: *Effective case history-taking gives the clinician a list of differential diagnoses by the end of the case history.*

Elements of Case History

The following elements should be included, but not limited to, in the case history of a pediatric eye examination: Chief complaint, birth history (prenatal, perinatal, and postnatal), developmental history, educational/social history, medical history and general health, family history, and ocular history. Previous special testing should be included if a child has a complex medical history. The clinician should use best judgment to determine whether developmental history is important after the child reaches first grade and can chose to omit detailed birth history questions. However, in cases of unusual refractive error, amblyopia, strabismus, learning or developmental delays, or potential binocular vision issues, history about pregnancy, birth, and developmental milestones should still be included.

1. **Chief Complaint/History of Present Illness**
   a. Open-ended question: "What brings you in today?"
   b. What are the associated factors affecting the chief complaint?
      - SOCRATES or FOLDARS/FOLDARQ acronyms are some of the many methods to probe details of the complaint
      - SOCRATES = Site, Onset, Characteristics, Radiation of Pain, Associated Features, Time Course, Exacerbating or Alleviating Factors, Severity (Oxford Medical Education, 2016)
      - FOLDARQ = Frequency, Onset, Location, Duration, Associated Factors, Relief, Severity/Quality (Dang, 2018)

Clinical Pearl: *Helpful Tips for Wording*

- Use wording for questions in relation to observed symptoms and not the diagnosis, such as: "When did you first notice her rubbing her eyes" rather than "When did her allergies start?"
- Use and document the caregiver's or patient's wording, rather than clinical language, when speaking with them and when documenting the history of present illness.
- Patients often do not have a sense of how long a problem has been occurring, or how long ago an event took place. The clinician can prompt the child with interval questions such as "6 months ago? 1 year ago? 5 years ago?" Do you think it was happening at her first birthday? This phrasing helps to provide a time range to give more helpful details.
- Some caregivers may be quite talkative to the point of taking up allocated examination time, sometimes with topics less relevant to what the clinician needs to know. In this instance, the clinician could ask the caregiver a few preliminary questions first to get started, and then during the 30-minute dilation window after drops are instilled, additional questions can be asked. Another strategy is to have the caregiver complete a history questionnaire during the examination of the independent child, to capture everything they want the clinician to know.

2. Birth History

Birth history is not as necessary in the case history of an elementary-aged or adolescent child. However, birth history is very important for an eye examination of an infant, toddler, and preschool-aged child, as the birth history can provide indicators for barriers to visual development.

1. Prenatal history: The relevant prenatal history is any serious illness or condition during pregnancy that may impact the child's vision, development, or general health. It includes in-utero exposure to tobacco, alcohol, or drugs. The clinician may want to ask this question in an open-ended manner instead of a direct query about smoking, alcohol, or drugs. Any hesitancy by the caregiver or an older pediatric patient may indicate issues such as alcohol or drugs that need further questioning with sensitivity.
2. Perinatal and Postnatal history
    i. Was there any history of pre-eclampsia or toxemia during pregnancy?
    ii. How was the delivery (e.g., breech birth, umbilical cord complication)?
        - What was the APGAR score?
3. Note about APGAR score: In 1952, Dr. Virginia Apgar at Columbia University published the APGAR score, which is the accepted standard of assessment for a newborn's health and/or need for resuscitation 1 minute and 5 minutes after delivery. The APGAR score assesses the following elements: heart rate, color, reflexes, muscle tone, and respiratory effort. Each element is given a score of 0, 1, or 2. Reassuring scores range from 7-10. These scores are also affected by gestational age, medications taken by the mother, birth weight, congenital conditions, and drug use or anesthesia (American Academy of Pediatrics, 2016).
4. If a caregiver does not remember the APGAR score, it was likely normal. Parents usually remember the developmental timelines or medical details that are abnormal.
    iii. How long was the pregnancy?
        - If premature, was oxygen treatment given? How long was the oxygen treatment, and does the caregiver recall if an eye exam was done before discharge from the neonatal intensive care unit (NICU)?

5. If the answer is yes for incubation/oxygen, the clinician should ask if parents recall if a follow-up eye appointment was scheduled. A recollection of a follow up likely indicates the presence of at least mild retinopathy of prematurity (ROP) or another condition meriting follow-up, such as high myopia or anisometropia.
6. If parents do not recall a follow-up eye appointment after NICU discharge, then it is likely there was no ROP.

Clinical Pearl: *For premature babies, the developmental milestones are based on their due date, not their birth date.*

3. Developmental History

a. Milestones (general): A key element of a developmental history is determining if a child is meeting age expected milestones. The presence of developmental delays can influence examination strategy and patient management. There are numerous milestones the clinician may inquire about as shown in Figure 2. At a minimum, eye care providers should ask about the major milestones of crawling, walking and language development. Additionally, the clinician may ask "are there any areas of development your pediatrician is concerned about". Most pediatricians take an in-depth developmental history which can be useful to the clinician. In multidisciplinary settings, this is easily reviewed in the shared electronic health record.
   i. Ask milestones based on the child's age (Figure 2).
   ii. For elementary-aged children, questioning should be focused on school performance and extracurricular activities/hobbies. It is fine to eliminate questions about developmental history, especially for a typical child who has reached first grade and up.
   iii. Ask if the child has received any Early Intervention services (Birth to age 3).

Clinical Pearl: *For a child with developmental delays, the best way to ask is with an open-ended question of what milestones the child has been working on recently, rather than asking at what point they have met certain milestones that they may not yet have achieved. Caregivers of children with special needs are often sensitive to answering that their child has not met any of the milestones asked directly by the clinician.*

Clinical Pearl: *If a child had speech therapy or physical therapy, the clinician could conclude that the child may have some developmental delay even if the parent does not remember the child's developmental milestone.*

b. Milestones (visual):
   i. Some age ranges for specific visual-neurological skills can be found in Figure 3. These are ranges and may vary with each child.
   ii. Visual development for young children can be surveyed by open-ended questions such as, "Have you noticed your baby grabbing for toys?" Figure 4 categorizes some visual milestones in groups for rapid recognition of milestone achievement.

Figure 2. Developmental milestones
(Adapted from Centers for Disease Control, 2021a)

Age	Gross Motor	Fine Motor	Language	Social
2 months	Raises chest off bed	Follows 180 degrees	Coos	Smiles
4 months	Picks head and chest up and rolls one way	Reaches for objects	Orients to voices	Initiates social interactions
6 months	Sits with support and rolls both ways	Transfers objects	Babbles	Recognizes unfamiliar people
12 months	Stands alone and walks while holding on	Releases an object	Single words	Imitates and cooperates with dressing
15 months	Walks well	Builds 2-block towers	10 word vocabulary	Begins to use cup
18 months	Runs, stoops, recovers	Builds 3-block towers and uses spoon	10-25 words and points to body parts	Words to communicate
2 years old	Walks up stairs and kicks ball	4-6 block towers and uses fork and spoon	2-word phrases and 50 word vocabulary	Removes clothes
3 years old	Rides tricycle and jumps from step	Copies circle	5-8 word sentences	Group play and shares
4 years old	Balance one foot and walks up and down stairs	Copies cross and catches ball	Intelligible speech	Dresses self and washes and dries hands
5 years old	Skips alternating feet and hops 10 times	Draws person with 6 body parts	Asks word meanings	Names 4 colors and plays by "the rules"

Figure 3. Visual development milestones
(Adapted from Boyd, 2020)

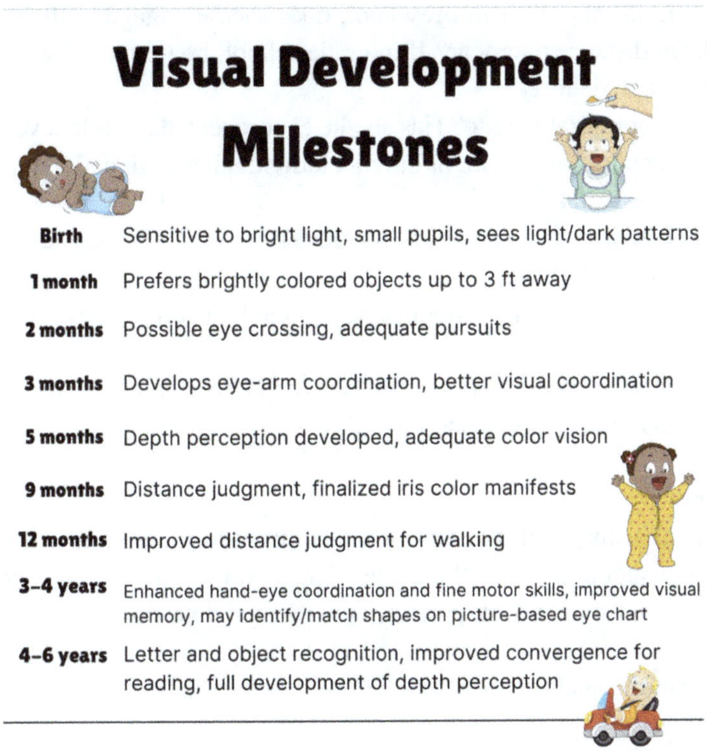

Figure 4. Developmental vision milestones from birth

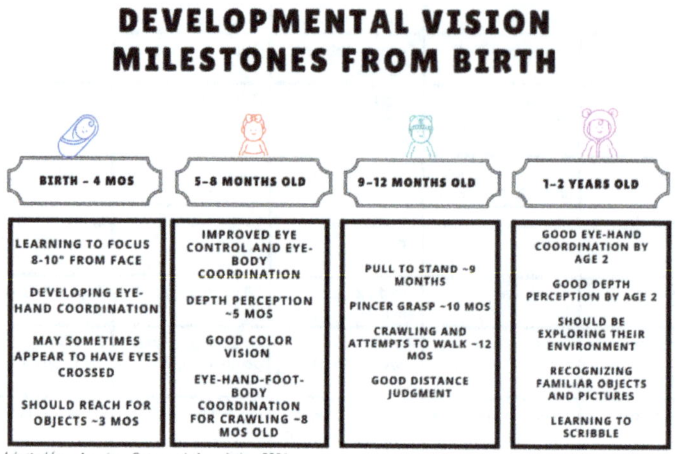

Adapted from American Optometric Association, 2021.

4. Educational/Social History

Case history for school-aged children and older should focus on their ability to focus and achieve tasks at school. In addition, they should be able to comfortably see objects and people at home and in social situations.

a. Are there any learning-related visual symptoms? For example, frontal headaches that are worst at the end of the day, avoids reading or near tasks. Short attention and focusing when reading.
b. How is child doing in school? If in preschool, does she/he engage with story time and visually demanding tasks at distance and near? If in grade school, how much does she/he like to read? Is the child reading on grade level?
c. Is child in the age-appropriate grade? Has she/he ever repeated a grade level? If yes, why?
d. Is child in a special education setting or have an individualized educational plan (IEP) or adjusted learning plan (such as a 504)?
e. What does the child do in her/his spare time? Include time spent outdoors and near work. (American Optometric Association, 2017)
f. How much total screen time in a 24-hour period (including cell phones, video games, computers, tablets, television, etc)?
g. Environmental History (especially important with chief complaints of itching, watering, eye rubbing, etc.). Ask about pets at home and type of housing.

5. Medical History

The patient's medical history is important for the clinician to assess ocular implications for the examination. The clinician should also ask the name of the child's pediatrician if not listed in the health record. The main categories to document pertinent positives and pertinent negatives are as follows:

a. Date of most recent medical examination
b. Major medical illnesses

c. History of surgeries or inpatient admissions
d. History of trauma
e. Reconciliation of medication list, including prescription and non-prescription drugs, as well as eye drops or ointments
f. Known drug, food, and environmental allergies

6. Review of Systems

Review of Systems (ROS) is a set of questions designed to screen for dysfunction in organ systems throughout the body. The ROS should be intentionally tailored to a patient's age, gender, risk factors, and medical history (Goldberg, 2018). A positive answer to a question necessitates further details to decide if further action is needed. For instance, a patient who has reported itchy eyes may report a long history of allergic dermatitis and knowing this detail could affect the management of the ocular itching.

There is confusion among health professionals about the best way to use ROS. While past criteria for coding medical exams included ROS elements, the complexity of a medical exam for billing purposes is now based on decision-making and risk level for the patient. Because using ROS as a screening tool can trigger a wave of further questions and/or testing (Goldberg, 2018), a more targeted approach of ROS questions can be more efficient and helpful to the clinician.

For a pediatric exam, the ROS translates to a case history interview with personal medical history, and the appropriate ROS items. Common pediatric conditions that may not naturally arise from patient responses include allergies and asthma. These are worth reviewing in the ROS. Asking the caregiver if a child with Down Syndrome has heart disease counts as asking about the cardiovascular system. A child with itchy eyes may have integumentary (skin) or general allergy conditions. In general, if the areas covered in section 5 above (medical history) are answered, the clinician should have enough of a history and ROS for a routine eye exam. Questions about health maintenance visits such as last physical or well-child visit may be included in this section as well.

Organ systems that may be reviewed in a routine comprehensive exam include the 15 systems listed below. Any conditions or symptoms in each category would be documented or reviewed, depending on whether the patient is new or established. It is not efficient for a clinician to review all 15 organ systems and is not a criterion of defining a comprehensive eye exam.

a. General
b. Vision
c. Head and Neck
d. Pulmonary
e. Cardiovascular
f. Gastrointestinal
g. Genitourinary
h. Hematology/Oncology
i. Obstetrics/Gynecology
j. Neurological
k. Endocrine
l. Infectious Diseases
m. Musculoskeletal
n. Mental Health

o. Skin and Hair

7. Ocular History

a. When was the last full eye exam for the child, or is this the first?
b. Has child ever worn glasses? How old are the current glasses? How often does child wear the glasses?
c. Has child ever worn contact lenses? (This question applies to older children.) If yes, how does she/he care for the contact lenses (e.g., disposal, hygiene, etc)?
d. Any observations of lazy eye or eye turns?

Clinical Pearl: *If a parent has noticed an ocular sign such as an eye turn, nystagmus, etc that is not manifesting during the exam, ask to show you a video, or to take a video and show it to you at the follow-up visit.*

8. Family Medical and Ocular History

Family medical history usually screens for cardiovascular disease or other hereditary conditions affecting the visual system. Family ocular history should rule out history of major childhood ocular conditions (Turbert, 2020). Positive family history for many of the items listed below could warrant further special testing.

a. Refractive error that onset early in life (screen for progressive myopia in family history)
b. Strabismus
c. Amblyopia
d. Glaucoma
e. Color Vision Deficiency
f. Blindness

Age-Specific Questions

When asking milestone questions, remember that each child develops at a different rate. Developmental milestone charts give approximate ages at which skills occur, but children may not necessarily follow these timelines to the exact age.

Clinical Pearl: *As significant screen time is more frequently a part of childhood; it is important to ask questions to assess if computer vision syndrome or dry eye will be a concern to address during the exam.*

1. Infants and Toddlers (Figure 5)

a. Case history will be directed at the parent and will center mostly on questions about the pregnancy, delivery, and developmental milestones. The clinician should be efficient and perform external observations of the child from a distance while discussing history with the caregiver.
b. Ask specific questions like whether the infant recognizes the caregiver's face, does she/he follow you or a preferred toy with their eyes? Reach for objects? Eyes cross?

Figure 5. Infant-toddler case history

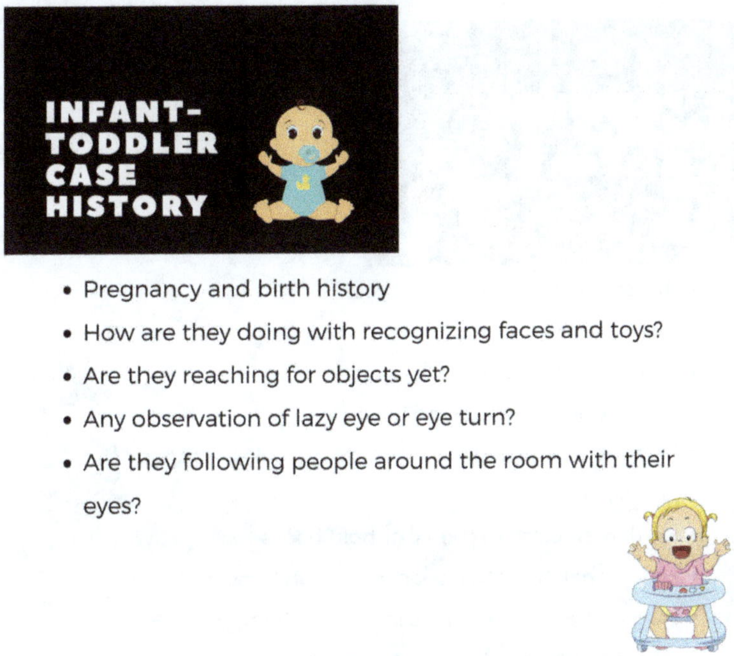

2. **Preschoolers (Figure 6)**
   a. Preschoolers are rapidly developing in many areas, including motor skills, hand-eye coordination, verbal skills, and social skills. Asking questions that focus on typical milestones for this age group allows the clinician to make connections to visual development and coordinate with other providers as appropriate.

3. **Elementary-aged Children (Figure 7)**
   a. School performance is a primary point of discussion for elementary-aged children, as well as any learning difficulties they may have. Questions regarding their visual habits are important to address, whether it is screen time, distance from screens and reading material, or complaints about fatigue after reading for several minutes.

4. **Adolescents (Figure 8)**
   a. Adolescents may be less responsive to questioning. Asking questions first about themselves and their preferences may help the clinician to establish a safe space for the teen to respond and to ask questions themselves. They may also be interested in contact lenses, and the clinician will need to assess the readiness of the child and the parent for this conversation and for the responsibility of contact lenses.

Figure 6. Preschool case history
(American Optometric Association, 2021a)

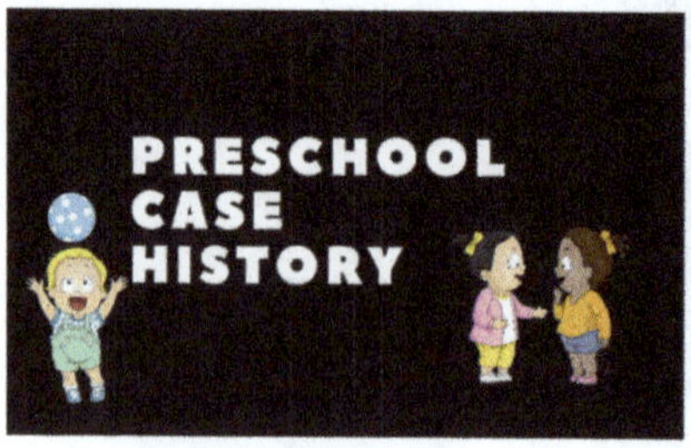

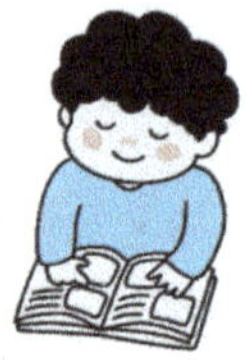

- Any sign of lazy or crossed eyes?
- Any squinting?
- Any sensitivity to light?
- Any frequent eye rubbing?
- How are they doing with recognizing colors, shapes and numbers?
- Do they sit close to the TV or hold books too closely?
- How is their attention span in relation to peers?
- How do they do with puzzles and building toys? Do you observe good hand-eye coordination at home?

Figure 7. Elementary-aged case history
(American Optometric Association, 2021b)

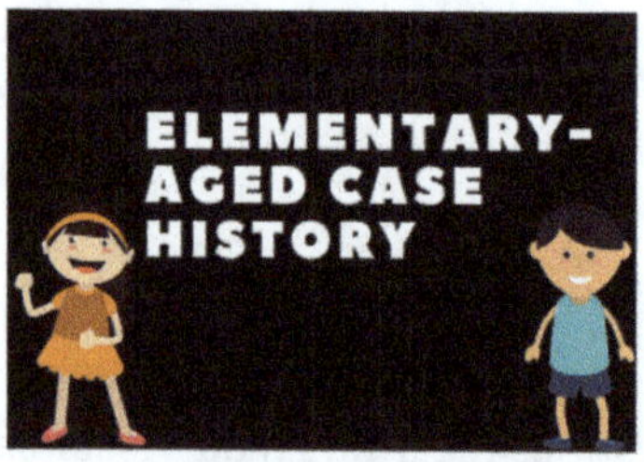

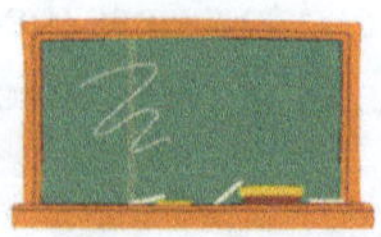

- 5-6 years old: Are they able to recognize objects and letters well?
- Able to read the whiteboard, computer screen, and books or tablets clearly?
- Any loss of place when reading, avoiding reading, or forgetting what was read?
- Do letters ever get mixed up, like "b" and "d"?
- Any sensitivity to light?
- Any frequent eye rubbing?
- How is performance at school?
- How is their attention span in relation to peers?
- Frequent headaches?
- Tilting the head or covering one eye?

Figure 8. Adolescent-aged Case History

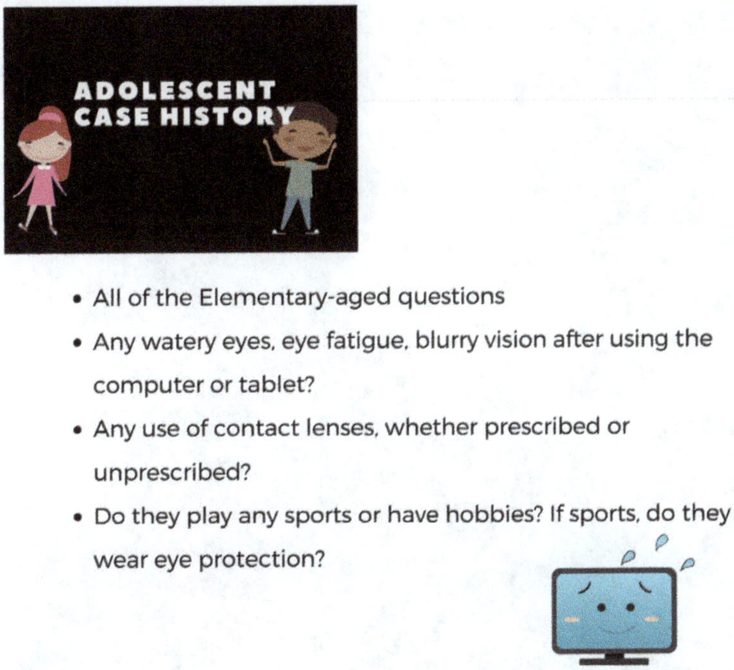

Case History for Children with Special Needs

Children with special needs have more complex case histories which necessitate the clinician's perceptiveness to verbal and nonverbal cues. It is vital for the clinician to assess the quality of history information the caregiver is providing. For instance, if the caregiver vaguely recalls that the child had eye surgery for a lazy eye, this would be important for the clinician to keep in mind when assessing the child's binocular status. In addition, for an effective and efficient appointment, the clinician will need to prioritize the medical conditions that are most likely to affect the visual system.

One way to do so in an efficient manner is to review all of the medical conditions according to the problem list in the electronic health record, but then to ask further detailed questions about the conditions that require more probing. An example of a line of questioning is as follows: "To confirm, besides Down Syndrome, a g-tube for enteral feeding, strabismus, amblyopia, and hypotonia, is there anything else that I've missed? Let's talk a little more about the strabismus and amblyopia. How is she doing with wearing her glasses? Do you notice whether her left eye is still turning, and how often does it turn?"

Before starting the actual physical exam, the clinician should ask the caregiver for advice on the best approach to the examination. Tips such as using a specific song or music genre, or playing the child's favorite videos, may assist with fixation and cooperation. Keep in mind children with special needs may have sensory issues and may not like to be touched or might be scared by clapping or loud noises. The clinician should not hesitate to ask for creative assistance from their caregiver.

Clinicians are often used to doing case history and exams in a certain manner. However, with children with special needs, it is important to be flexible with all elements of the appointment. Before calling in the patient, it may be helpful to observe the child in the waiting room to assess what she/he is playing

Figure 9. Child with special needs and clinician interacting during an eye exam

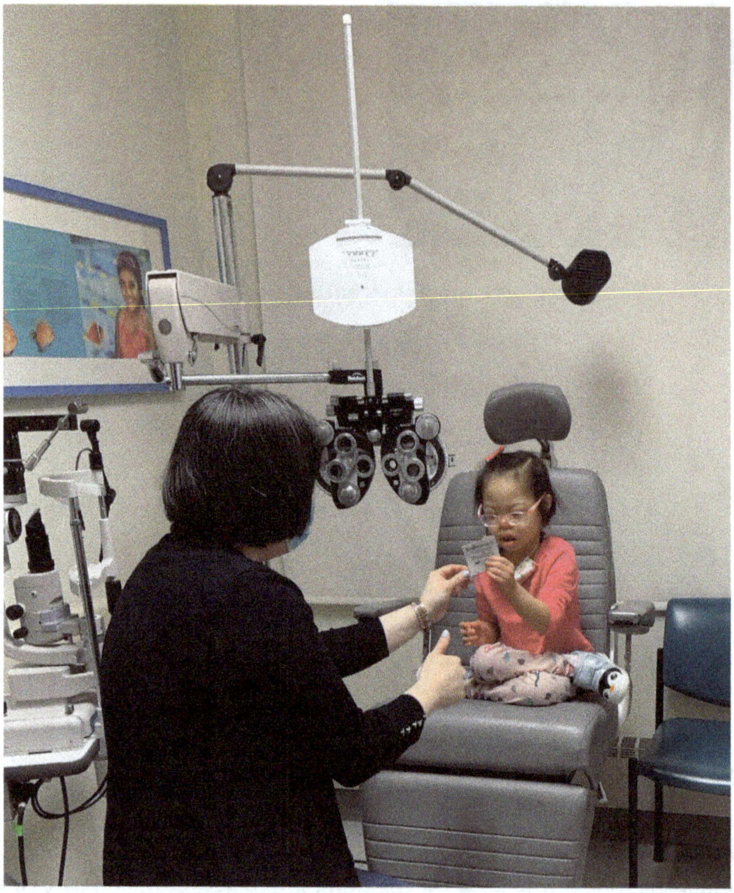

with, reading, using an electronic device, exploring the room, looking at the caregiver, or communicating in a specific manner. These observations may serve as helpful insights for navigating the examination once the child is in the room. The clinician should always stay positive during the examination. Children with special needs often do not respond well to negative reinforcement, but redirection and enthusiastic positive reinforcement are usually welcome (Figure 9).

A clinician should be aware of best practices guidelines for referring to children with special needs. There are those who identify with person-first language, and others who identify with identity-first language. Person-first language uses the person before the diagnosis while speaking, while identity-first language uses the diagnosis/condition first before the person (Centers for Disease Control, 2021b). This can be confusing for healthcare professionals because some health communities have strong emotional connections with how they are identified, especially if their identity pertains to how they interact with the world. Those in the Down Syndrome community generally follow person-first guidelines. A girl with Down Syndrome should not be referred to as "the Downs girl," but rather "the girl who has Down Syndrome." The term "Downs" has negative connotations to those with Down Syndrome because it does not take into account the many other facets of their individuality.

Autism and deafness are examples for which some may prefer identity-first language, rather than person-first language, which is often the recommended guideline for healthcare professionals (Brown,

2011). An example of person-first language is "the boy who has autism," and an example of identity-first language is "the autistic person." Person-first has been more at the forefront because people have not wanted to have their condition define their identity. However, there are those who believe that identity-first language implies that their condition is a negative state of being, which is not true to them. One should always start with referring to the individual by name first, followed by person-first language. It is also appropriate to ask the patient or caregiver about their preference.

Summarizing the Exam and Setting Expectations

While conventional eye exams begin with case history, the pediatric eye care provider-should not feel restricted to performing the case history first and then the exam.

At the end of the case history, the clinician should summarize to the caregiver the chief complaint and other issues that will be examined. The clinician should then state what will come next in the exam to the caregiver, taking care to use the caregiver's wording, and avoid alarming the child. For example, the clinician can say "So now that we have discussed how your eyes have been very itchy, we are going to check how your eyes see the letters on the chart, and then I will take a closer look at your eyes with some lights." For some children, once physical contact takes place between the clinician and the child, crying ensues, and it may be more difficult for the clinician and caregiver to discuss findings at the end. By summarizing expectations and the path of the exam, patient education and treatment instructions may happen more efficiently.

Figure 10. Pediatric case history elements for eye care

Pediatric Case History Elements for Eye Care

- Position at child's level, make eye contact
- Observe child behaviors during case history
- Create rapport with the child and caregiver first
- Practice active listening
- Ask history questions:
  - Chief Complaint/History of Present Illness
  - Birth History
  - Developmental History
  - Social/Educational History
  - Medical History
  - Review of Systems
  - Ocular History
  - Family Medical and Ocular History
- Age-Specific Questions
- Summarize history and set exam expectations

CONCLUSION

A good case history is a critical foundation for the rest of the examination. This chapter has outlined the tips for success during the history-taking so that the examination can be effective and efficient (Figure 10). The examination procedures should proceed based on the direction indicated by the chief complaint and other factors elicited by the comprehensive case history. Taking a detailed history can happen throughout the examination as needed. While practicing active listening and repeating back a summary of information, the caregiver and patient feel heard and become active members in the management plan. General knowledge of milestones and age-appropriate interests can help to establish rapport and accomplish the clinician's goals of assessing age-appropriate visual development and visual performance.

REFERENCES

American Academy of Pediatrics. (2006). Committee on Fetus and Newborn, American College of Obstetricians and Gynecologists and Committee on Obstetric Practice. The Apgar Score. *Pediatrics, 117*(4), 1444–1447. PMID:16585348

American Optometric Association. (2017). *Comprehensive Pediatric Eye and Vision Examination: Evidence-based clinical practice guideline.* https://www.aoa.org/AOA/Documents/Practice%20Management/Clinical%20Guidelines/EBO%20Guidelines/Comprehensive%20Pediatric%20Eye%20and%20Vision%20Exam.pdf

American Optometric Association. (2021a). *Preschool vision: 2 to 5 years of age.* https://ww1.aoa.org/healthy-eyes/eye-health-for-life/preschool-vision?sso=y

American Optometric Association. (2021b). *School-aged vision: 6 to 18 years of age.* https://www.aoa.org/healthy-eyes/eye-health-for-life/school-aged-vision?sso=y

Boyd, K. (2020, July 8). *Vision development: Newborn to 12 months.* American Academy of Ophthalmology. https://www.aao.org/eye-health/tips-prevention/baby-vision-development-first-year

Brown, L. (2011). *Identity-first language.* Autistic Self Advocacy Network. https://autisticadvocacy.org/about-asan/identity-first-language/

Centers for Disease Control. (2021a). *CDC's developmental milestones.* https://www.cdc.gov/ncbddd/actearly/milestones/index.html

Centers for Disease Control. (2021b). *Communicating with and about people with disabilities.* https://www.cdc.gov/ncbddd/disabilityandhealth/materials/factsheets/fs-communicating-with-people.html

Dang, V. T. (2018, August 1). *Identifying ocular allergy.* Optometric Management. https://www.optometricmanagement.com/issues/2018/august-2018/identifying-ocular-allergy

Goldberg, C. (2018). *Practical guide to clinical medicine.* UCSD School of Medicine and VA Medical Center. https://meded.ucsd.edu/clinicalmed/ros.html

Keifenheim, K. E., Teufel, M., Ip, J., Speiser, N., Leehr, E. J., Zipfel, S., & Herrmann-Werner, A. (2015). Teaching history taking to medical students: A systematic review. *BMC Medical Education, 15*(1), 159. doi:10.118612909-015-0443-x PMID:26415941

Oxford Medical Education. (2016). *History Taking—Overview.* https://www.oxfordmedicaleducation.com/history/medical-general/

Peterson, M. C., Holbrook, J. H., Von Hales, D., Smith, N. L., & Staker, L. V. (1992). Contributions of the history, physical examination, and laboratory investigation in making medical diagnoses. *The Western Journal of Medicine, 156*(2), 163–165. PMID:1536065

Rosenberg, E. E., Lussier, M. T., & Beaudoin, C. (1997). Lessons for clinicians from physician-patient communication literature. *Archives of Family Medicine, 6*(3), 279–283. doi:10.1001/archfami.6.3.279 PMID:9161356

Turbert, D. (2020). Vision Development: Childhood. *American Academy of Ophthalmology.* https://www.aao.org/eye-health/tips-prevention/children-vision-development

World Health Organization. (2021). *Adolescent Health.* https://www.who.int/health-topics/adolescent-health#tab=tab_1

KEY TERMS AND DEFINITIONS

504 Plan: A tailored plan for a child whose disability does not qualify for an IEP, but still needs special supports and resources to help them to succeed in elementary or secondary education.

Adolescent: A child approximately between the ages of 10-19 years of age, with 3 major stages during this time period--early, middle, and late adolescence (World Health Organization, 2021).

Case History: An intentional interview of a patient and/or caregiver, performed by a clinician with the goal of performing a medical evaluation. This includes the history of present illness, social history, medical history, developmental history, family history, and ocular history.

Developmental Milestone: A skill or behavior that is generally expected by a certain age as part of normal development.

Elementary-Aged Child: A child usually between 5 to 11 years of age and refers to grades kindergarten (K) through grade 5 or 6.

Identity-First Language: Making reference to a person with their condition listed first, such as "Deaf person."

Individualized Educational Program (IEP): A tailored plan for a child with an eligible disability to provide for specialized instruction, supports, and resources to help the child to thrive in elementary or secondary education.

Infant: This refers to children anywhere from birth to 1-year-old.

Perinatal: The period immediately before and after birth; the definition can vary to include the time period starting at 154 days gestation and lasting through 7 days after birth.

Person-First Language: Making reference to a person with the person first and then condition, such as "person with Down Syndrome."

Postnatal: The period from birth until a baby is 6 weeks old.

Prenatal: The period between conception and birth.

Preschooler: A child between 3-5 years of age who has not yet attended kindergarten.

Toddler: This refers to the age group of a child about 12 to 36 months old.

Section 2
Examination

A pediatric comprehensive eye examination consists of several components, ranging from visual acuity, stereopsis, and binocularity to ocular health. The following chapters will cover in detail the examination of color vision, stereopsis, visual acuity, visual field, pupil, ocular motility, refraction, binocularity, accommodation, anterior segment, and posterior segment. Additionally, this book includes sections specifically on the use of diagnostic agents, slit lamp examination, direct ophthalmoscopy, and indirect ophthalmoscopy with special emphasis in children. A focus on the special needs of premature infants, management of ocular emergencies, and children with myopia are also covered. Clinical pearls are provided within each chapter for a more efficient and effective exam, including modifications to enable a successful eye exam in children of all ages and cognitive abilities.

Chapter 2
Testing Color Vision in Children

Kristen L. Kerber
New England College of Optometry, USA

ABSTRACT

It is important to screen for acquired or hereditary color vision defects as early as possible. Color vision is a critical part of the early learning experience, and children who have color deficiencies may have difficulties compared to their peers if there is color-based schoolwork. It becomes important for career interests/goals for older children as some jobs may require normal color vision. Hereditary red-green deficiencies are X-linked and therefore affect approximately 8% of males and less than 1% of females. Acquired color vision defects and blue-yellow defects are rare in the pediatric population; therefore, these conditions will be discussed minimally in this chapter. Infants are able to discern color by 2-3 months of age, but accurate color naming may not develop until 4-6 years of age. Screening tests are sensitive, fast, and easy to administer. If a deficiency is suspected through screening, further testing must be evaluated in order to determine the type and severity of the color vision defect. Color vision is typically tested starting at age 3 years and up.

INTRODUCTION

Color vision rapidly develops in the first few months postnatally (Brown, 1990); however, color naming and discrimination relies on cognitive development occurring in the first few years of life. For this reason, color vision testing is typically started with children aged 3 years and older and is not indicated in infants or toddlers. Many color vision tests and screeners are difficult for this young age, therefore adaptions using recognizable shapes are used. Since acquired color vision defects and blue-yellow defects are rare in children, this chapter will concentrate on congenital red-green defects. The objective of this chapter is to guide the pediatric clinician in the types of color vision tests available and their procedures.

DOI: 10.4018/978-1-7998-8044-8.ch002

BACKGROUND

It is important to identify children with color vision defects at a young age. Color vision defects are not uncommon. Hereditary red-green deficiencies are X-linked, and therefore are present in approximately 8% of males and less than 1% of females. Early learning experiences (such as toys, décor, schooling, etc.) assume normal color vision, but children with color vision defects may have early academic difficulties if there is color-dependent schoolwork or activities. It becomes more important to identify color vision deficiency with increasing age as it may affect career choices later in life.

There are multiple color vision test options available to pediatric eye care practitioners. Typically, a screening test is chosen to differentiate those with normal color vision from those with color vision deficiency. Those with deficiencies may be further evaluated to identify the type and severity. Often, complete evaluation cannot be performed until the child is old enough to complete more intricate tests such as hue discrimination, disc comparison, or the anomaloscope. Screening younger children is often accomplished with Color Vision Test Made Easy (CVTME) and the Hardy-Rand-Rittler (HRR) pseudoisochromatic plates. Older children can be tested with Ishihara test plates. Digital color vision tests are also becoming more readily available. A full discussion of each is provided in this chapter.

GENERAL GUIDELINES FOR PEDIATRIC COLOR VISON TESTING

1. Typical test distance is 75cm (Carlson, 2004; National Research Council (US) Committee on Vision, 1981), but the examiner can permit young children to move closer to better engage visual attention or facilitate a motor/tracing response.
2. Color vision screening is more accurate when conducted in natural daylight or with a CIE Standard Illuminant C lamp (Birch, 2001). These lamps mimic average daylight's spectral distribution. Incandescent stand lamps are strongly discouraged during color vision screening as deutans will often perform better and may even pass screening testing when completed in this lighting.
3. Present the color vision test plates perpendicular to the line of sight.
4. Be prepared to shift to a developmentally easier test method. For example, if a school age child unexpectedly cannot correctly name numbers, shift to a tracing method. Note that the font used for some color vision numbers can be confusing to children.
5. Binocular color vision testing is standard. Consider monocular color vision testing if ocular disease is suspected.
6. It is important that children do not touch the pages in the color vision test books and the pages are not exposed to direct sunlight as it ruins the printed color. If the tracing method is employed, have children trace with a small paint brush or cotton tip applicator.
7. If the clinician suspects the child is failing the test because of poor cooperation, consider asking the parent to administer the test.
8. It is helpful to have printed information available for children who test positive for color vision deficiency.
9. It is common for parents to need reassurance that their child is not color-blind.

PSEUDOISOCHROMATIC PLATES (PIPS)

PIPs are relatively inexpensive. Each plate consists of colored dots in a mosaic pattern which create letters, numbers, shapes, or lines. Patients with abnormal color vision will either not see the target, or see a different target compared to those with normal color vision. Each book comes with an answer key outlining what a patient with normal color vision will see compared to those with abnormal color vision. Below, several PIP tests are discussed.

Ishihara

Ishihara PIPs (Figure 1) are the most commonly used color vision test plates in eye clinics. They are red-green color deficiency screening tests that can classify basic defects. They do not screen for blue-yellow defects. There are two versions: one with 24 plates and a more concise version with 14 plates. Waggoner's Pseudoisochromatic Plates Ishihara Compatible (PIPIC) is similar but can screen for both red-green and blue-yellow defects.

Equipment:

- Ishihara book

Figure 1. Ishihara test plates. Note the font and spacing of '29' can be confusing to a young child (left plate)

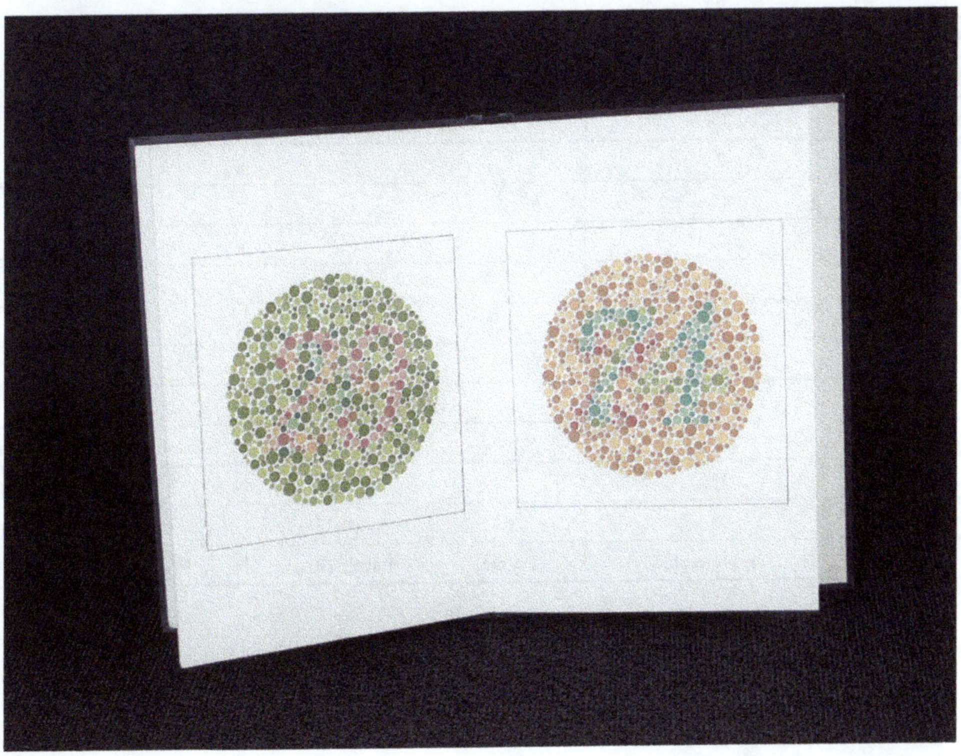

Procedure:

Step 1: Hold the PIPs at 75cm from the patient and slightly tilted so the plates are perpendicular to the line of sight. It is best viewed with diffuse natural daylight

Step 2: Ask the child to name each number, but if the patient is shy or nonverbal then they may trace it to complete the test

Step 3: The first plate is visible to all children regardless of their color vision status. If a child with satisfactory visual acuity does not identify this plate it renders the test unreliable

Step 4: For the 14-plate edition, the patient must get 10 correct to pass (plates 12-14 may be omitted if only trying to establish normal vs. abnormal color vision)

Step 5: If using the 24-plate edition, plates 1-17 are administered to children who can recognize numbers. 13 correct out of 17 is required to pass. If a patient cannot identify numbers, plates 18-24, which contain traceable curving lines, may be administered.

Clinical Pearl: *The traceable lines in the Ishihara PIP have been shown to be invalid in the preschool age group (Haegerström-Portnoy, 1990).*

Table 1. Ishihara answer key. "x" denotes plate cannot be read. Parentheses indicate they may be read, but not as clear

<table>
<tr><th>Plate Number</th><th>Normal</th><th colspan="4">Red-Green Deficient</th></tr>
<tr><td>1</td><td>12</td><td colspan="4">12</td></tr>
<tr><td>2</td><td>8</td><td colspan="4">3</td></tr>
<tr><td>3</td><td>5</td><td colspan="4">2</td></tr>
<tr><td>4</td><td>29</td><td colspan="4">70</td></tr>
<tr><td>5</td><td>74</td><td colspan="4">21</td></tr>
<tr><td>6</td><td>7</td><td colspan="4">x</td></tr>
<tr><td>7</td><td>45</td><td colspan="4">x</td></tr>
<tr><td>8</td><td>2</td><td colspan="4">x</td></tr>
<tr><td>9</td><td>x</td><td colspan="4">2</td></tr>
<tr><td>10</td><td>16</td><td colspan="4">x</td></tr>
<tr><td>11</td><td>Traceable Line</td><td colspan="4">x</td></tr>
<tr><td colspan="2" rowspan="2"></td><th colspan="2">Protan</th><th colspan="2">Deutan</th></tr>
<tr><td>Strong</td><td>Mild</td><td>Strong</td><td>Mild</td></tr>
<tr><td>12</td><td>35</td><td>5</td><td>(3) 5</td><td>3</td><td>3 (5)</td></tr>
<tr><td>13</td><td>96</td><td>6</td><td>(9) 6</td><td>9</td><td>9 (6)</td></tr>
<tr><td>14</td><td>2 lines traceable</td><td>Purple</td><td>Purple (Red)</td><td>Red</td><td>Red (Purple)</td></tr>
</table>

Color Vision Test Made Easy® (CVTME)

CVTME (Figure 2) is a color vision screening tool without classification ability (only normal vs. abnormal) that is widely used in pediatric eyecare. It does not classify the type or the severity. It is typically used in preschool age children. It is a PIP test with more easily recognizable shapes and pictures for children. There are two parts. The first consists of circle, square, and star targets that may be named or traced. Part two is made for less responsive patients and consists of a picture of a boat, house and dog. There are 10 plates in the first part. Part two contains only 3 plates which is appropriate for the short attention span of some young children. The part two test items are larger than the part one test items which further serves to capture the attention and cooperation of immature children. CVTME was determined to be 100% compatible with the Ishihara PIPs (Cotter, 1999).

Equipment:

- CVTME book

Figure 2. CVTME test plate

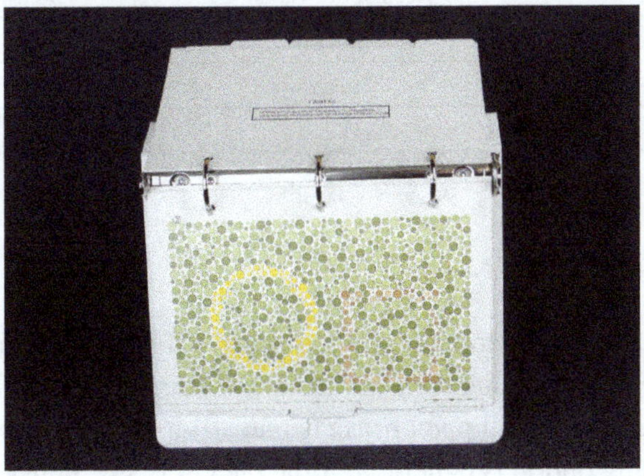

Procedure:

Step 1: Review the possible shapes with the child to aid in understanding of the test

Step 2: Hold the cards at 75cm and perpendicular to the line of sight

Step 3: The first plate is the test plate and visible to all children

Step 4: If the child is shy, some practitioners may ask the children to find or trace the ball (circle) on each page. Thus, a child with red-green deficiency will successfully trace a circle on plates 3-5 demonstrating understanding of the test. If using this method, showing the child plates 3-5 first, a color deficient child will begin with 3 successful attempts

Step 5: The patient must get 8 of the 9 test plates correct to pass

Table 2. CVTME part 1 answer key

Plate Number	Normal Individual	Red-Green Deficient Individual
1	Circle, Square	Square
2	Circle, Star	Star
3	Square, Circle	Circle
4	Circle, Square	Circle
5	Square, Circle	Circle
6	Square, Circle	Square
7	Circle, Square	Nothing
8	Circle, Star, Square	Nothing
9	Star, Circle	Nothing

Table 3. CVTME part 2 answer key. Note: Shapes may vary slightly depending on version purchased

Plate	Normal Individual	Red-Green Deficient Individual
A	Boat	Nothing
B	House	Nothing
C	Dog	Nothing

Hardy-Rand-Rittler (HRR)

The HRR color vision test can detect and classify red-green defects in addition to blue-yellow defects. Therefore, it can be helpful in identifying congenital and acquired color vision defects. It has the advantage of child friendly shapes and a mini paint brush (Figure 3) for children to trace the shapes in lieu of a verbal response. The tracing option is beneficial if the patient is shy, non-verbal, or speaks a different language than the clinician. This test is best administered with CIE source C lamps, but if not available, indirect natural daylight is a close approximation. The first four plates are demonstration plates to confirm child's understanding of the test. The next six screening plates are used to separate normal from those with defective color vision.

Equipment:

- HRR book
- Small paint brush

Procedure:

Step 1: Hold the book approximately 75cm from the patient, perpendicular to their line of sight

Step 2: Present the demonstration plates number 1 - 4. Ask the child to report what is seen on each page. The child may trace the plates with the paint brush

Step 3: If the child fails the demonstration plates, they may be malingering or not cooperating because of apprehension or confusion. Stop the test and do not continue to Step 4

Figure 3. HRR test plate (#15 pictured) and paintbrush

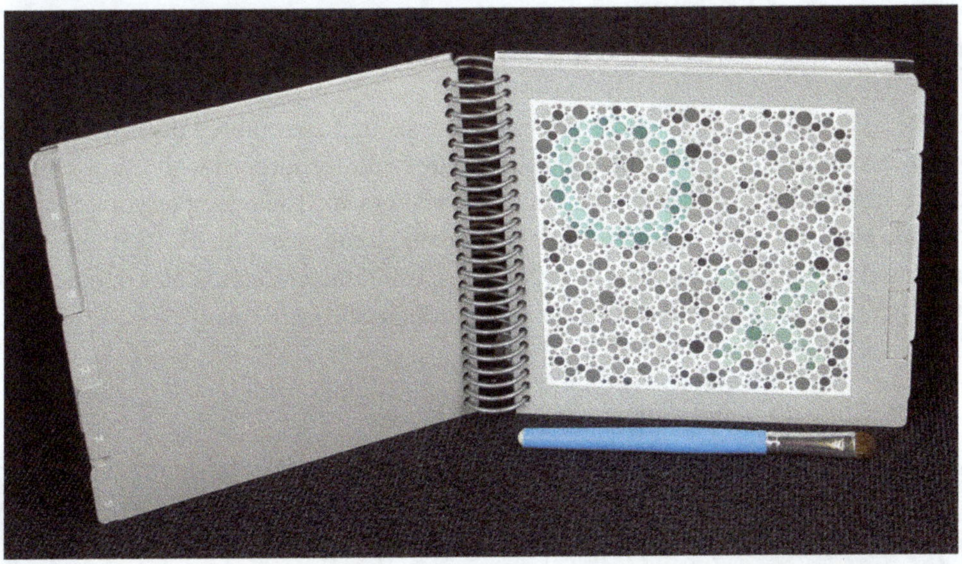

Step 4: If the patient can complete the demonstration plates, continue with the remaining plates. If child fails the six screening plates, there are 14 subsequent plates to diagnose the extent and type of defect

- If plates 5-6 are missed, a blue-yellow defect is suspected. If plates 7-10 are missed, a red-green defect is suspected. Only plates 11-20 are shown below to concentrate on red-green defects (Table 4)
- If plates 11-15 are missed in any capacity, the defect is mild. If 16-18 are missed, the defect is moderate. Lastly, if 19-20 are missed, the defect is severe (Table 5)

Table 4. Hardy-Rand-Ritter (HRR) plates answer key

Plate Number	Answer Key
1-4	DEMO Plates – not scored
5	O, X
6	O,
7	X,
8	O,
9	O
10	X

Table 5. HRR diagnostic plates answer key for plates 11-20. Plates 21-24 are to further classify blue-yellow defects

Plate Number	Protan	Deutan
11	O	
12		X
13		
14	O	X
15	X	O
16		O
17	O	
18		X
19	X	O
20	O	

HUE DISCRIMINATION ARRANGEMENT TESTS

Farnsworth Panel D 15 (FD15) and Farnsworth Munsell 100 (FM100)

FD15 and FD100 are hue discrimination arrangement tests that use colored discs to assess color discrimination and extent of color confusions. These tests are typically not used with young children as they require concentration and higher levels of cognitive development. There are preset reference discs and the patient must place the discs in a gradual color changing sequence. The FD15 (Figure 4) is shorter and typically used for industrial classification purposes. Children with mild color deficiencies can still pass this test, but those with moderate to severe color deficiencies will fail.

Figure 4. FD15 testing discs and storage box

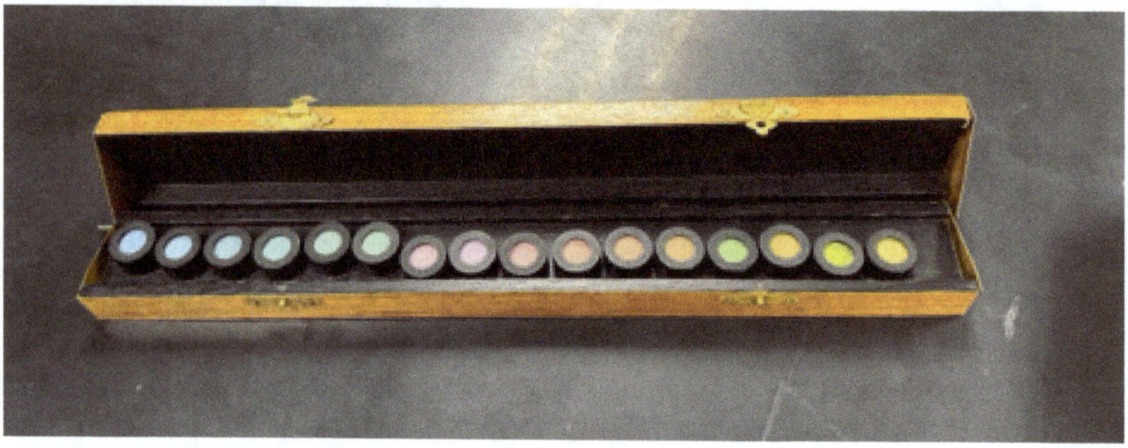

The FM100 (Figure 5) is similar in presentation to the FD15, but uses 100 discs that the patient is asked to place in a gradual color changing sequence. Due to the length of the test, typically taking 15-30 minutes to administer, the FM100 test is typically reserved for junior high or high school children with color vision deficiency to support vocational counseling.

ANOMALOSCOPE

The anomaloscope (Figure 6) is the gold standard for color vision testing. However due to the high cost and limited availability, this instrument is most used in research and academic settings (Birch, 2001; National Research Council (US) Committee on Vision, 1981). The anomaloscope is the only test that identifies the abnormal retinal pigment (protan v. deutan) *and* determine the number of functioning pigments (dichromacy v. trichromacy). The use of the instrument requires extensive examiner training and is not typically administered to children under 8 years old due to the cognitive and attentional demands.

Figure 5. FM100 testing discs and storage boxes

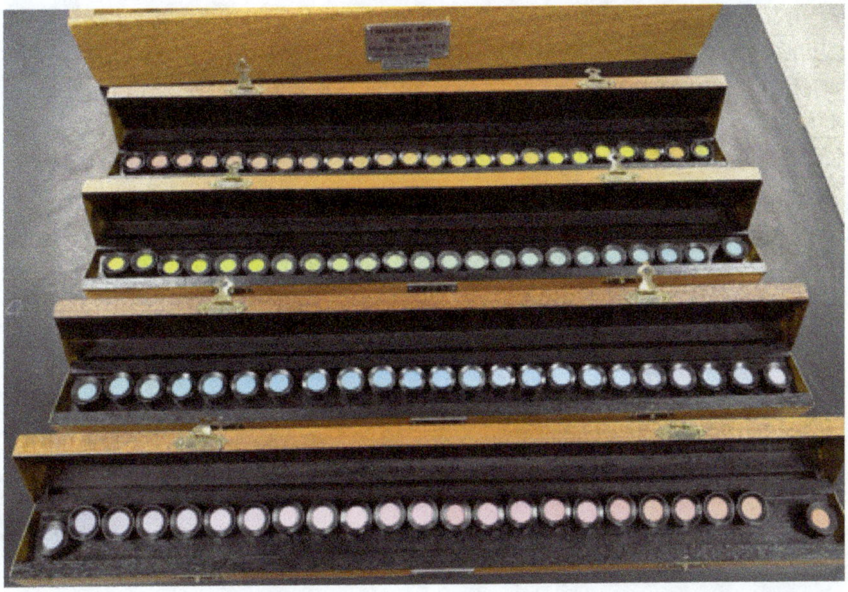

Figure 6. Neitz anomaloscope

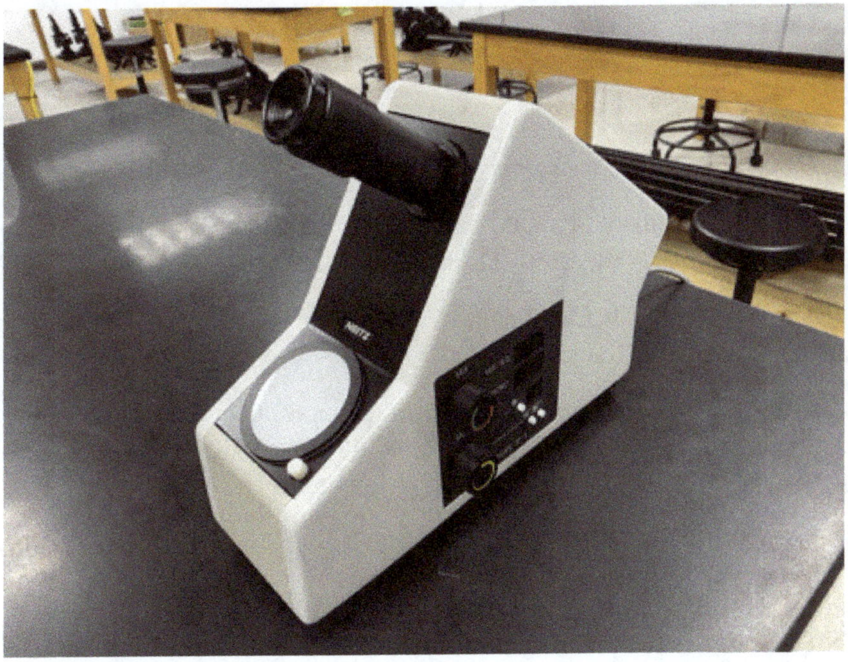

Digital Color Vision Tests

Digital color vision tests are gaining popularity. In a small study conducted by van Staden et al. (2018), an online Ishihara test on color-blindness.com was able to discern between normal and deficient color vision patients but did not identify the extent of the defect accurately. Waggoner Computerized Color Vision Test (CCTV) at TestingColorVision.com has shown promise when studied by the United States Navy, showing better sensitivity and specificity than Ishihara PIPs, and equal to that of the Nagel anomaloscope (Picken, 2014). An important consideration using digital tests is whether the test's reliability or validity can be affected by the monitor's resolution and calibration. Glare from room lighting or computer screens must also be considered. More research is needed to test digital color vision test's validity.

CONCLUSION

It is important for the eye care provider to identify children with color vision defects as early as possible. If a child fails an initial color vision screening test, it is beneficial to perform repeat testing in order to confirm the color vision deficiency. Equally important is educating patients, teachers, and parents regarding potential limitations in school or in future career paths. Fortunately, there are many options for the practitioner to screen both younger and older children. These different options allow the practitioner to adapt to both the age and ability of the patient.

REFERENCES

Birch, J. (2001). *Diagnosis of defective colour vision* (2nd ed.). Butterworth-Heinemann.

Brown, A. M. (1990). Development of visual sensitivity to light and color vision in human infants: A critical review. *Vision Research, 30*(8), 1159–1188. doi:10.1016/0042-6989(90)90173-I PMID:2205977

Carlson, N. B., Kurtz, D., Heath, D., Capone, R. C., & Watanabe, R. K. (2004). Clinical procedures for ocular examination (3rd ed.). McGraw-Hill.

Cotter, S. A., Lee, D. Y., & French, A. L. (1999). Evaluation of a new color vision test: "color vision testing made easy. *Optometry and Vision Science*, *76*(9), 631–636. doi:10.1097/00006324-199909000-00020 PMID:10498004

Duckman, R. H. (2006). *Visual development, diagnosis, and treatment of the pediatric patient*. Lippincott Williams & Wilkins.

Haegerström-Portnoy, G. (1990). Color Vision. In A. A. Rosenbloom & M. W. Morgan (Eds.), *Principles and Practice of Pediatric Optometry* (pp. 449–466). J.B. Lippincott Company.

Home Vision Care. (1994). *Color vision testing made easy*. Terry L. Waggoner.

Kanehara & Co. Ltd. (1997). The series of plates designed to test for colour-deficiency. Tokyo, Japan: Shinobu Ishihara.

National Research Council (US) Committee on Vision. (1981). *Procedures for Testing Color Vision: Report of Working Group 41*. Washington, DC: National Academies Press (US). Available from: https://www.ncbi.nlm.nih.gov/books/NBK217823/

Picken, D., Mann, W., & Rings, M. (2014). *Validation of a computerized color vision test* [Paper presentation]. *Aerospace Medical Conference*, San Diego, CA.

Richmond Products. (2002). *H.R.R. Pseudoisochromatic Plates*. Author.

Van Staden, D., Noor Mahomed, F., Govender, S., Lengisi, L., Singh, B., & Aboobaker, O. (2018). Comparing the validity of an online Ishihara colour vision test to the traditional Ishihara handbook in a South African university population. African Vision and Eye Health, 77(1). doi:10.4102/aveh.v77i1.370

KEY TERMS AND DEFINITIONS

Anomaloscope: The gold standard for color vision testing using an anomaloscope, a device in which knobs are used to match two colored areas in both color and brightness. Well-known brands in the United States include Nagel, Neitz, and Pickford-Nicolson.

Color Vision Test Made Easy (CVTME): A pseudoisochromatic plate test that is typically used in preschool age children due to its easily recognizable shapes and pictures. It only classifies between normal and abnormal color vision, not the type of severity.

Farnsworth: A type of hue discrimination arrangement test using colored discs in a gradual color changing sequence. The Farnsworth Panel D 15 (FD15) is the shorter version (compared to the Farnsworth Munsell 100).

Farnsworth Munsell: A type of hue discrimination arrangement test using colored discs in a gradual color changing sequence. The Farnsworth Munsell 100 (FM100) is typically used in older children or adults due to the length of the test.

Hardy-Rand-Rittler (HRR): A pseudoisochromatic plate test that can classify both red-green and blue-yellow defects, as well as the severity. It has child friendly shapes.

Ishihara: A pseudoisochromatic plate test that screens for red-green deficiencies using predominantly numbers that may be more difficult for younger children or illiterate patients.

Pseudoisochromatic Plates (PIPs): A category of color vision tests containing colored dots in a mosaic pattern.

Red-Green: The most common inherited color vision defect grouping both protan and deutan defects together.

Waggoner: Dr. Terrace L. Waggoner, renowned color vision expert who has developed both print and digital pseudoisochromatic plate color vision tests.

Chapter 3
Testing Stereopsis in Children

Kristen L. Kerber
New England College of Optometry, USA

ABSTRACT

Stereopsis develops very early in life and is thought to be present in a normally developing child by six months of age. In order to develop stereopsis, multiple components of visual development must be intact including visual acuity and bifoveal fixation. Stereopsis is the most sensitive way to assess sensory fusion but can be unreliable in very young age groups due to difficulty understanding the test or instructions. It is best to choose an option with global stereopsis (high level cortical stereo), as local stereopsis may overestimate ability due to available monocular cues. Global is created using random dot stereograms (RDS) – computer-generated patterns to create a stereoscopic form, while local contains line stereograms which create horizontal retinal image disparity giving the perception of depth. Stereopsis can be affected by strabismus, amblyopia, and other binocular vision dysfunctions that interfere with visual efficiency (especially in school-age children). The chapter discusses the most commonly used clinical tests of global and local stereopsis.

INTRODUCTION

Stereopsis testing is a way to quantify the smallest retinal image disparity that provides depth perception. Both visual acuity and ocular alignment must be within normal ranges in order for stereopsis to develop (Schnell, 2020). There are two types of stereopsis that are found in the tests described in this chapter: global and local. When possible, it is best to test global stereopsis, which requires high level cortical stereopsis provided only from bifoveated images. Local stereopsis however, may be elicited using monocular cues (i.e., motion parallax) to detect disparity. Stereopsis testing is most useful in detecting amblyopia and/or strabismus. In older children, it may also aid in detecting or monitoring other binocular dysfunctions affecting sensory or motor function. This chapter will discuss the most commonly used clinical stereo tests of global and/or local stereopsis.

DOI: 10.4018/978-1-7998-8044-8.ch003

BACKGROUND

Testing stereopsis in young children is important for assisting in the identification and progression of conditions such as amblyopia, strabismus, and significant refractive error. In older children, it can be additive in detecting or monitoring other types of binocular vision disorders that can affect visual efficiency. Global stereopsis is a random dot stereogram (RDS) that is composed of computer-generated dots giving rise to stereoscopic forms if bifoveally fixated. RDS testing can quickly rule out most strabismus, including microtropias. There are no monocular cues to aid in detection. Local stereopsis on the other hand is a line stereogram using horizontal retinal disparity to elicit the perception of stereopsis. Local stereopsis can be detected through monocular cues, therefore making it less robust in detecting amblyopia and strabismus. It is important for the clinician to minimize the use of these cues by having the patient and stereo book remain still. Stereopsis norms increase with age as well as reliability in these tests (Pai, 2012; Tarczy-Hornoch, 2008). Table 1 outlines general norms for stereoacuity by age.

Table 1. Stereoacuity norms by age

Age (years)	Norm (sec of arc)
3-4	150
4-5	70
5-8	40
11+	20

(Schnell, 2020)

Clinical Pearl: *Some children will need more time to perceive stereopsis targets (especially global); clinicians should be encouraging to garner the child's interest in finding the hidden items.*

Random Dot E

This 2-alternative-forced-choice test uses random-dot stereograms to test global stereopsis. It is sometimes used in vision screenings as it has been shown as an effective screening for amblyopia and refractive error. Conditions that have "coarse" stereopsis (such as anisometropic amblyopes, monofixators and microstrabismics) will not be able to pass this test. It is a great tool for not only screenings, but examinations in young children.

The set of testing plates include a blank, an embossed or model E, and a stereopsis E (Figure 1). The blank plate contains a random-dot stereogram that appears as a random assortment of dots. The model E is visible by all individuals regardless if they have stereopsis. The last plate contains a random-dot stereogram that shows the letter E to individuals wearing polarized glasses who have stereopsis. It is the only stereopsis test not conducted at a near point distance.

Equipment

1. Pediatric polarized glasses
2. Random Dot E plate (blank, demo, and test plates)

Procedure

Step 1: Place polarized glasses on the child's face for the entire duration of the test. Show the Model E and ask what child sees. If child does not know letters, ask if she/he sees a shape or picture on the card. If child can appreciate that something is on the card, proceed to step 2.

Step 2: Present the blank plate next to the Model E (equidistant apart so as not to influence the child). If the child can detect the Model E, proceed to step 3. If child cannot, she/he will likely randomly choose which card has the letter or shape (~50% chance).

Clinical Pearl: *a child who is malingering will likely choose the blank card with every presentation.*

Step 3: Once the examiner is confident the child understands the pretest, the stereo E plate and blank are presented 4 times. If the child can get a minimum of 3 out of 4 correct, she/he has stereopsis at that test distance. The preferred test distance is at 5 feet (1.5 meters), as this distance can identify children who have small angle strabismus, amblyopia, and/or significant refractive error. At 5 feet, the stereo E is 168 seconds of arc (Schnell, 2020).

Clinical Pearl: *testing a child at a closer distance first will often improve confidence and performance at 5 feet.*

Advantages

1. Presented at different distances and positions so that the correct responses cannot be memorized.
2. Nonverbal or shy children are able to point to the correct plate.
3. Malingers can be detected using this test as a 4/4 wrong answer indicates the patient is likely not guessing (as you would expect about a 50:50 ratio).

Figure 1. Random Dot E testing plates

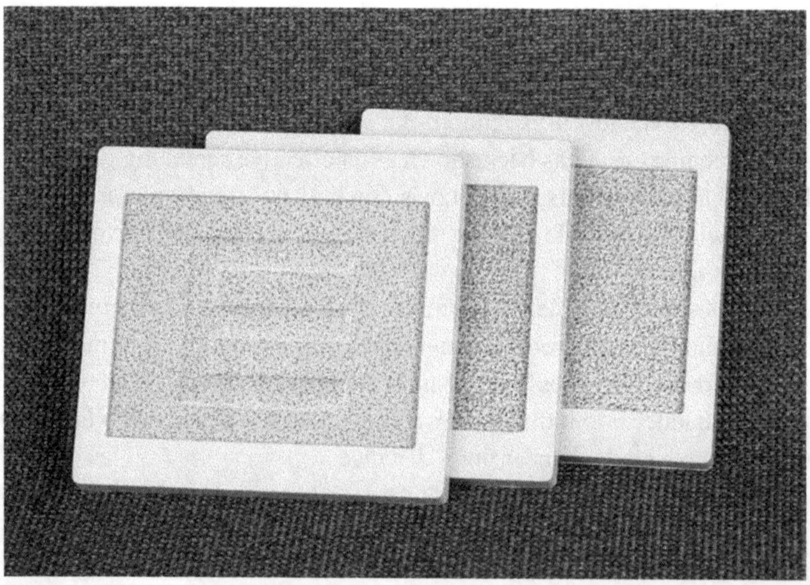

Preschool Assessment of Stereopsis with a Smile (PASS)

PASS is a global stereopsis test created to improve testability in younger children and is similar in presentation and design (2-alternative-forced-choice) to the Random Dot E described above. The smiley face target is thought to be more child friendly than the E. This test is presented at 40cm, a closer distance than Random Dot E which may keep children more engaged in the procedure. There is a blank, a demo card with a blue smiley face seen by all children, and four stereopsis cards (60, 120, 240 and 480 seconds of arc) (Figure 2). The procedure is the same as the random dot E (child must correctly identify 3 out of 4 presentations before the next level stereopsis can be used).

Figure 2. PASS testing plates

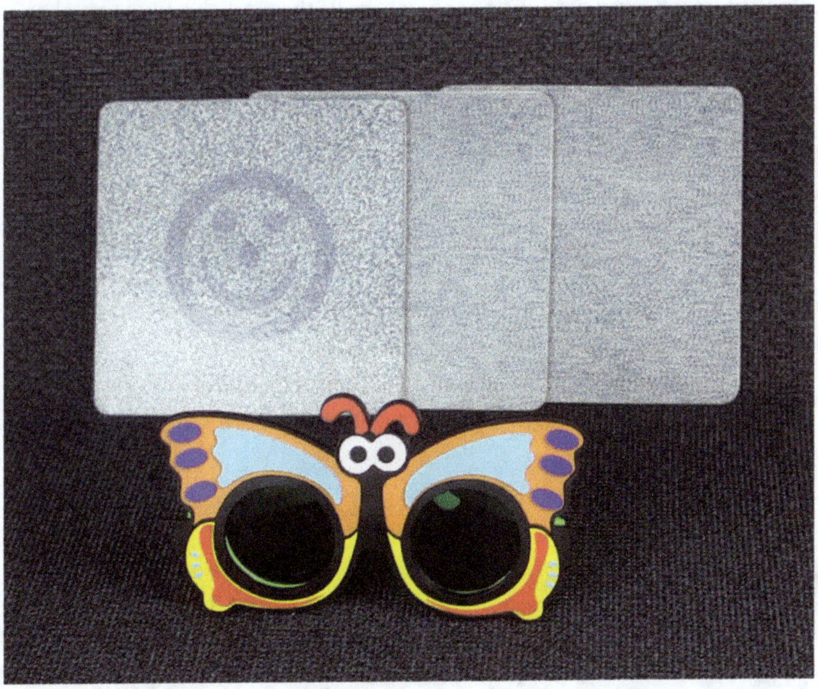

Equipment

1. Pediatric polarized glasses
2. PASS Plates (Blank, demo, and four test plates)

Procedure

Step 1: Place polarized glasses on the child's face for the entire duration of the test. Show the demo PASS plate and ask what she/he sees. If child can appreciate that something is on the card, proceed to step 2

Step 2: Present the blank plate next to the demo plate (equidistant apart so as not to influence the child). If the child can detect the blue smiley face, proceed to step 3. If child cannot, she/he will likely randomly choose which card has the smiley face (~50% chance)

Clinical Pearl: *a child who is malingering will likely choose the blank card with every presentation.*

Step 3: Once the examiner is confident the child understands the pretest, the 480" stereo smile plate and blank are presented 4 times at 40cm. If the child can get a minimum of 3 out of 4 correct, proceed to the next level of stereopsis. If the child cannot get at least 3 presentations correct, record the level of the previous plate

Randot Preschool Stereoacuity Test

This test of global stereopsis uses random dot stereograms of kid friendly shapes (i.e., heart, elephant, car, etc.) (Figure 3). There are three sets ranging from 800 to 40 seconds of arc. For each level of stereopsis there are two-dimensional black and white test shapes on the left-hand side of the booklet and random dot presentations on the right-hand side. For each set, only three of the four test shapes are located on the random dot stereogram side, leaving one blank square.

Equipment

1. Pediatric polarized glasses
2. Randot Preschool book

Procedure

Step 1: Place polarized glasses on the child and hold the book at 40cm (16in)
Step 2: Have the child name each black and white test picture
Step 3: Ask the child to find three of those pictures on the random dot stereogram side
Step 4: The child must get 2 of the 3 shapes to move onto the next level

Figure 3. Randot Preschool stereoacuity test

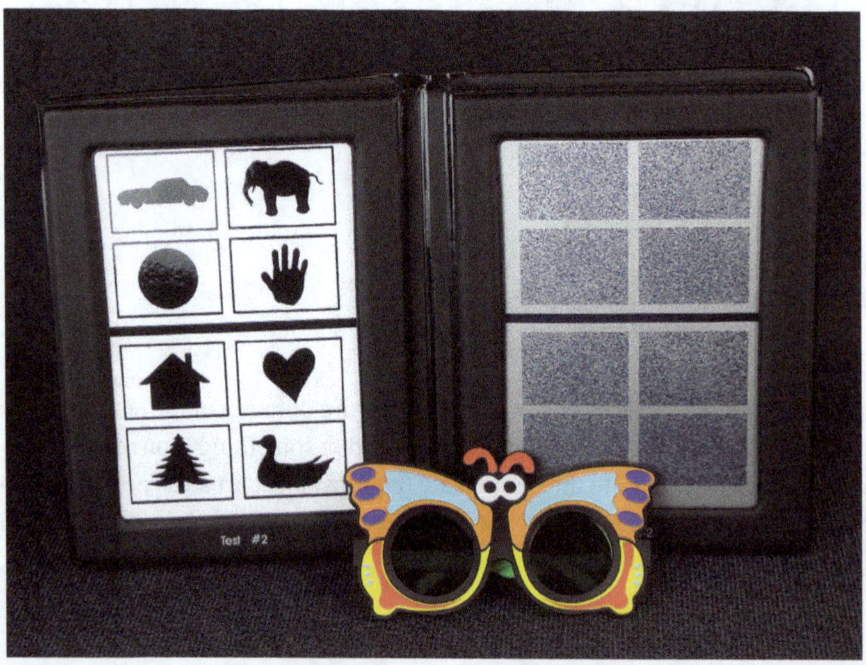

Lang Stereo Test

Two versions of Lang stereo test plates are available with differing 3D objects. Lang Stereotest I (Figure 4) has a star, cat, and car (600-1,200 seconds of arc), while Lang stereo test II displays a moon, truck and elephant (200-600 seconds of arc). Lang Stereotest II also has a star that can be viewed monocularly for demo purposes. Each shape has a different level of stereopsis. The greatest advantage of this screening test is that polarized glasses are not needed. This is particularly useful in children who are resistant to wearing polarized glasses. For shy or nonverbal children, the examiner may ask if they see one of the shapes and ask the child to point to it. This can also be used with infants by holding it up and watching for the child to attempt to grab the shapes.

Equipment

1. Lang stereo card(s)

Procedure

Step 1: Hold the test plate at 40cm (16in) perpendicular to the line of sight
Step 2: Ask the child if he or she sees any shapes on the plate
Step 3: Once a 3D object has been named, ask the child to look for additional shapes and to describe them

Figure 4. Lang Stereopsis

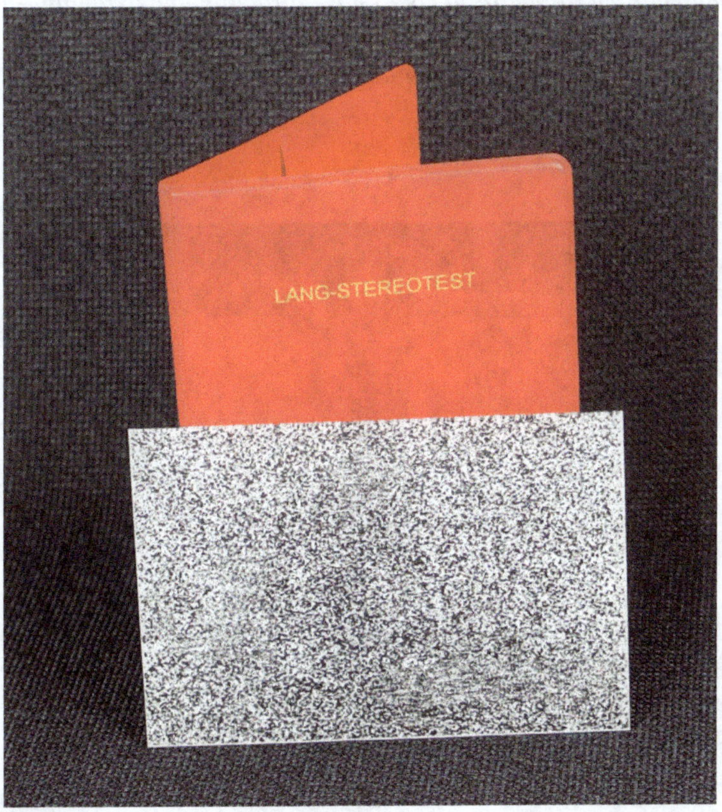

Titmus Fly or Butterfly

The Titmus test contains the well-known fly (Figure 5) which tests gross stereopsis (3000 seconds of arc). The butterfly is also commonly seen in place of the fly in some books. This booklet has local stereopsis, therefore patients with course stereopsis may do well on this test through monocular cues such as motion parallax. There are three sections: the fly/butterfly, animals, and circles.

Equipment

1. Pediatric polarized glasses
2. Titmus stereo book

Procedure

Step 1: Place polarized glasses on the child and hold the stereo book at 40cm (16in)

Step 2: Direct attention to the large stereo fly or butterfly and ask the child to grab or pinch the wings. A child who sees the animal "floating" will grab the wings *above* the booklet. A child who does not see the wings floating will likely just touch the book's surface

Step 3: There are three rows containing five local stereo animals each, with only one animal that appears to float off the page. To pass all three rows, patients must have 100 seconds of arc

Step 4: Lastly, direct the child to the circles. In each group of four, one is made of disparate stimuli which causes it to "float" above the page. This local stereo measures up to 20 seconds of arc

Clinical Pearl: *Young children are more likely to have difficulty understanding the circles. One way to engage the child in the circles may be to use instructions that may be familiar to them through other toys. For example, "which circle looks like a button you can push?"*

Figure 5. Titmus Fly

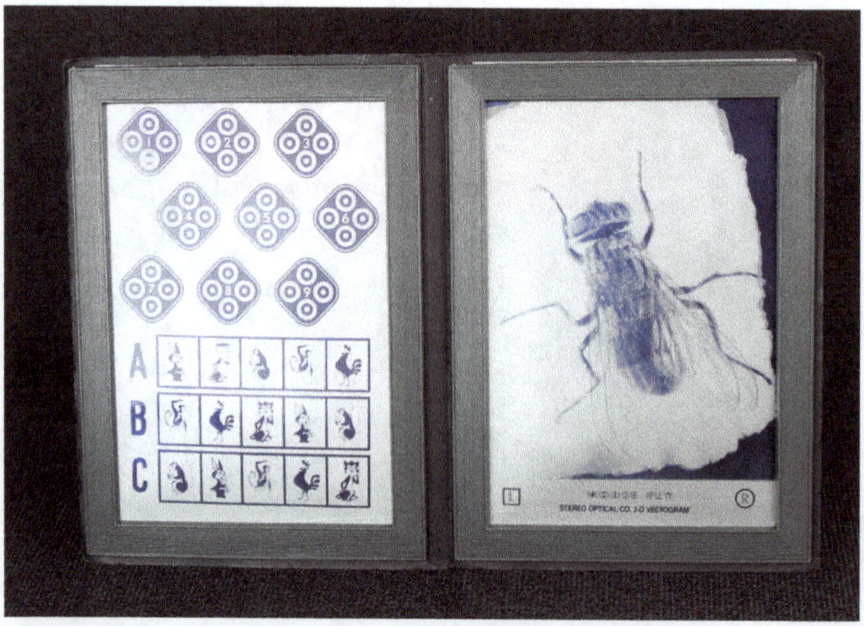

Randot with Global Stereo Shapes

These are some of the most common stereo booklets used for older children and adults. Depending on the version of the book, it varies in how much of the testing is global or local stereopsis. One disadvantage is that there are many targets presented at once which may confuse young children. The original book (Figure 6) contains random dot stereograms (250 and 500 seconds of arc) on the right-hand side, utilizing kid friendly shapes. On the left, it contains the animals and circles described as above in the Titmus Fly book. Studies show that most typically developing preschool children will have stereopsis of 70 seconds of arc on the Randot circles, while typically developing school-age children will have 40-50 seconds of arc (Kulp, 2005).

The Random Dot 2 book (Figure 7) uses Lea symbols for the global section as well as replacing the animals. Similar to the original version, the right-hand side is global while the left-hand side is local stereopsis. The newer Random Dot 3 (Figure 8) has the same targets as Random Dot 2, but *all* targets are global stereopsis. Lea matching symbols can be utilized for nonverbal patients, or the examiner can ask them to find and point to a certain shape (i.e., "Where is the circle?").

Equipment

1. Pediatric polarized glasses
2. Randot book

Procedure

Step 1: Place polarized glasses on the child and hold the stereo book at 40cm (16in)

Step 2: Direct the child towards the global symbol boxes containing easily recognizable shapes. Ask her/him to describe the shapes seen. These tests at the level of 500 and 250 seconds of arc for the original book and up to 125 seconds of arc in versions 2 and 3

Step 3: If using the original, move onto the local stereo animals. If using version 2 or 3, begin with the Lea symbols shapes on the bottom and ask the child which one appears to be floating in each row

Step 4: Lastly, direct the child to the circles (local if using the original or version 2, global if using version 3)

Frisby Stereotest

This stereotest is unique in the sense that it uses real depth, therefore no polarized glasses are needed. This is accomplished using clear plates that have the target and its surround printed on opposite sides of the plate (Figure 9). There are three test plates varying in thickness to change the depth tested. A greater range of depth can be created by varying test distance from 30-150cm (5-600 seconds of arc). Each plate contains four boxes, only one of which will have the stereo target. Patients with poor stereopsis will not be able to observe the target. If the examiner has no stereopsis, the correct square can be determined using the corner "studs". The stud nearest the stereo target square is flat which can be discriminated from the other corners by touch.

Figure 6. Original Randot with global stereo shapes, local animals and circles

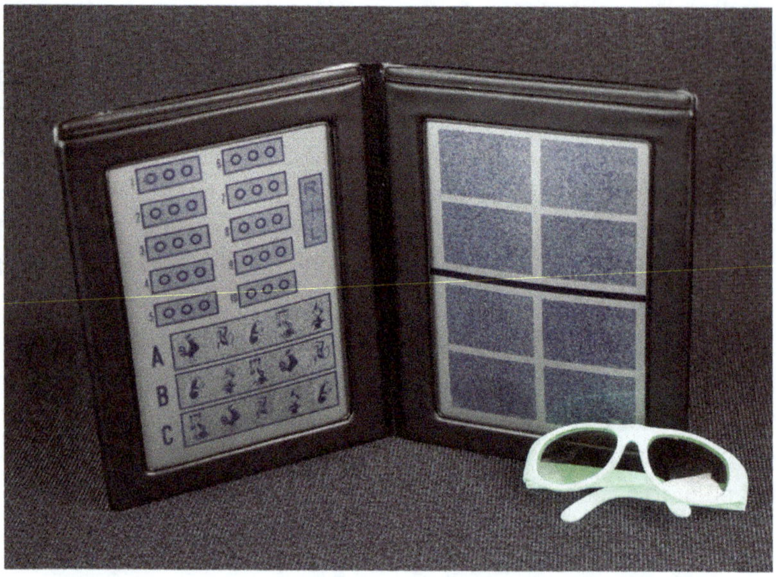

Figure 7. Randot 2 with global stereo shapes, local Lea symbols and circles

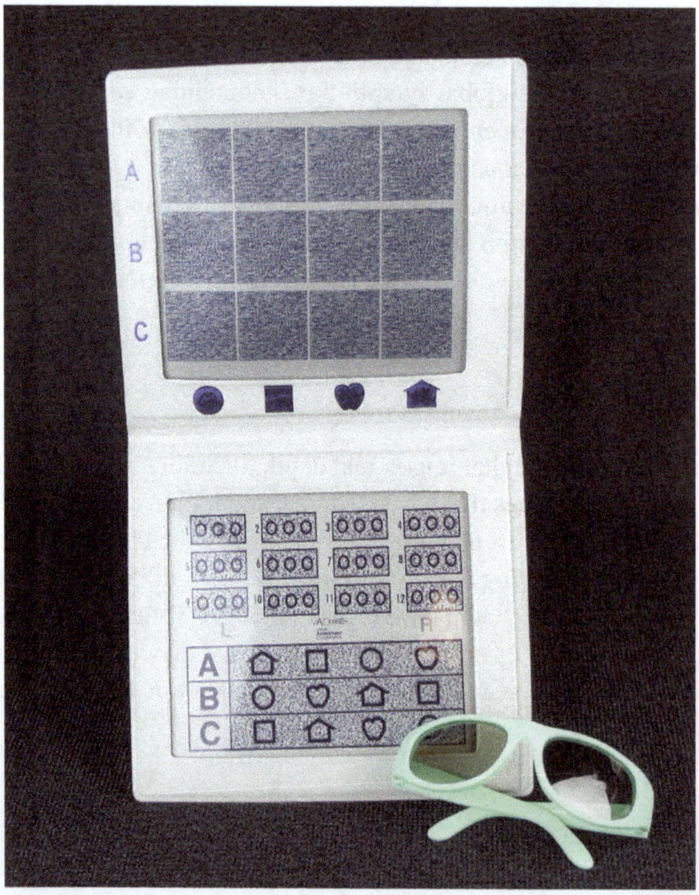

Figure 8. Randot 3 with global stereo shapes, Lea symbols and circles

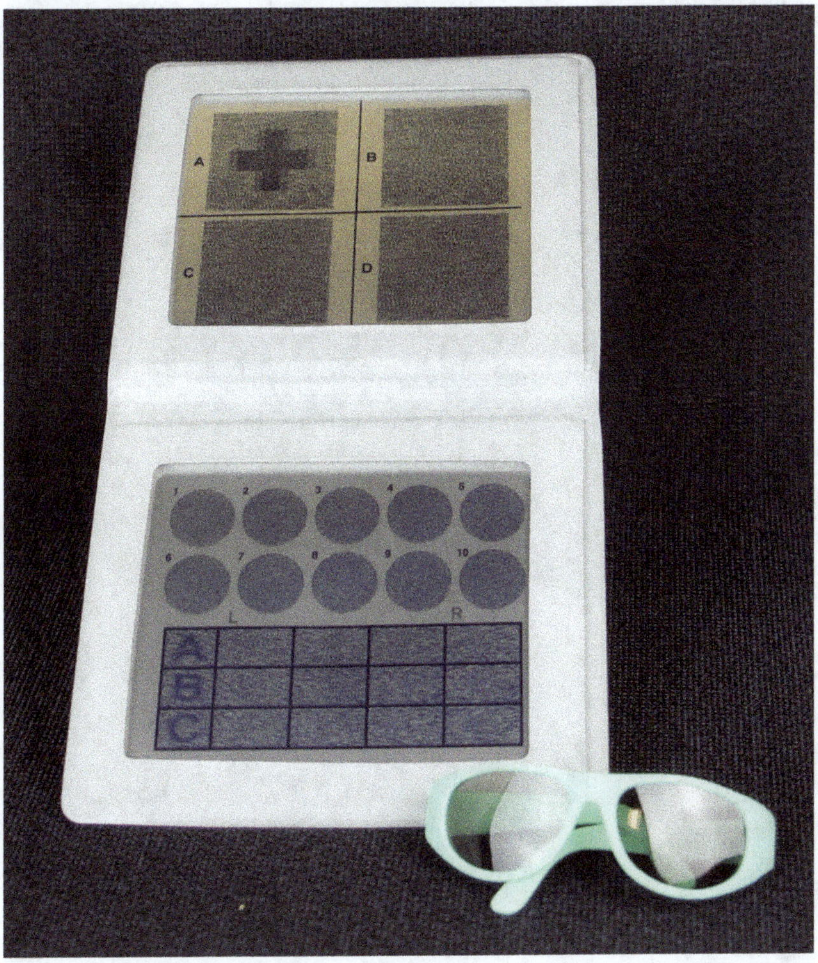

Equipment

1. Frisby stereo box and 3 test plates

Procedure

Step 1: Position child at the desired test distance (typically at 40cm for the initial testing) and instruct to keep head still

Step 2: The test plate is held on the edge of the folded down flap of the Frisby storage box, with its top edge held just a few inches above the flap. The plate should be square to the child's line of sight and held still

Clinical Pearl: *Do not hold the plate flat against the white box flap while testing as shading cues may reveal the stereo target to individuals with no stereopsis. This however can be useful to demo the target so the patient knows what they are looking for. Motion parallax can also be used to demo the target by twisting the plate back and forth.*

Step 3: Starting with the thickest plate, ask the child to identify the square that has a circle "sticking out" or creating a "hole". This orientation is determined by which side of the plate is facing the child

Step 4: The target is considered seen if the child can guess the correct location at least three out of four presentations

Figure 9. Frisby stereo test

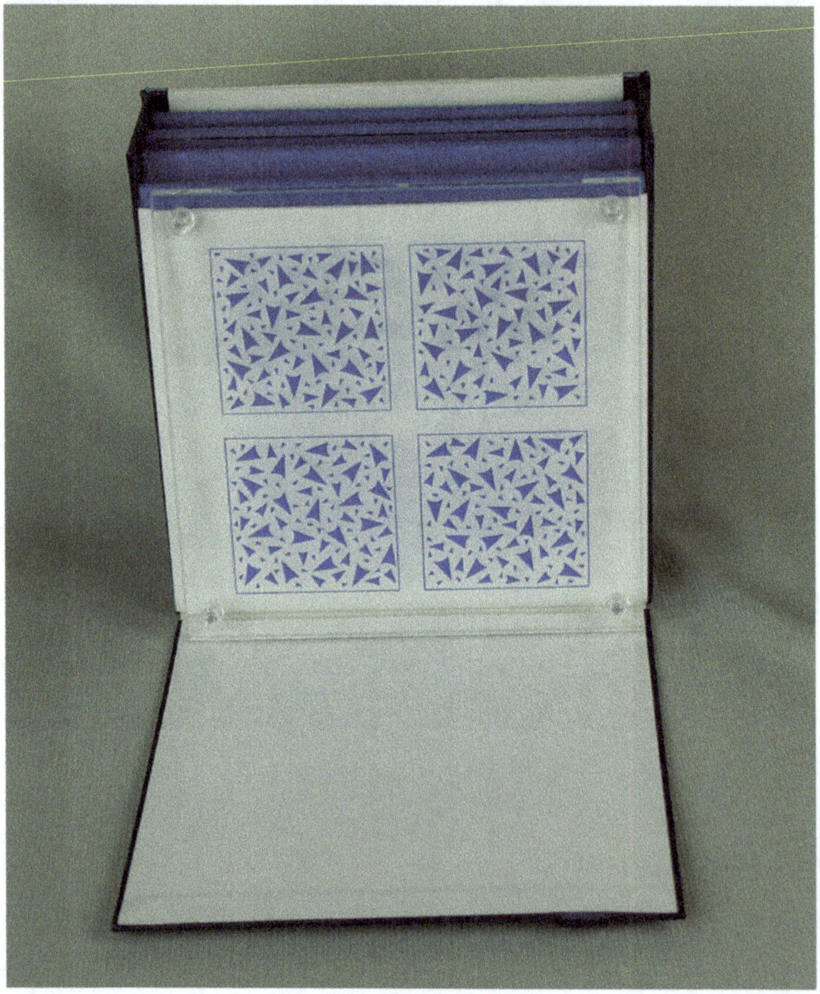

CONCLUSION

Stereopsis testing is vital in the detection and monitoring of strabismus and amblyopia. It is also helpful in monitoring visual efficiency-related conditions in older children.

REFERENCES

Kulp, M. T., & Mitchell, G. L. (2005). Randot stereoacuity testing in young children. *Journal of Pediatric Ophthalmology and Strabismus, 42*(6), 360–364. doi:10.3928/01913913-20051101-05

Pai, A. S.-I., Rose, K. A., Samarawickrama, C., Fotedar, R., Burlutsky, G., Varma, R., & Mitchell, P. (2012). Testability of refraction, stereopsis, and other ocular measures in preschool children: The Sydney Paediatric Eye Disease Study. *Journal of AAPOS, 16*(2), 185–192. https://doi.org/10.1016/j.jaapos.2011.09.017

Schnell, P. H., Taub, M. B., & Duckman, R. H. (Eds.). (2020). *Visual development, diagnosis, and treatment of the pediatric patient* (2nd ed.). Wolters Kluwer.

Tarczy-Hornoch, K., Lin, J., Deneen, J., Cotter, S. A., Azen, S. P., Borchert, M. S., Wang, Y., Varma, R., & Multi-Ethnic Pediatric Eye Disease Study Group (2008). Stereoacuity testability in African-American and Hispanic pre-school children. *Optometry and Vision Science: Official Publication of the American Academy of Optometry, 85*(3), 158–163. https://doi.org/ doi:10.1097/OPX.0b013e3181643ea7

ADDITIONAL READING

Afsari, S., Rose, K. A., Pai, A. S., Gole, G. A., Leone, J. F., Burlutsky, G., & Mitchell, P. (2013). Diagnostic reliability and normative values of stereoacuity tests in preschool-aged children. *The British Journal of Ophthalmology, 97*(3), 308–313. doi:10.1136/bjophthalmol-2012-302192

Stereo Optical Company, Inc. (2009). *Randot® Preschool Stereoacuity Test.* Eileen Birch.

KEY TERMS AND DEFINITIONS

Frisby: A stereopsis test using real depth due to transparent plates of varying thicknesses.

Global: A type of stereopsis test using random dot stereograms which make it only achievable in a patient with bifoveal fusion and high-level cortical stereopsis.

Lang: A stereopsis test that uses kid friendly shapes and does not need to utilize stereo glasses.

Local: A type of stereopsis test that uses horizontal retinal image disparity to create the appearance of depth; monocular cues may be used to pass these tests.

PASS: Preschool Assessment of Stereopsis with a Smile (PASS) is a type of stereopsis test that uses kid friendly smiley faces.

Random Dot: Computer-generated dots giving rise to stereoscopic forms if bifoveally fixated.

Randot: A registered trademark of Stereo Optical Company, Inc. This is a commonly used, shortened term for "Random Dot."

Titmus: A type of stereopsis test that is known for its large animal fly.

Chapter 4
Pediatric Visual Acuity Testing

Gayathri Srinivasan
New England College of Optometry, USA

ABSTRACT

Visual acuity measurement is an essential component of any eye exam. In adults and older children, letter-based acuity (i.e., recognition acuity) is commonly used to measure vision. However, in infants and toddlers, performing traditional visual acuity testing is nearly impossible. Instead, modified optotypes such as gratings and pictures are shown to observe the young child's visual behavior. Additionally, there are objective visual acuity methods that negate the need for observing visual behavior. For the practicing clinician, the choices are many and can be confusing. With new commercial products coming into the market every day, it is nearly impossible to comprehensively cover each one of them. Instead, in this chapter, commonly used and/or studied visual acuity tests are covered. For each test, the set-up, procedure, documentation, and scientific evidence supporting or negating its use are discussed.

INTRODUCTION

Visual acuity is one of the commonly measured visual functions as part of a pediatric eye examination. It is the ability of the visual system to identify a target or resolve spatial details of a target. The threshold for identifying a target is defined as recognition acuity (i.e., recognition of letters or shapes) and the threshold for resolving spatial details within a target is defined as resolution acuity (i.e., resolving the thickness of the black bars in a black and white grating). Development of vision has been studied using behavioral observations and electrophysiological studies. Robert Fantz, a psychologist, formalized the use of pattern stimuli (black and white gratings on a gray background) to understand the looking behavior of infants called forced preferential looking (FPL) ((Fantz, 1963; Frantz et al., 1962). Data obtained from FPL experiments show that the monocular grating acuity at 1 month of age (about 1 cycle/degree (cpd), approximate Snellen equivalent 20/600) develops rapidly in the first year reaching about 6 cpd at 1 year of age (Snellen equivalent 20/100), followed by a gradual increase until reaching adult-like acuity (25 cpd, Snellen equivalent 20/25) at 5 years (Mayer et al., 1995). Similarly, the mean recognition acuity (using picture-based optotypes) reaches 20/25 by 4 years of age. Additionally, electrophysiological studies

DOI: 10.4018/978-1-7998-8044-8.ch004

using visually evoked potential (VEP), using a bold pattern stimulus such as a square-wave grating, also show a rapid development of grating acuity in the first 6 months that continues during the second half, reaching adult-like levels by 1 year of age, which is earlier than FPL techniques (Norcia & Tyler, 1985).

While letter-based charts can be used to measure visual acuity in older children (6 years and above), modified charts containing shapes, or finite number of letters, are used in toddler and preschool children to improve testability. In infants and toddlers, since communication is challenging, clinicians rely on other techniques such as behavioral observations (observing the infant looking behavior towards the visual stimuli) or objective technique such as VEP to measure visual acuity. While VEPs are not frequently used in clinic, behavioral observations are and demand significant examiner experience to accurately interpret results. Since there are significant methodological differences between these methods, direct comparison of visual acuity across these methods is discouraged. Despite these challenges, visual acuity measurement is integral to a pediatric eye exam for several reasons, the most important being the detection of unilateral or bilateral amblyopia. Defined as a developmental disorder affecting spatial vision with a prevalence of 1-3% (Webber & Wood, 2005), amblyopia is characterized by reduced visual acuity in one or both eyes and is the common cause of reduced vision in children, and can impact other visual functions such as accommodation, binocular function, contrast sensitivity and reading performance (Kelly et al., 2015; McKee et al., 2003; Weakley, 2001). Without early intervention, visual acuity loss remains even if spectacle correction is provided later. Since visual acuity is the current clinical standard for diagnosing amblyopia, it is important for clinicians to be familiar with clinical visual acuity tests in children. Additionally, understanding visual acuity norms in children can help clinicians differentiate reduced vision from age-expected vision. This chapter covers the various qualitative and quantitative visual acuity tests for infants, toddlers, and preschoolers.

VISUAL ACUITY TESTING IN INFANTS AND TODDLERS

Tests that are suitable for infants and toddlers require minimal or no verbal response from the child and depend on either the clinician's observation of visual behavior to the stimulus presented, or the utilization of instrumentation to measure visual acuity (e.g., VEP). While most tests allow the clinician to make qualitative measures of visual acuity, some do not and are qualitative.

Clinical Pearl: *Several studies have shown that children have better acuities with grating than recognition acuity (Friendly et al., 1990; Kushner et al., 1995; Mayer, 1986; Mayer et al., 1984; Rydberg et al., 1999). In particular, grating acuity overestimates vision in strabismic amblyopia (Kushner et al., 1995). For this reason, Snellen equivalents (provided in the accompanying test manuals of grating acuity tests) are not used for clinical interpretation and instead the grating acuity is recorded in cycles per cm (c/cm) or cycles per degree (cpd).*

All quantitative tests discussed in this section measure grating acuity except for Cardiff test.

The quantitative and qualitative procedures discussed in this section are:

- **Qualitative vision assessment of fixation pattern**
  - Fix and Follow (monocular fixation pattern)
  - Fixation preference test (binocular fixation pattern)

- **Quantitative vision assessment**
    - **Preferential Looking Tests**
        - Teller Acuity Card (TAC)
        - Lea gratings/Patti Stripes
        - Cardiff test
- **Objective tests**
    - Optokinetic Nystagmus (OKN)
    - Visually Evoked Potential (VEP)

QUALITATIVE VISION ASSESSMENT OF FIXATION PATTERN

A quick way to evaluate an infant's vision is observing whether the infant prefers to fixate with one eye over the other (i.e fixation preference). The rationale is that in amblyopia, infants will prefer to fixate with the non-amblyopic eye, and conversely, infants without amblyopia will show no preference for either eye. However, a population-based study (Cotter et al., 2009) that compared letter-based acuity test (ex: HOTV test) with the fixation preference test showed that fixation preference test had poor sensitivity and specificity in detecting interocular difference in visual acuity in 30 to 72-month-old children with amblyogenic risk factors. Therefore, the fixation preference method is not recommended as a sole assessment tool for detecting amblyopia in preverbal children. Rather, other quantitative tests should be administered to quantify vision when possible.

Fix and Follow (Monocular Fixation Pattern)

Procedure
Step 1: The examiner sits in front of the infant in a well-lit room
Step 2: The examiner presents an appropriate target (such as a small toy) at 40 cm

Clinical Pearl: *The squeaky sounds from auditory toys (Figure 1) should not be enabled during testing to ensure that visual information from the target alone is used to evaluate the ability to fixate and follow.*

Step 3: Occlude the infant's non-tested eye with the hand or thumb and slowly move the target (about 2cm per second) in the cardinal gaze positions (i.e up, down, up and right, up and left, down and right, and down and left)
Step 4: Observe the fixation ability and accuracy as the target is slowly moved in all directions. It might be necessary to guide the infants' attention back to the target if there is fixation loss during testing.
Step 5: Repeat testing with the other eye.
Step 6: Infants with poor vision in the tested eye may resist occlusion of the non-tested, better seeing eye. In such circumstances, it is worthwhile to repeat Steps 2-4 to ensure repeatability of results.

Clinical Pearl: *If there is uncertainty about whether the infant is fixating on the target, the examiner can move the target slightly to one side and observe whether there is a concordant pursuit movement.*

Figure 1. Examples of fixation toys used to garner a child's attention

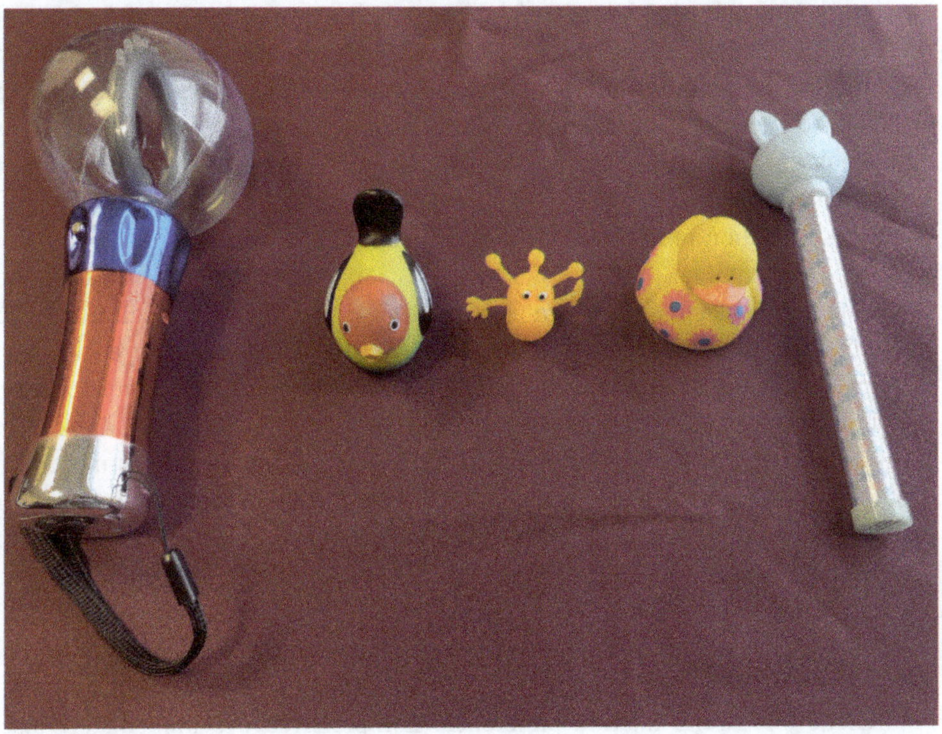

Interpretation:

1. The expected response is steady fixation and accurately following the target in all directions.
2. Consistent response to occlusion of the non-tested eye might indicate poor vision in the tested eye.

Fixation Preference Test (Binocular Fixation Pattern)

The procedure to evaluate binocular fixation pattern depends on whether there is a manifest deviation.

In a young child with no strabismus or small angle strabismus (<10pd), a dissociative vertical prism is used, and the test is called the induced tropia test (ITT).

In a young child with strabismus >10pd, the dissociative prism is not used, and instead the standard fixation preference test (SFPT) is used.

Induced Tropia Test

Procedure

Step 1: The clinician sits in front of the child in a well-lit room and holds an accommodative target at 40cm

Step 2: A 10pd (base up or base down) prism is placed in front of one eye while the patient's attention is directed to the near target

Step 3: The clinician observes which eye is fixating on the target. If there is no fixation preference, the examiner will observe spontaneous alternation of fixation between the eyes

- For example, when 10BD is held in front of the right eye, vertical diplopia is induced with the top image seen by the right eye and the bottom image seen by the left eye. The first movement expected is for both eyes to move up (eyes move towards the apex of the prism). If there is no fixation preference of the right eye, the eyes will move down and then up again spontaneously to alternate fixation between the images seen by each eye. The testing is repeated with the prism over the left eye to confirm whether the fixation preference is reproducible. If so, testing stops here.
- If there is a fixation preference of the right eye (the eye behind the prism), both eyes will move up and continue to stay up. The test is repeated with the prism over the left eye. Sometimes, the switching of prism from one eye to the other can result in a switch in fixation preference, wherein, now with the prism over the left eye, both eyes will move up and continue to stay up. If this is observed, this is considered no fixation preference, although it did not happen spontaneously as described above.
- If, however, one eye was consistently preferred even after the prism is moved to the other eye, the examiner should then occlude the preferred eye and force the non-preferred eye to assume fixation. The preferred eye is then uncovered to see how long the non-preferred eye continues maintaining fixation on the target (Figure 2).

Step 4: Grade the fixation preference

- Several grading systems have been proposed to describe fixation preference (Sener et al., 2002; Wallace, 2005; Wright et al., 1981):
  - Grade 0 - Strong fixation preference (non-preferred eye immediately loses fixation when the preferred eye is uncovered)
  - Grade 1 - Holds fixation momentarily (non-preferred eye holds fixation for 1-2 seconds, but loses before the blink)
  - Grade 2 - Holds fixation well (non-preferred eye holds fixation through a blink
  - Grade 3 - No fixation preference – free alternation of fixation between the eyes

Standard Fixation Preference Test

This test is administered in children with strabismus (>10pd) to describe their fixation pattern.

Procedure

Step 1: The clinician presents a target with accommodative detail at 40cm and directs the child's attention to it.

Step 2: If constant unilateral strabismus is present, it is expected for the non-strabismic eye (preferred eye) to assume fixation and maintain fixation in which case, the preferred eye is occluded and non-preferred eye is forced to assume fixation as detailed in the ITT and the same grading system is used to describe fixation preference.

Step 3: If alternating strabismus or intermittent strabismus is present, observe if there is spontaneous alternation of fixation between the eyes.

Step 4: Record:

- Fix, Follow, and Maintain (FFM) with each eye; no resistance to occlusion; Grade 3 fixation preference binocularly

- Fix and Follow OD; Resisted occlusion of the right eye; Grade 0 fixation preference OD binocularly.

Figure 2. Illustration of the fixation preference test

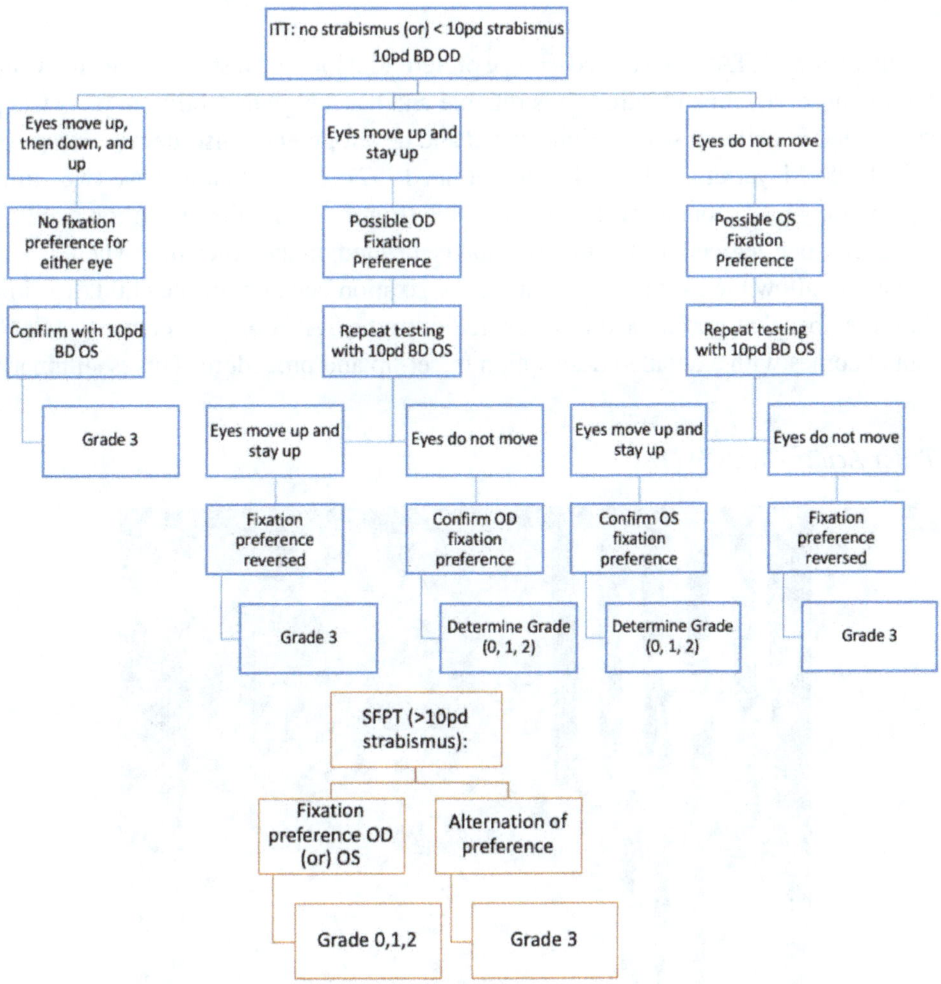

QUANTITATIVE VISION ASSESSMENT

Preferential Looking Tests

Preferential looking tests (PLT) involve simultaneous presentation of two stimuli - a patterned stimulus and gray background, both of which have equal average luminance. Some tests contain gratings for the pattern (ex: TAC, Lea gratings) while other tests (ex: Cardiff acuity test) contain popular pictures that are recognizable by children. Regardless, all these tests contain coarser (low resolution acuity) to finer levels (high resolution acuity) of patterns. The clinician presenting the stimuli should be masked to the position of the pattern to minimize bias. At threshold, the pattern and the gray background will not be distinguishable for the child and therefore a preference towards the pattern stimulus will not be observed. These tests can be used in infants and toddlers as well as in individuals with disabilities. Each of these tests are reviewed separately below.

Teller Acuity Cards

The Teller Acuity Cards™ (TAC) is a forced-choice preferential looking test developed to evaluate resolution acuity in infants and young children. It is reliable and has a high testability in pediatric population and has been studied in children with various visual and developmental disorders (Courage et al., 1994; Dobson et al., 1995; Mayer et al., 1995; Preston et al., 1987). The test cards have two stimuli (square wave grating and gray background) printed on one side (Figure 3) and the resolution acuity (cycles per cm (cpcm) or cycles per degree (cpd)) and test distance printed on the other side. There is a small peephole in the center to allow the examiner to observe the fixation behavior of the child. It is important for clinicians to remember that grating acuity measured with the TAC does not convert to Snellen acuity. The test manual comes with a detailed description of set-up and procedure. This is summarized below.

Figure 3. Teller Acuity Cards™ (TAC)

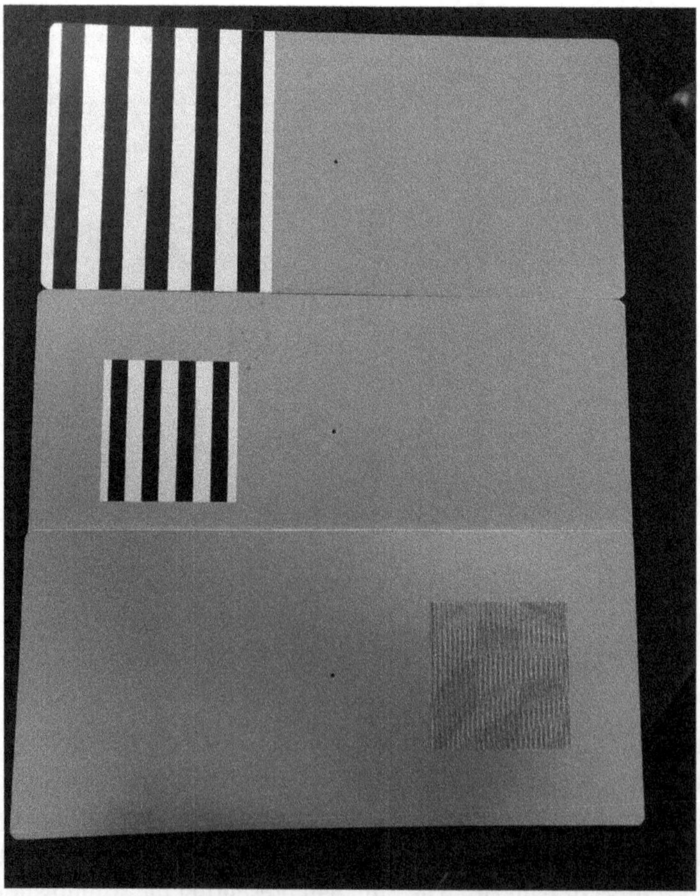

Set-Up

1. The child is seated on the attendant's lap or alone if older, at the test distance from the examiner.
2. Normal room illumination is adequate for testing. If needed, additional illumination should be directed towards the ceiling and not directly on the card.
3. The card should be held vertically and not tilted since this can vary its luminance.

Clinical Pearl: *In patients with esotropia or horizontal nystagmus, the card can be held vertically to allow easy observation of eye movements. In such instances, it is recommended that the card be held in the patient's lower field.*

4. There are 16 test cards in a full set with spatial frequencies ranging from 0.23 cpcm to 38.0 cpcm. The grating side on 0.23 cpcm card (i.e "Low vision card") goes from top to bottom (Figure 3, top card). The full set also contains a gray card.
   a. Note: The spatial frequency difference between the cards is half an octave. One octave is halving or doubling of a spatial frequency.
   b. Note: The left-right position of the grating should be varied so that both the examiner and the child can anticipate the grating position in the next card.
5. The "Start Card" is one that most children with normal eyes should see. The following guideline is recommended, as shown in Table 1.
6. The test distance varies based on the child's age as shown in Table 2.

Table 1. Teller Acuity Cards guideline for start card based on age. Source: TAC II Reference and Instruction Manual. Stereo Optical Co., Inc

Age	Start Card
<6 months (or) any child with visual impairment	0.64 cpcm
6 to 18 months	1.3 cpcm
>18 months	2.4 cpcm

Table 2. Teller Acuity Cards guideline for test distance based on age. Source: TAC II Reference and Instruction Manual. Stereo Optical Co., Inc

Age	Test Distance
Birth to 6 months	38 cm (15 inches)
7 months - 3 years	55 cm (21.7 inches)
> 3 years	84 cm (33 inches)
Children with visual impairment	19 cm (7.5 inches) or 9.5 cm (3.7 inches)

Clinical Pearls:

- *The test distance should be maintained throughout testing.*
- *If a different test distance is used for one eye, grating acuity calculation should be performed separately for each eye based on the test distance used.*
- *If 55cm test distance is used, the card itself can be used as a tool for monitoring test distance since the length of the card is 55cm.*
- *Since testing is done at near distance, the resulting acuity is not sensitive in detecting refractive errors such as mild or moderate myopia.*

7. The testing area should be quiet and free from distractions. It is recommended that other individuals (ex: clinicians and attendants) not gather around the examiner, which can be distracting for the child.
8. The test card stack should be arranged such that the grating side of the card is face-down and not visible to the examiner.

Procedure:

Step 1: The clinician attracts the child's attention straight ahead with a toy and shows the "Start Card" followed by the blank card. This step allows the child to familiarize with the grating and the examiner to observe the fixation pattern of the child

Step 2: The next finer grating card is presented, and the child's fixation is observed

Step 3: Each card is presented *at least* twice. Before the second presentation, the card is rotated 180 degrees

Clinical Pearls on minimizing examiner bias:

1. *The examiner should not look at the orientation of the grating between presentations at each acuity level.*
    - *Only when the examiner is confident about his/her observation, can they look at the position of the grating. If the examiner is uncertain, the testing is repeated by rotating the card and the masking is maintained.*
2. *During each presentation, the examiner should avoid looking at the attendant holding the child who might glance towards the side of the grating.*

Step 4: Once the clinician is confident about the fixation pattern of the child, the next card is presented

Step 5: The cards can be presented in 1 octave steps (every other card) for coarser gratings and if the clinician is confident about his/her judgement

Step 6: At threshold level, since the fixation behavior may be unclear, multiple presentations are needed and the card is presented in 0.5 octave steps (every card)

Step 7: The acuity card that yields the last reliable response is identified as the grating acuity.

- Common fixation behaviors when the grating is seen:
    - In infants, a quick gaze shift towards the side of the grating can be observed. In toddlers, pointing, touching or a verbal response can be observed.
- Common behaviors when the grating is not seen:
    - In infants who cannot see the grating side, a random scanning of the card, looking away from the card or refusal to see the card can be observed.

Step 8: Record the results

- The results should include the acuity level and the test distance. Acuity is recorded in cpd. Note: Although Snellen equivalents are provided, there are not equivalent to grating acuity.

Clinical Pearl: *At 55cm (about 2 feet), the number of cpcm is equal to the number of cpd. If testing is done at 1 ft, then the number of cpd is half of that at 2 feet distance.*

Interpretation of Results:

- Acuity norm charts are available for monocular and binocular viewing conditions.
- These charts contain upper and lower prediction limits (99% and 95%) based on age and viewing distance.
- Acuity below the 99% prediction limit should occur only once in 200 times and acuity below 95% prediction limit should occur only about 2 to 3 times every 100 times.
- If the patient's acuity falls within 0.5 octave (1 card) from the age expected norm, it is considered marginal and should be verified with re-testing.
- One octave (2 cards) or more difference between eyes is considered significant.

Lea Gratings/Patti Stripes

These are two modified preferential looking tests to evaluate how patients respond to grating stimuli. The difference between these tests and the TAC is that they use paddles to present the gratings. The test kit contains a gray paddle and several grating paddles in different spatial frequencies (Figure 4). They are less expensive than the TAC and easily portable. However, they are studied less extensively in comparison.

Procedure

Step 1: Cover one eye with a patch

Step 2: The typical test distance is 57cm. However, the test distance can be varied (i.e. 28cm, 43cm, 57cm, 85cm, 115cm) to engage and maintain visual attention. These test distances are multiples of 57cm and makes the calculation of cycles per cm (cpcm) easy. For example, 1 cpcm grating at 57cm is 0.5 cpcm at 28cm and 2 cpcm at 115cm

Clinical Pearl: *In young infants and in patients with disabilities, it is helpful to test at farther test distances to not encroach their personal space.*

Step 3: Unlike the TAC, the gray side and grating side are separated individually as separate cards. This means that it might be difficult to mask the examiner's face, which can be a source of distraction. For this reason, it is recommended that the background (including the examiner's clothing) be neutral to avoid distraction

Step 4: Start with a coarse grating. The paddles can be presented in a few ways:

- Present the gray and grating paddle (one held in each hand) simultaneously side by side (as done with the TAC) and observe the fixation response.
- Hold the two paddles together in one hand, with the gray paddle facing the patient, and then separate them sideways/vertically in the same speed.
    - If the child can see the moving grating, he/she will follow it
    - In the child has difficulty processing visual motion, he/she might saccade to the grating after movement is stopped instead of following it while moving

Step 5: Repeat at least once more to ensure the response is repeatable. Once a reliable response is observed, show every other grating, and use this staircase procedure to obtain threshold grating level. It might be necessary to show the next card in succession when approaching threshold levels

Step 6: Repeat with the other eye.
Step 7: Record the results

- OD- 2 cpcm grating at 57cm testing distance; OS – 1 cpcm grating at 57 cm testing distance.

Figure 4. Patti Stripes™ (top) and Lea Gratings (bottom)

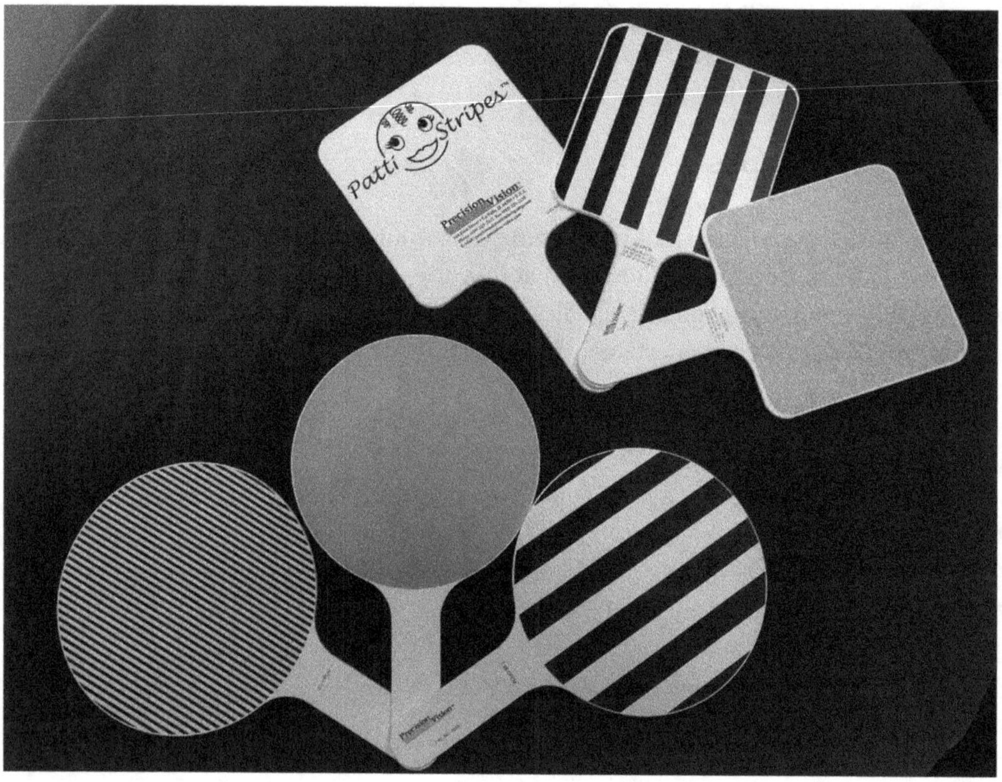

Cardiff Acuity Test

The Cardiff test is another preferential looking test developed to assess vision in young children with cognitive impairment. Instead of using gratings, this test uses familiar shapes (ex: boat, fish, duck, apple, etc.,) that are outlined by a white band (Figure 5) and flanked by black lines that have the same average luminance as the grey background. The thickness of the white lines will decrease with finer acuity levels. At threshold, the picture side and the grey side of the card will look no different from each other as if it vanished from the card (i.e., vanishing optotypes). These pictures are printed on one side of grey cards with the other side being blank. There is no peephole in the center for the examiner to observe the patient's response and the cards can only be presented vertically. Twelve acuity levels tested are from 20/160 to 20/12.5 for testing distance of 1m, with three cards available for each acuity level. If presented at a shorter distance (ex: 50cm), the range of acuity measured changes (i.e., 20/320 - 20/25). Table 3 provides the Cardiff test expected visual acuities by age.

Procedure

Step 1: Typical testing distance is 1m

Step 2: Start with a coarse acuity and present the card at the child's eye level. It is important for the clinician to be masked to the location of the picture

Step 3: All three cards must be presented for each acuity before going to the next higher level

Step 4: The child's acuity is the level with which at least 2 of the 3 cards are identified correctly

Step 5: Since older children can point to and/or name the pictures while infants cannot, to ensure consistency of the observed response across age groups, only the eye movements are used to determine the acuity level

Step 6: Record the results

- Use the logMAR (Minimum Angle of Resolution) or Snellen acuity as described in the back of test cards

Figure 5. Cardiff Acuity Cards - Boat (left, 0.8 logMAR at 1m distance); Fish (right, 0.4 logMAR at 1m distance)

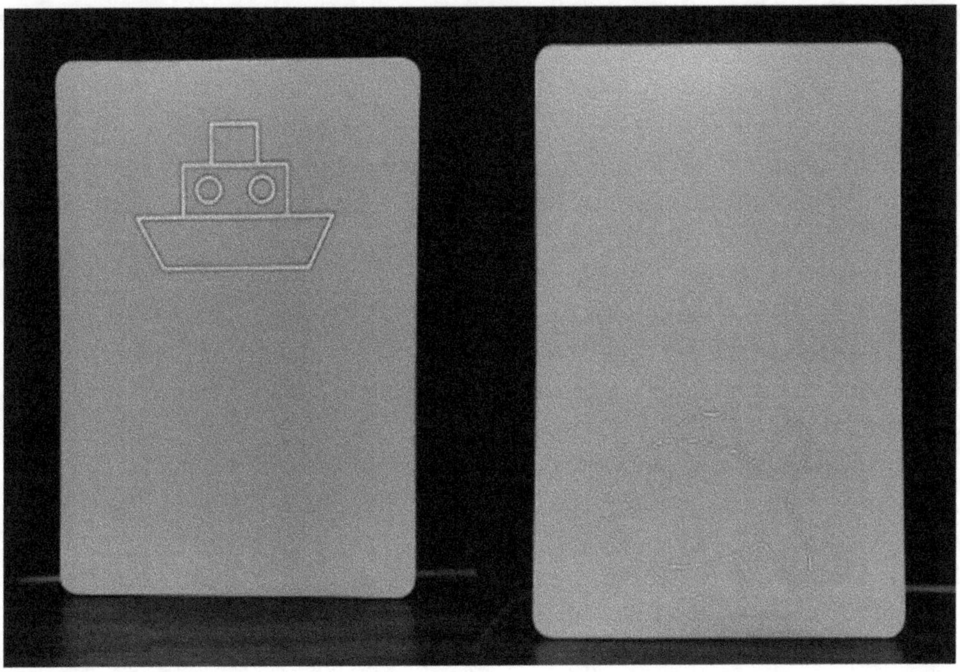

Table 3. Cardiff acuity test expected visual acuities by age in a typically developing child

Age (months)	Binocular VA	Monocular VA
12-17.9	20/160 to 20/40	20/160 to 20/50
18-23.9	20/80 to 20/25	20/100 to 20/25
24-29.9	20/50 to 20/25	20/63 to 20/25
30-36	20/40 to 20/20	20/40 to 20/20

(Adapted from Adoh & Woodhouse, 1994)

OBJECTIVE VISUAL ACUITY ASSESSMENT

Two common objective methods to evaluate visual acuity in young children include Visually Evoked Potential (VEP) and Optokinetic Drum (OKN). They do not necessitate a behavioral response from the child.

Visual Evoked Potential (VEP)

Visual evoked potentials are electric signals in the visual cortex generated by visual stimulation which are captured using electrodes attached to the scalp. The two main types of visual stimuli used for generating a VEP are (a) unpatterned light flash (flash VEP) and (b) patterned stimuli. Although patterned stimuli have more clinical utility, flash VEP can be helpful in situations such as media opacity, impaired vision, and difficulty sustaining attention with pattern stimuli. A checkerboard pattern containing alternate black and white squares is commonly used in pattern VEP to measure visual acuity. The pattern can be reversed at a specific reversal rate without changing the average luminance in pattern-reversal VEP. The spatial frequency of this pattern can be varied, and the response amplitude is measured to obtain visual acuity. The spatial frequency that yields zero amplitude response is obtained by plotting a regression fit (Leat et al., 2009).

Procedure

Step 1: The contact points for the electrodes are cleaned properly

Step 2: Three electrodes are placed as per the 10-20 guidelines (American Clinical Neurophysiology Society, 2006)

- Reference electrode on the forehead
- Ground electrode at the vertex
- Active electrode at about 2cm above the tip of the occipital protuberance (inion)

Step 3: Sit the child at a comfortable distance from the pattern stimulus and refractive correction (if needed) is worn

Step 4: The stimulus is presented on a screen and the response is amplified and averaged

Step 5: The procedure can also be performed one eye at a time

Interpretation of Results:

- The typical pattern-reversal VEP result is a waveform with three notable components (Figure 6). The first negative peak (N1 or N75) followed by a positive peak (P1 or P100) and a second negative peak (N2 or N135).
- Of clinical interest is the amplitude and latency of the P100. Expected P100 latency in adults is around 100ms and in infants this latency reaches adult-like levels at around 4 months (McCulloch et al., 1999; McCulloch & Skarf, 1991; Moskowitz & Sokol, 1983).
- In infants, the mean visual acuity increased from 4.5 cpd in 1-month-olds to about 20 cpd in 8-13-month-olds (Norcia & Tyler, 1985). Another study showed that visual acuity at 1 year of age was within one octave of adult acuity (Skoczenski & Norcia, 1999).

Figure 6. Pattern VEP waveforms from a healthy 38-year-old male using a 64x64 stimulus. OD - Right eye, OS - Left eye, OU - Both eyes
Image credit: Dr. Christopher Borgman, Southern College of Optometry, Memphis, Tennessee

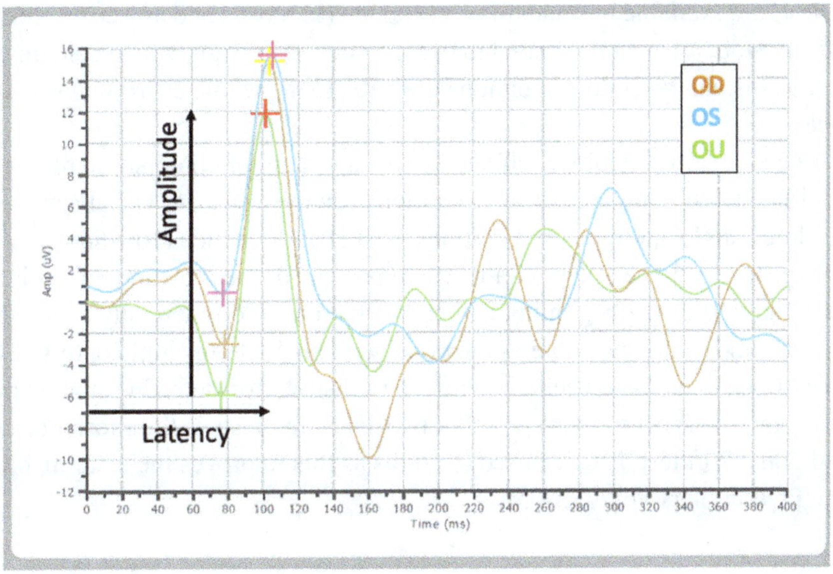

Optokinetic Drum (OKD)

The use of optokinetic nystagmus (OKN) elicited by a moving grating (such as the commercially available optokinetic drum (OKD) can also be used to measure grating acuity in infants (Dobson & Teller, 1978; Gorman et al., 1957). OKN is a reflexive eye movement generated to see a moving stimulus while the head is stationary. The OKN is composed of two eye movements that vary in speed - a slow component towards the direction of the rotation of the moving stimulus and a fast saccade in the opposite direction. The stimulus used in the rotating drums can either be gratings or other patterns such as pictures.

Procedure
Step 1: The drum is held either horizontally or vertically in front of the child and rotated slowly
Step 2: If the child can see the stimulus, OKN response will be observed
Step 3: When a grating is used, the spatial frequency can be increased until OKN is no longer observed

VISUAL ACUITY IN PRESCHOOL CHILDREN

In children between 3-5 years of age, letter-based charts with matching cards (e.g., HOTV) or picture-based charts with matching cards (e.g., Lea symbols, Patti Pics) are used to measure threshold visual acuity. In addition to these tests of recognition acuity, tests of resolution acuity (e.g., Broken Wheel test) are also available for this population. However, owing to the high testability in preschool children (Kulp 2004; Cotter 2007), the HOTV optotypes and Lea symbols are commonly used clinically and in research studies. The use of matching cards is particularly helpful in 3 to 4-year-old children. The advantages of HOTV and Lea symbol optotypes include calibration based on logMAR scale, standardization of optotypes (they have left/right symmetry and are equally discriminable) (Hyvarinen et al., 1980; Committee on Vision, 1980), and come with matching cards which allows a child to respond by matching the optotypes. Both tests are available in standard print version (Figure 7) and as a computerized version. In the standard print version, it is recommended to use the booklet version, which contains a single acuity level in each page to sustain the child's attention compared to the whole chart with several acuity levels visible all at once.

When measuring recognition acuity in children, it is important for clinicians to remember the impact of crowding on visual acuity. Single letter presentations can overestimate visual acuity, particularly in amblyopia. Therefore, single optotype presentations must always include crowding bars. When a single line of optotypes (generally 5 characters in a line) are presented, the crowding effect is present for the middle characters and not for the beginning and end of the line. Commercially available Lea symbols test and HOTV test booklets are available as crowded versions for both single optotype (or) single line presentations. These versions have been shown to be sensitive for detecting amblyopia (Graf et al., 2000). Another important aspect of these preschool visual acuity tests is the shorter test distance (10ft) compared to traditional 20ft test distance used in adults as this improves the test reliability and repeatability (Vision in Preschoolers Study, 2005).

Figure 7 - Lea Symbols (left) and HOTV (right) logMAR charts with corresponding matching cards in the bottom

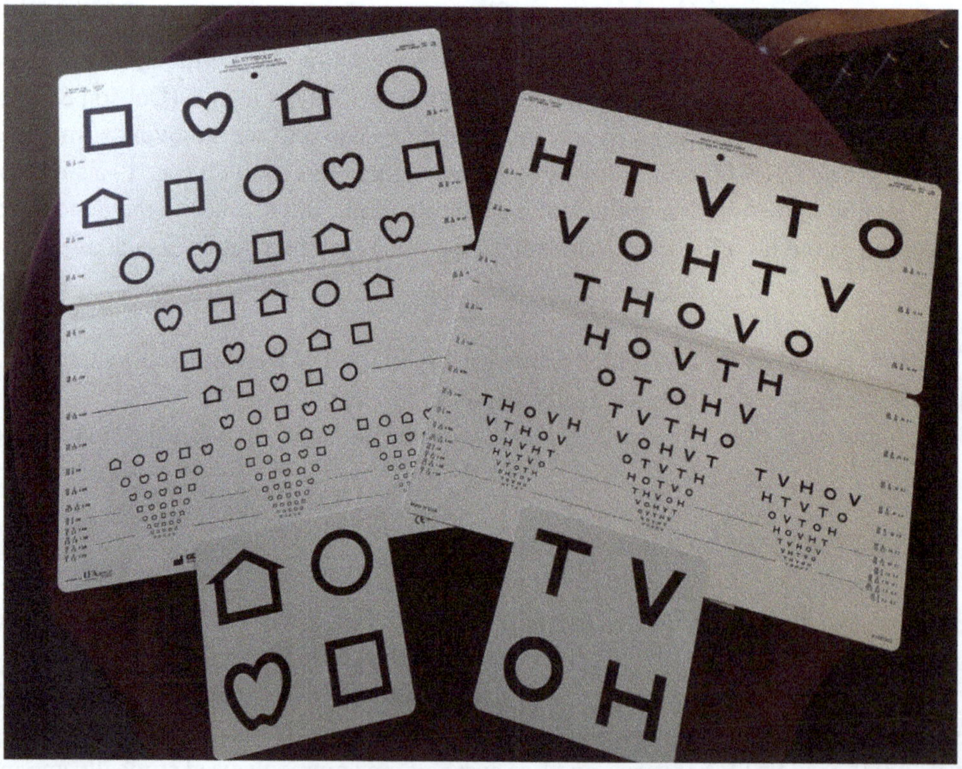

The qualitative recognition and resolution acuity procedures discussed in this section are:

- **Recognition Acuity:**
    - **Picture-based Optotypes:**
        - Lea Symbols
        - Patti Pictures
        - Allen Pictures
    - **Letter-based Optotypes:**
- HOTV
- **Resolution Acuity:**
    - Broken Wheel Test

Lea Symbols

Procedure

Step 1: The test plates contain four recognizable symbols: a house, apple, circle, and square

Step 2: Have the child hold the matching card. The clinician points to each shape and asks the child to identify the shape name, or alternatively ask the child to call out the names of each shape

- The use of a test card increases the testability in preschool children compared to verbal identification of targets (Fern & Manny, 1986; Friendly, 1978; Hedin et al., 1980).

Clinical Pearl: *If the child is unable to name shapes, matching shapes should be encouraged.*

Step 3: The distance chart is presented at 10 ft (3m). A suprathreshold target (ex: 20/120) is used as a starting point

Step 4: With both eyes open, the child is asked to match or call out the large optotypes. The optotype can be pointed to, if needed. Care must be taken to not break the crowding bars. The electronic versions come with a provision to insert an arrow below the optotype that is to be identified.

Step 5: Once the child understands the task and can identify optotypes correctly, monocular testing should be performed

Step 6: For occlusion, adhesive patches are a foolproof way to ensure each eye is fully covered. Commercially available occluder glasses (Figure 8) are advantageous if the child is resistant to the adhesive patches

Clinical Pearl: *When a hand is used as an occluder, the palm should be used to fully cover the eye instead of the fingers.*

Step 7: With one eye covered, testing proceeds to the next line if at least three of the five symbols are correctly identified. As smaller letter sizes are presented, frequently, a single optotype are presented instead of a whole line to sustain attention on the task.

Clinical Pearl: *Crowding bars should be used around single optotypes to not overestimate visual acuity (Figure 9).*

Step 8: The visual acuity is the last (smallest) line with 3 out of 5 symbols correctly identified
Step 9: Testing is repeated with the other eye

Figure 8. Occluder glasses for the right and left eye
(From Good-Lite®)

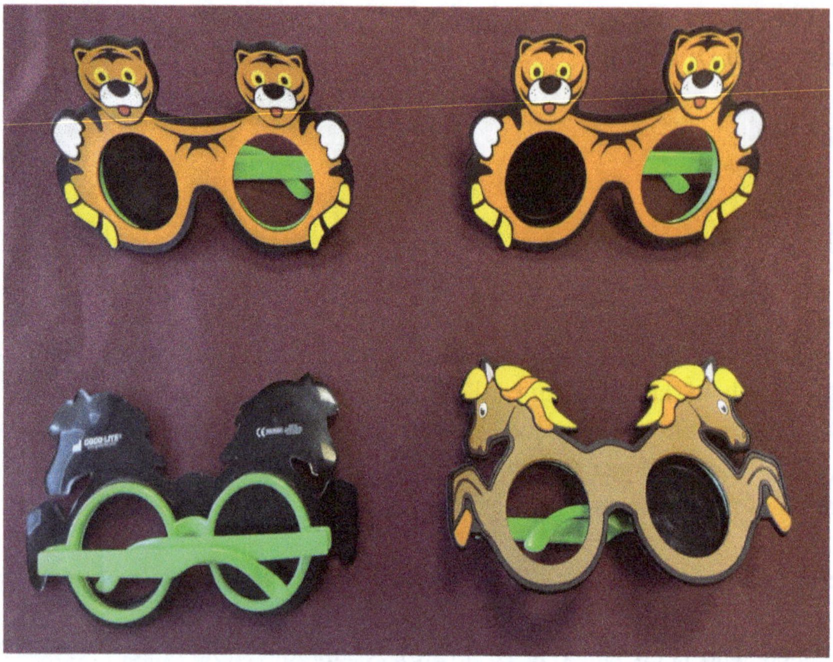

Figure 9. Crowding bars surrounding a letter optotype

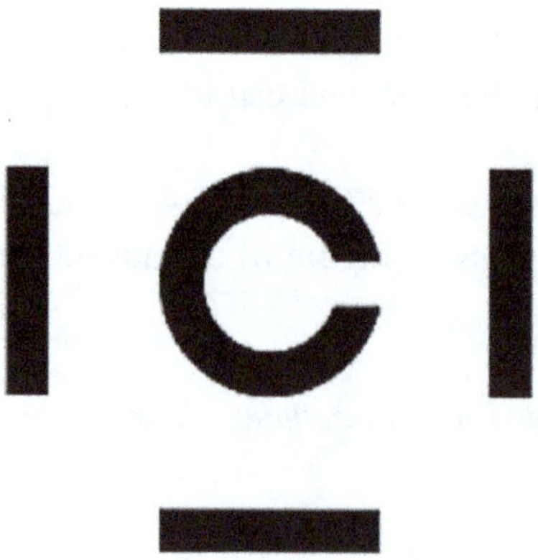

Patti Pics

The set up and procedure is the same as described under Lea Symbols. The only difference is that the addition of a fifth shape on the test plates (house, apple, circle, square, and *star*). This reduces the guess rate to 20% compared to 25% with Lea Symbols.

Allen Pictures

The Allen pictures include some recognizable childhood items such as a birthday cake and a Christmas tree but also include out of date pictures such as a landline telephone. These optotypes are not standardized because they are recognizable even when blurry (therefore not sensitive for measuring visual impairment) and have been found to overestimate visual acuity compared to standard clinical tests. Despite these significant limitations, they are commonly utilized because of their availability in projector charts. The clinician is discouraged from using this test for visual acuity measurements in children.

HOTV

The set up and procedure is the same as described under Lea Symbols. The target contains four upper case alphabets namely H, O, T, and V. The test kit comes with a matching card to assist with the matching response.

Broken Wheel Test

This is a forced choice test that measures resolution acuity. Using the Landolt C as the optotype, the child is presented with two cards for each acuity level, each containing a car with two wheels (Figure 10). One of the cars has two full wheels and the other has two broken wheels (the Landolt C). The child is asked to either point to or verbally identify the card containing the broken wheels.

Procedure

Step 1: The testing distance is 10 ft (3m)

Step 2: A suprathreshold target is presented and the child is asked to identify the card with the broken wheel. This pretest is repeated a few times to ensure that the child understands the task. The examiner shuffles the cards between each presentation.

Step 3: Each acuity level is tested 4 times and if correct responses are obtained three out of four times (75% success), testing continues to the next smaller level. If more than one incorrect response is obtained, the preceding level with the 75% success rate is documented as the acuity level

Figure 10. Three different acuity levels in the Broken Wheel Test

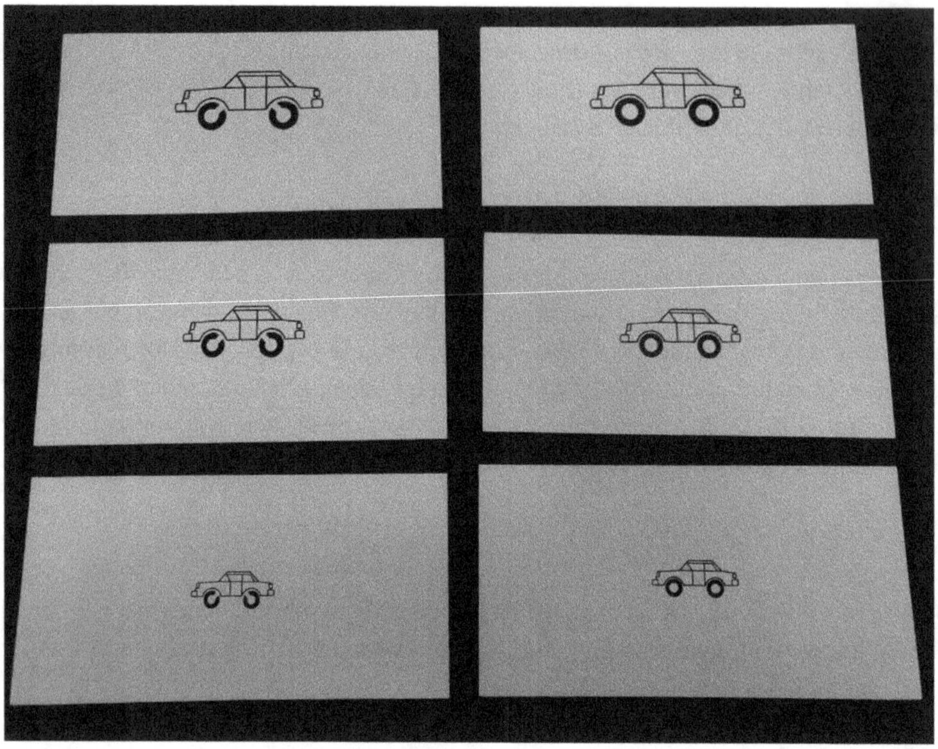

ADULT VISUAL ACUITY CHARTS FOR USE IN OLDER CHILDREN

Snellen, Early Treatment of Diabetic Retinopathy Study (ETDRS

A vast majority of children 6 years and older should be testable with adult visual acuity charts such as the Snellen, or the Early Treatment of Diabetic Retinopathy Study (ETDRS) chart. Although these charts produce repeatable results in children, adult-level acuities are not reached with the ETDRS chart until adolescent years (Dobson et al., 2009).

CONCLUSION

Visual acuity is the key diagnostic measure for the detection of amblyopia in children. As the infant's vision and cognition matures, a variety of test stimuli are utilized clinically to measure vision. Becoming familiar with these testing methods helps the clinician to administer age-appropriate tests. Additionally, it is important for the clinician to distinguish between what type of acuity is measured with each test method (e.g., resolution versus recognition acuity) and to exercise caution in comparing the results of these very different acuity types.

REFERENCES

Adoh, T. O., & Woodhouse, J. M. (1994). The Cardiff acuity test used for measuring visual acuity development in toddlers. *Vision Research, 34*(4), 555–560. doi:10.1016/0042-6989(94)90168-6 PMID:8303838

American Clinical Neurophysiology Society. (2006). Guideline 9B: Guidelines on visual evoked potentials. *Journal of Clinical Neurophysiology, 23*(2), 138–156. doi:10.1097/00004691-200604000-00011 PubMed

Committee on Vision. (1980). Recommended standard procedures for the clinical measurement and specification of visual acuity. Report of working group 39. Assembly of Behavioral and Social Sciences, National Research Council, National Academy of Sciences, Washington, D.C. *Advances in Ophthalmology, 41*, 103–148. https://www.ncbi.nlm.nih.gov/pubmed/7001873 PMID:7001873

Cotter, S. A., Tarczy-Hornoch, K., Song, E., Lin, J., Borchert, M., Azen, S. P., & Varma, R. (2009). Fixation preference and visual acuity testing in a population-based cohort of preschool children with amblyopia risk factors. *Ophthalmology, 116*(1), 145–153. doi:10.1016/j.ophtha.2008.08.031 PMID:18962921

Courage, M. L., Adams, R. J., Reyno, S., & Kwa, P. G. (1994). Visual acuity in infants and children with Down syndrome. *Developmental Medicine and Child Neurology, 36*(7), 586–593. doi:10.1111/j.1469-8749.1994.tb11895.x PMID:8034120

Dobson, V., Clifford-Donaldson, C. E., Green, T. K., Miller, J. M., & Harvey, E. M. (2009). Normative monocular visual acuity for early treatment diabetic retinopathy study charts in emmetropic children 5 to 12 years of age. *Ophthalmology, 116*(7), 1397–1401. doi:10.1016/j.ophtha.2009.01.019 PMID:19427702

Dobson, V., Quinn, G. E., Tung, B., Palmer, E. A., & Reynolds, J. D. (1995). Comparison of recognition and grating acuities in very-low-birth-weight children with and without retinal residua of retinopathy of prematurity. Cryotherapy for Retinopathy of Prematurity Cooperative Group. *Investigative Ophthalmology & Visual Science, 36*(3), 692–702. PMID:7890499

Dobson, V., & Teller, D. Y. (1978). Visual acuity in human infants: A review and comparison of behavioral and electrophysiological studies. *Vision Research, 18*(11), 1469–1483. doi:10.1016/0042-6989(78)90001-9 PMID:364823

Fantz, R. L. (1963). Pattern Vision in Newborn Infants. *Science, 140*(3564), 296–297. doi:10.1126cience.140.3564.296 PMID:17788054

Fern, K. D., & Manny, R. E. (1986). Visual acuity of the preschool child: A review. *American Journal of Optometry and Physiological Optics, 63*(5), 319–345. doi:10.1097/00006324-198605000-00003 PMID:3717284

Frantz, R. L., Ordy, J., & Udelf, M. (1962). Maturation of pattern vision in infants during the first six months. *Journal of Comparative and Physiological Psychology, 55*(6), 907–917. doi:10.1037/h0044173

Friendly, D. S. (1978). Preschool visual acuity screening tests. *Transactions of the American Ophthalmological Society, 76*, 383–480. https://www.ncbi.nlm.nih.gov/pubmed/754379 PMID:754379

Friendly, D. S., Jaafar, M. S., & Morillo, D. L. (1990). A comparative study of grating and recognition visual acuity testing in children with anisometropic amblyopia without strabismus. *American Journal of Ophthalmology, 110*(3), 293–299. doi:10.1016/S0002-9394(14)76347-0 PMID:2396655

Gorman, J. J., Cogan, D. G., & Gellis, S. S. (1957). An apparatus for grading the visual acuity of infants on the basis of opticokinetic nystagmus. *Pediatrics, 19*(6), 1088–1092. PMID:13441362

Graf, M. H., Becker, R., & Kaufmann, H. (2000). Lea symbols: Visual acuity assessment and detection of amblyopia. *Graefes Archive for Clinical and Experimental Ophthalmology, 238*(1), 53–58. doi:10.1007004170050009 PMID:10664053

Hedin, A., Nyman, K. G., & Derouet, B. (1980). A modified letter matching chart for testing young children's visual acuity. *Journal of Pediatric Ophthalmology and Strabismus, 17*(2), 114–118. doi:10.3928/0191-3913-19800301-13 PMID:7391898

Hyvarinen, L., Nasanen, R., & Laurinen, P. (1980). New visual acuity test for pre-school children. *Acta Ophthalmologica, 58*(4), 507–511. doi:10.1111/j.1755-3768.1980.tb08291.x PMID:7211248

Kelly, K. R., Jost, R. M., De La Cruz, A., & Birch, E. E. (2015). Amblyopic children read more slowly than controls under natural, binocular reading conditions. *Journal of American Association for Pediatric Ophthalmology and Strabismus, 19*(6), 515–520. doi:10.1016/j.jaapos.2015.09.002 PMID:26610788

Kushner, B. J., Lucchese, N. J., & Morton, G. V. (1995). Grating visual acuity with Teller cards compared with Snellen visual acuity in literate patients. *Archives of Ophthalmology, 113*(4), 485–493. doi:10.1001/archopht.1995.01100040107035 PMID:7710400

Leat, S. J., Yadav, N. K., & Irving, E. L. (2009). Development of visual acuity and contrast sensitivity in children. *Journal of Optometry, 2*(1), 19–26. doi:10.3921/joptom.2009.19

Mayer, D. L. (1986). Acuity of amblyopic children for small field gratings and recognition stimuli. *Investigative Ophthalmology & Visual Science, 27*(7), 1148–1153. https://www.ncbi.nlm.nih.gov/pubmed/3721793 PMID:3721793

Mayer, D. L., Beiser, A. S., Warner, A. F., Pratt, E. M., Raye, K. N., & Lang, J. M. (1995). Monocular acuity norms for the Teller Acuity Cards between ages one month and four years. *Investestigative Ophthalmology & Visual Science, 36*(3), 671-685. https://www.ncbi.nlm.nih.gov/pubmed/7890497

Mayer, D. L., Fulton, A. B., & Rodier, D. (1984). Grating and recognition acuities of pediatric patients. *Ophthalmology, 91*(8), 947–953. doi:10.1016/S0161-6420(84)34209-9 PMID:6493704

McCulloch, D. L., Orbach, H., & Skarf, B. (1999). Maturation of the pattern-reversal VEP in human infants: A theoretical framework. *Vision Research, 39*(22), 3673–3680. doi:10.1016/S0042-6989(99)00091-7 PMID:10746137

McCulloch, D. L., & Skarf, B. (1991). Development of the human visual system: Monocular and binocular pattern VEP latency. *Investigative Ophthalmology & Visual Science, 32*(8), 2372–2381. https://www.ncbi.nlm.nih.gov/pubmed/2071348 PMID:2071348

McKee, S. P., Levi, D. M., & Movshon, J. A. (2003). The pattern of visual deficits in amblyopia. *Journal of Vision (Charlottesville, Va.), 3*(5), 380–405. doi:10.1167/3.5.5 PMID:12875634

Moskowitz, A., & Sokol, S. (1983). Developmental changes in the human visual system as reflected by the latency of the pattern reversal VEP. *Electroencephalography and Clinical Neurophysiology*, *56*(1), 1–15. doi:10.1016/0013-4694(83)90002-0 PMID:6190626

Norcia, A. M., & Tyler, C. W. (1985). Spatial frequency sweep VEP: Visual acuity during the first year of life. *Vision Research*, *25*(10), 1399–1408. doi:10.1016/0042-6989(85)90217-2 PMID:4090273

Preston, K. L., McDonald, M., Sebris, S. L., Dobson, V., & Teller, D. Y. (1987). Validation of the acuity card procedure for assessment of infants with ocular disorders. *Ophthalmology*, *94*(6), 644–653. doi:10.1016/S0161-6420(87)33398-6 PMID:3627713

Rydberg, A., Ericson, B., Lennerstrand, G., Jacobson, L., & Lindstedt, E. (1999). Assessment of visual acuity in children aged 1 1/2-6 years, with normal and subnormal vision. *Strabismus*, *7*(1), 1–24. doi:10.1076tra.7.1.1.656 PMID:10401500

Sener, E. C., Mocan, M. C., Gedik, S., Ergin, A., & Sanac, A. S. (2002). The reliability of grading the fixation preference test for the assessment of interocular visual acuity differences in patients with strabismus. [JAAPOS]. *Journal of American Association for Pediatric Ophthalmology and Strabismus*, *6*(3), 191–194. doi:10.1067/mpa.2002.122364 PMID:12075297

Skoczenski, A. M., & Norcia, A. M. (1999). Development of VEP Vernier acuity and grating acuity in human infants. *Investigative Ophthalmology & Visual Science*, *40*(10), 2411–2417. https://www.ncbi.nlm.nih.gov/pubmed/10476810 PMID:10476810

Vision in Preschoolers Study. (2005). Preschool vision screening tests administered by nurse screeners compared with lay screeners in the vision in preschoolers study. *Investigative Ophthalmology & Visual Science, 46*(8), 2639-2648. doi:10.1167/iovs.05-0141

Wallace, D. K. (2005). Tests of fixation preference for amblyopia. *The American Orthoptic Journal*, *55*(1), 76–81. doi:10.3368/aoj.55.1.76 PMID:21149113

Weakley, D. R. Jr. (2001). The association between nonstrabismic anisometropia, amblyopia, and subnormal binocularity. *Ophthalmology*, *108*(1), 163–171. doi:10.1016/S0161-6420(00)00425-5 PMID:11150283

Webber, A. L., & Wood, J. (2005). Amblyopia: Prevalence, natural history, functional effects and treatment. *Clinical & Experimental Optometry*, *88*(6), 365–375. doi:10.1111/j.1444-0938.2005.tb05102.x PMID:16329744

Wright, K. W., Walonker, F., & Edelman, P. (1981). 10-Diopter fixation test for amblyopia. *Archives of Ophthalmology*, *99*(7), 1242–1246. doi:10.1001/archopht.1981.03930020116012 PMID:7259597

KEY TERMS AND DEFINITIONS

20/20 Vision: The ability to see a target clearly at 20 feet which an average person can also see at 20 feet. Similarly, 20/40 vision means that the target was seen clearly at 20 feet whereas an average person can see that same target from 40 feet distance. This is the Snellen denomination.

Amblyopia: Unilateral or bilateral reduction in vision in an otherwise structurally intact eye caused by abnormal visual experience in early life.

Crowding: The impaired ability to visually detect objects in a clutter as opposed to when presented in isolation.

LogMAR: Logarithm of the Minimum Angle of Resolution (logMAR). LogMAR charts have logarithmic progression of optotype spacing within each line and between lines.

Minimum Angle of Resolution (MAR): Angular size of a letter in minutes of arc. It is calculated by dividing the Snellen denominator by the numerator. The MAR conversion for 20/20 is 1' (1 minute of arc).

Recognition Acuity: The ability to recognize optotypes such as letters, numbers or pictures.

Resolution Acuity: The ability to resolve spatial details within a target, such as detecting the gap in a Landolt C.

Chapter 5
Testing Visual Fields in Children

Jacky K. W. Kong
New England College of Optometry, USA

ABSTRACT

Visual fields in the pediatric population are an essential part of the eye exam that remain challenging to even the most experienced clinicians. Becoming educated in the multiple ways a child's visual field can be tested regardless of age and cognitive and physical abilities will allow the clinician to gain better insight into the child's function and in some cases, allow the clinician to identify pathological or neurological anomalies in the visual pathway. Gross visual field or functional visual field extent can be estimated by tests such as confrontation visual field testing, finger counting field testing, and white sphere kinetic perimetry. For threshold measurements of a child's visual fields, the Goldmann perimeter, or the more advanced computerized tests such as the Humphrey perimeter, Octopus perimeter, or frequency doubling technology perimeter can be used. Modifications can be made to certain tests to better suit the child's cognitive and physical abilities. The chapter covers different methods of visual field testing specific for the pediatric population.

INTRODUCTION

Visual field testing should be a part of a comprehensive pediatric eye examination to detect for any functional deficits in the patient's field of view. Visual field defects can be caused by, but is not limited to, multiple genetic disorders, trauma, and/or complicated birth. Knowledge of the visual field of children with suspected visual pathway disorders is, therefore, crucial for a number of reasons. Visual field tests in children can indicate whether the clinician should refer the child for diagnostic imaging (Chou & Digre, 1999; Molia et al., 1996; Suharwardy & Elson, 1997) and can also contribute to decisions regarding treatment (Kim et al., 2008; Wild et al., 2007). Characterization of the visual field is also crucial in establishing appropriate educational approaches and remediation services that take visual field loss into account. However, visual field assessment in children remains challenging in part because it requires a certain level of attention and cognition on the child's behalf.

DOI: 10.4018/978-1-7998-8044-8.ch005

On occasion, especially with low functioning, multiply impaired children, the goal of a visual field test is generally not to find out what their threshold of sensitivity is, but where in their field of view do they have attention and where in their field of view will they respond to the visual stimuli. This is important because in instances where, for example, a wheelchair bound nonverbal and multiply impaired child is in a classroom, instruction and recommendations can be given to the teacher (or other care takers) to present learning material to the child within the spatial confines of the child's estimated binocular field extent. This will undoubtedly enhance the child's learning and engagement within the classroom environment. Knowledge of the visual field will also be helpful if the patient is working with an orientation mobility specialist because different strategies can be employed in training in order to overcome the visual field deficit(s) found.

This chapter covers different methods of visual field testing specific for the pediatric population.

BACKGROUND

Children with physical or developmental disabilities are at a significantly increased risk of visual acuity deficits, visual field defects, or a combination of both (Van den Broek et al., 2006; Warburg, 1994). Examples of these include pre- or post-natal injury as a result of perinatal hypoxic-ischemic brain injury or because of complications of hydrocephalus, systemic infections, traumatic brain injury, retinopathy of prematurity, optic nerve damage, progressive retinal degeneration, or tumors of the optic chiasm. (Gilbert et al., 2003; Rahi & Gilbert, 2005).

When it comes to visual field testing in children we can divide it up into two different types: the traditional methods and the modified methods.

Traditional Visual Field Methods

The traditional methods are effective for children that are able to respond to instructions and give accurate feedback. These are straightforward in testing and interpretation of the results are relatively easy. Tests that fall under this category include confrontation visual field test, finger counting visual field test, Goldmann perimetry, frequency doubling technology perimetry, and automated perimetry such as the Humphrey Field Analyzer and Octopus 900.

Modified Visual Field Methods

The modified methods are usually reserved for children that are unable to respond either verbally, or physically (pointing, gesturing, or pressing buttons). These children also do not follow instructions well. Modified methods of perimetry takes the traditional methods and re-adapts the tests to be used for the child being tested. It takes some experience to administer the test and interpretation may not be straight forward. Modifications cannot be made to all tests but can be made to the following: confrontation visual field test, finger counting visual fields, Goldmann perimetry and Octopus perimetry.

White Sphere Kinetic Perimetry

An additional method of visual field testing is called white sphere kinetic perimetry. This is one of the more common preferential looking methods that is used to obtain a visual field analysis of children with multiple disorders. These children are often lower functioning individuals. Usage of this technique is common in clinical research but has limited uses in everyday clinical care due to its difficulty to set up and time to administer.

It is important to consider the child's cognitive ability in determining what type of visual field test is most appropriate. It is recommended to select the most complex testing that matches the child's cognitive and physical capabilities. Monocular testing of visual fields should be attempted. However, if unable then binocular visual field testing is acceptable.

Clinical Pearl: *For monocular visual field testing, use of a plastic eye patch is preferred because alcohol or other cleaning agents will evaporate and dry quickly. Use of a cloth or fiber like eye patch will result in the absorption of alcohol or cleaning agent if not evaporated or dried completely before use, it may also sting the eye.*

CONFRONTATION VISUAL FIELD TEST

Advantages

- Easy to administer and low-cost screening method that is able to pick up substantial visual field loss.

Disadvantages

- Requires child to sit upright and be able to follow basic directions.
- Dependent on examiner having a normal visual field for comparison.

Equipment

1. Fixation target. Typically, a small white sphere with a diameter that is 3 mm or less mounted on a stick. Modifications may need to be made to capture child's attention. An example of that is to change the central and peripheral target to 1-inch sized finger puppets.
2. Occluder or eye patch

Procedure

Step 1: Glasses should be removed, but if the refractive error is high, it can be left on
Step 2: Occlude one eye either with an eye patch or an occluder

Clinical Pearl: *If child refuses occlusion, perform the test binocularly.*

Step 3: Position yourself approximately 50 cm in front of the child and at similar eye level
Step 4: Present two targets, one central target and one peripheral target. The central target is where the child is to be fixating on at all times, and the peripheral target is placed outside of both the child's and the examiner's field of views

Clinical Pearl: *Ensure that the central fixation target is the same or similar to the peripheral target. In some instances, if the central target is larger, brighter, and easier to see versus the peripheral target, it may attract visual attention away from the peripheral target leading to an underestimation of the child's visual field.*

Step 5: Slowly move the peripheral target towards the child and the examiner's line of sight. Once the peripheral target is seen or noticed by the child, instruct him or her to verbalize it

Clinical Pearl: *If child is nonverbal, the examiner will have to diligently watch for gaze redirection from the central target to where the peripheral target is. When using gaze redirection to determine visual field extent, it is important to test the appropriate locations multiple times in random order to establish statistical confidence.*

Step 6: Repeat step 5 to test the eight locations at each of the four visual field meridians (Figure 1) (Carlson & Kurtz, 2016)
Step 7: Switch the occlude or eye patch to the other eye. Repeat steps 4-6
Step 8: Document the results

1. If the field is normal, it can be documented as such
2. If there are restrictions, document the location/quadrant of where the restriction is located

Figure 1. Illustration of the eight locations, marked with X, at each of the four visual field meridians to be tested in each eye

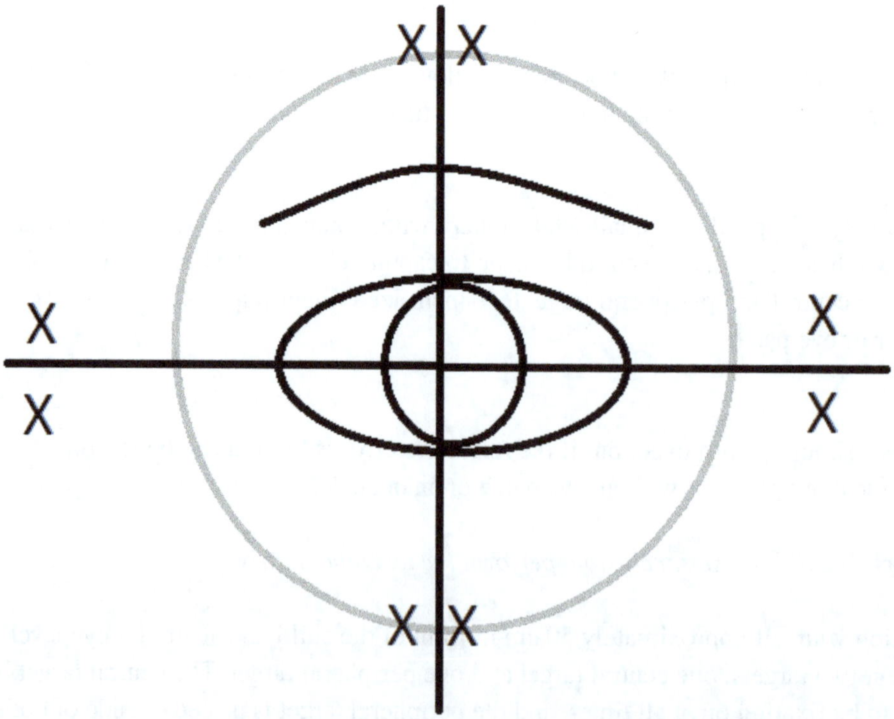

FINGER COUNTING FIELD TEST

Advantages

- Easy to administer and low-cost screening method that is included in the entrance exam of a typical comprehensive eye exam.

Disadvantages

- The number of digits on a hand are limited and subject to guessing.

Equipment

1. Occluder or eye patch

Procedure

Step 1: The examiner is seated at approximately 1 meter from the child and at eye level

Step 2: Glasses should be removed. Occlude one eye with either an occluder or an eye patch

Step 3: The fixation target is the examiner's eye directly across from the child. While the child is fixated on the examiner's eye, let the child know you will hold up either one, two, or four fingers in the periphery

Clinical Pearl: *Instead of finger counting, the examiner can also make use of finger movements and ask the child to state if he or she notices it.*

Step 4: On each side of the four visual field meridians (for a total of eight test locations) the examiner's fingers are presented as far out as to the extent of where the examiner thinks he or she can see them (refer to Figure 1 for test locations).

Step 5: Switch the occluder or eye patch to the other eye. Repeat steps 3 and 4

Step 6: Document the results

1. If the field is normal, it can be documented as such
2. If there are restrictions, document the location/quadrant of where the restriction is located

GOLDMANN PERIMETRY

Goldmann manual kinetic perimetry (GKP) had been the gold standard for visual field assessment up to the modern era of computerized static perimetry (Anderson, 1987).

Advantages

- Results are consistent and provides an in-depth visual field analysis.
- Is a standard method of perimetry for typically developing children from age 4-5 years (Mayer & Fulton, 2004) and is also successful for some older children with physical and developmental disabilities.

Disadvantages

- Difficult to administer and requires practice and training.
- Children with developmental and physical disabilities cannot meet the test requirements of holding the chin and forehead on a rest, fixating on a small dot in the perimeter center, and pressing a buzzer to indicate peripheral light detection.

Equipment

1. Goldmann perimeter
2. Occluder or eye patch

Procedure

Step 1: Glasses should be removed, but if the refractive error is high, it can be left on
Step 2: Occlude one eye either with an eye patch or an occluder

Clinical Pearl: *If child refuses occlusion, perform the test binocularly to obtain a measurement of binocular functional field extent.*

Step 3: Position the child's chin comfortably on the chin rest, and forehead against the forehead rest
Step 4: Instruct the child to fixate on the small dot in the perimeter center, and to respond by pressing the buzzer to indicate detection of a peripheral light. Remind the child to always look at the center light, and if there is a light in his/her side vision, to respond by pressing the buzzer once.

Clinical Pearl: *If the child's head can fit within the measuring dome, but is unable to respond by pressing the buzzer, an alternative method of estimating the visual field extent is by observing for a reflexive-looking behavior to the peripheral targets. The child's eye movements can be observed through the telescope located in the backside of the perimeter (Figure 2).*

FREQUENCY DOUBLING TECHNOLOGY (FDT) PERIMETRY

FDT perimetry consists of identifying a low spatial, high temporal frequency stimulus that is presented in different locations of the patient's field of view. This test can be easily administered to anyone that is able to follow instructions to fixate on a target and to press a button when the stimuli is noticed.

"The targets are imaged at optical infinity; thus, patients should wear their distance corrected lenses while performing the test (bifocals and progressive are acceptable). The large low spatial frequency targets are not significantly affected by refractive errors up to 6 D, so optimal near correction is not needed" (Zeppieri, 2008).

Advantages

- Easy to administer.
- FDT has been demonstrated to be quite effective and reliable in children over the age of 10 years (Kocabeyoglu et al., 2013) when a qualitative assessment is needed.

Figure 2. Back side of the Goldmann perimeter. The telescope for viewing patient fixation is in the center (marked by white letter "T")

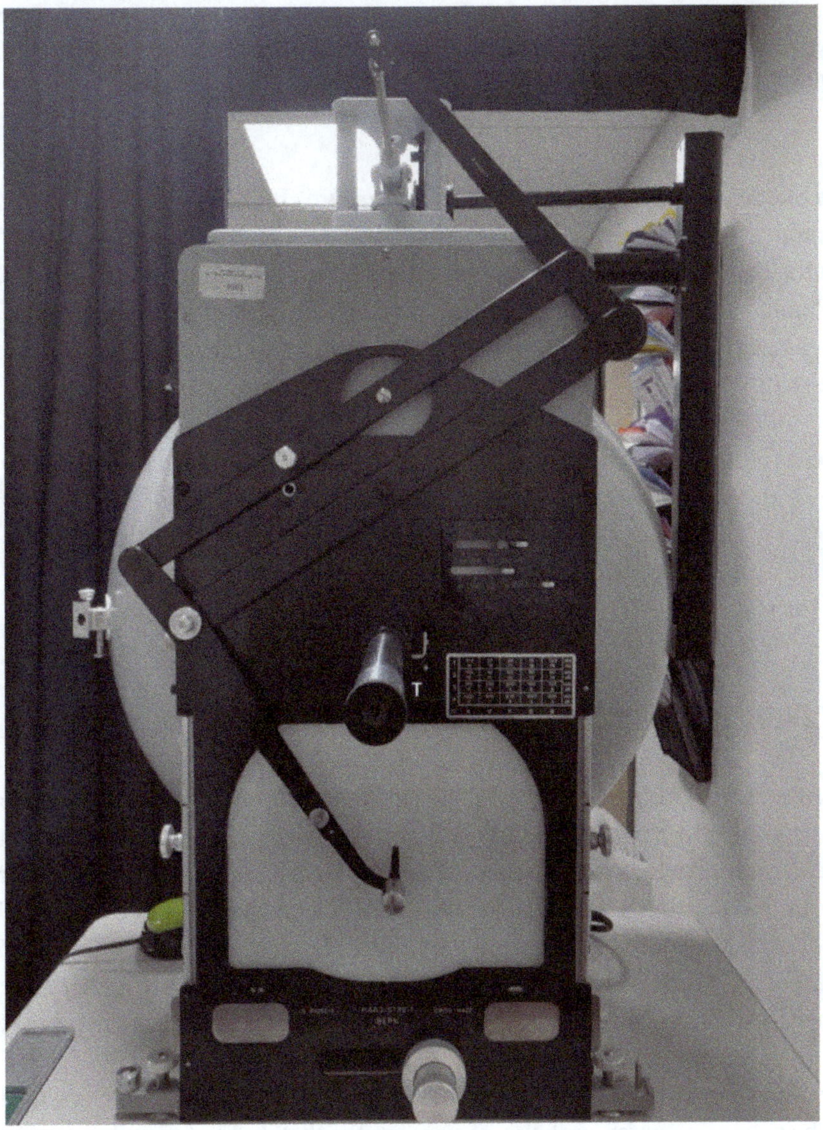

Disadvantages

- High cognitive function of the child is required due to its non-examiner dependent nature.
- Results are compared with the device's normative database, which may not yield statistically meaningful analysis in children under 18 years of age.

Equipment

1. FDT perimeter
2. Occluder or eye patch

Procedure

Step 1: Child wears habitual correction for the test, if needed.

Clinical Pearl: *Correction is not necessary if refractive error is between -2.00 D to + 2.00 D for threshold testing, and -6.00 D to +6.00 D for screening testing (Spry, et al., 2008)*

Step 2: Occlude one eye

Step 3: Position forehead against the forehead rest and ensure child can see all four corners of the screen to ensure proper positioning

Step 4: Instruct the child to fixate on the central target and to respond by pressing the button if a target appears. Remind the child to press the response button right after the appearance of the target. The child can get familiarized with the test by responding to the sample targets that are projected during the set-up.

Clinical Pearl: *The child should be told that if the background or vision suddenly appears to be fading, a few eye blinks or eye movements will allow things to reappear as normal.*

Step 5: Switch the occluder or eye patch to the other eye. Repeat steps 3 and 4

Step 6: Record the results

HUMPHREY FIELD ANALYZER PERIMETRY

The Humphrey field analyzer is an automated static perimetry. Humphrey field analyzer perimetry is one of the most widely used auto-perimetry for clinical visual field testing in adults. Main usage is to test for any visual field changes under the circumstances of neurological disorders, retinal disorders, or glaucoma.

In general, four main testing algorithms are used: SITA standard 24-2 or 30-2, which tests up to 24 degrees and 30 degrees, respectively, out from the central field; and SITA Fast 24-2 or 30-2, which is a faster version of the SITA standard and is comparable in its effectiveness (Heijl & Patella, 2002). These tests are static perimetric tests, meaning the peripheral target is fixed and not moving (Heijl & Patella, 2002).

For computerized automated perimetry tests, the target size can be changed to ensure detection within the confines of the patient's isopter, without influencing the threshold of visual/spatial sensitivity which is determined by stimulus illumination. An absolute visual field defect is recorded when no awareness is detected under conditions of the appropriate stimulus size and maximum stimulus brightness.

The Humphrey field analyzer perimetry is generally reserved for children able to take instructions from the examiner. The child also needs to tolerate ocular occlusion with an eye patch because for Humphrey perimetry, all SITA standard and SITA fast testing must be done monocularly for the analysis to be meaningful.

Advantages

- Moderately easy to administer.
- Results are very consistent and provides in-depth visual field analysis.

Figure 3. Front side of Goldmann perimeter

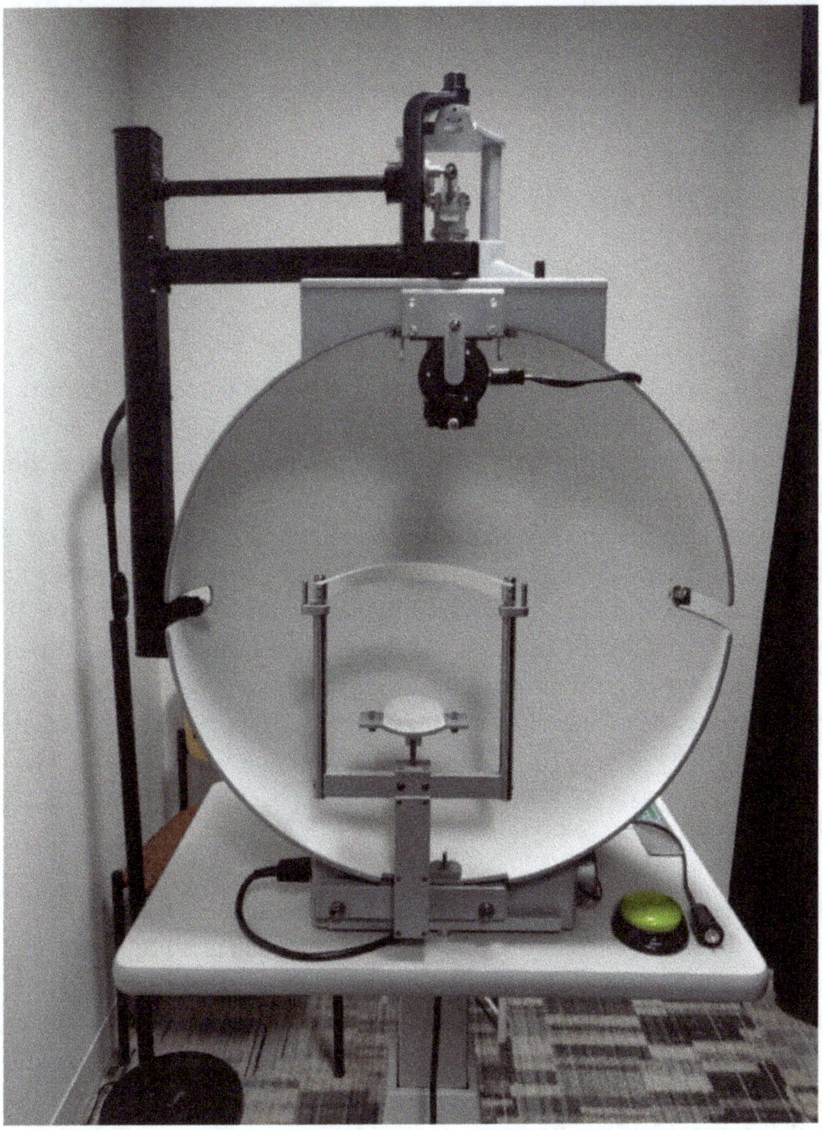

Disadvantages

- Humphrey Field Analyzer Perimetry is a difficult test for any young child. It requires high cognition, good motor control, adequate physical stamina, and most importantly good attention and cooperation.
- Normative database is based on a sample size with age range of between 17 to 89 (Heijl et al., 1987). Therefore, data obtained may not have any statistical significance if the child is younger than 17 years of age.

Clinical Pearl: *With automated perimetry methods it would not be possible to determine statistical significance of the results because there are no normative data to compare with if the patient is under 18. It is, however, important for the clinician to conduct a qualitative analysis based off the threshold data acquired through testing, paying special attention to any longitudinal changes.*

Equipment

1. Humphrey field analyzer perimeter
2. Occluder or eye patch

Procedure

Step 1: Occlude one eye

Step 2: Place the child's spectacle correction into the lens holder (spectacle correction should not be worn because they can cause false defects)

Step 3: Situate the child's head slowly within the dome where the chin is resting comfortably on the chin rest and the forehead is on the forehead rest

Step 4: Select the appropriate test. Follow the screen instructions to adjust and calibrate

Step 5: Instruct the child to press the clicker whenever there is a peripheral stimulus noticed

Step 6: Watch the screen display of the eye to monitor the fixation. Remind the child to remain fixated on the central target. Any loss of attention will result in unreliable results. Turn off the blind spot monitor if too much eye or head movement is occurring

Step 7: When completed, switch the occluder to the other eye. Repeat steps 4 - 6 for the other eye

OCTOPUS PERIMETRY

The Octopus 900 perimeter is a versatile computerized perimeter that can perform both static and kinetic testing. This is one of the newer devices out on the market manufactured by Haag Streit. It is structurally similar to that of Goldmann Kinetic perimeter and Humphrey Field Analyzer perimetry whereby the child is situated on a chin/forehead rest in front of a white dome. The Octopus 900 can perform the standard 30-2, 24-2, and 10-2 static testing and has a customizable kinetic testing similar to that of Goldmann Kinetic Perimeter.

The Octopus 900 perimeter is an alternative to the Goldmann perimeter (which is no longer manufactured) where manual kinetic perimetry can be performed digitally. The digital display allows customization of target size, speed, and intensity. Stimuli can be presented manually by using a mouse to guide the test points. There is a trial lens calculator that assists with determination of the proper lens to use for testing, based on the distance refractive correction (Racette, et al.,2016)

Advantages

- Moderately easy to administer.
- Results are very consistent and provides in-depth visual field analysis.
- Has an automatic gaze tracking and adjustment feature helpful for a moving child.
- Can be performed on children as young as five years old (Patel et al., 2015).

Figure 4. Patient side of FDT perimeter

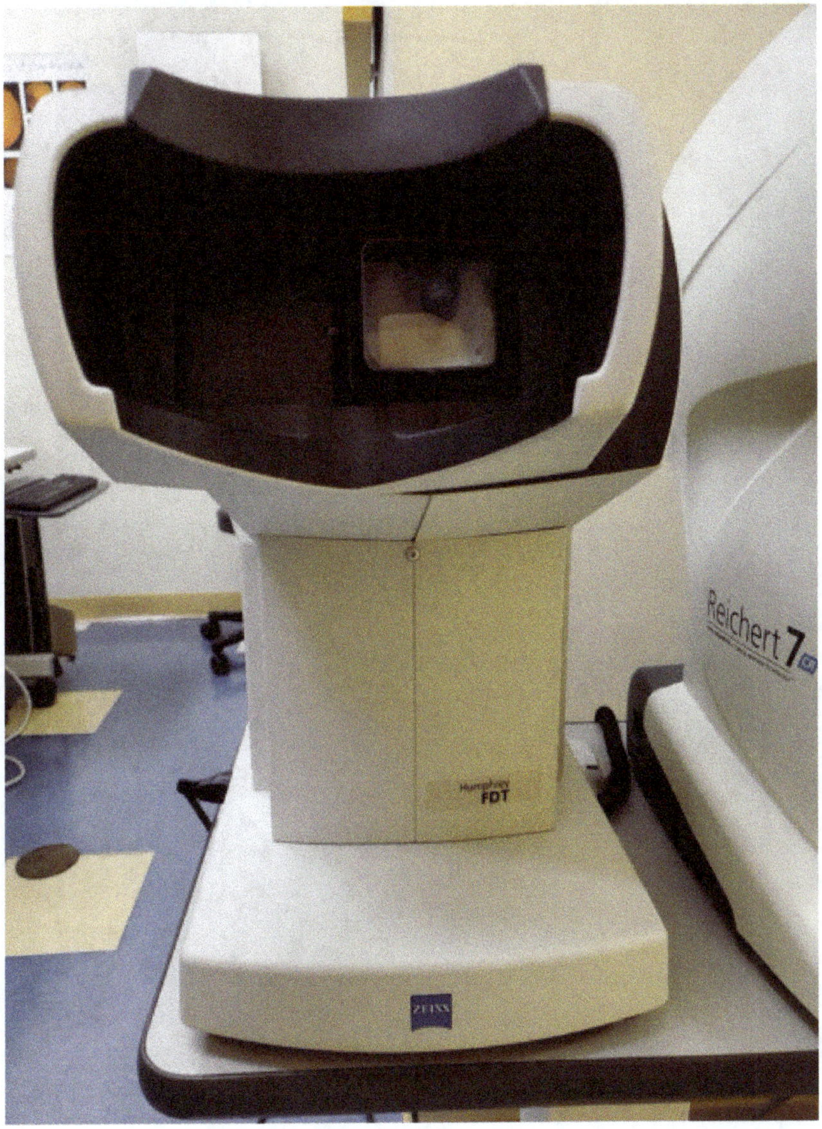

Disadvantages

- This is a difficult test for a young child. It requires high cognition, good motor control, adequate physical stamina, and most importantly good attention and cooperation.

Clinical Pearl: *With automated perimetry methods, it would not be possible to determine statistical significance of the results because there are no normative data to compare with if the patient is under 18. It is, however, important for the clinician to conduct a qualitative analysis based off the threshold data acquired through testing, paying special attention to any longitudinal changes.*

Figure 5. Examiner side of FDT perimeter

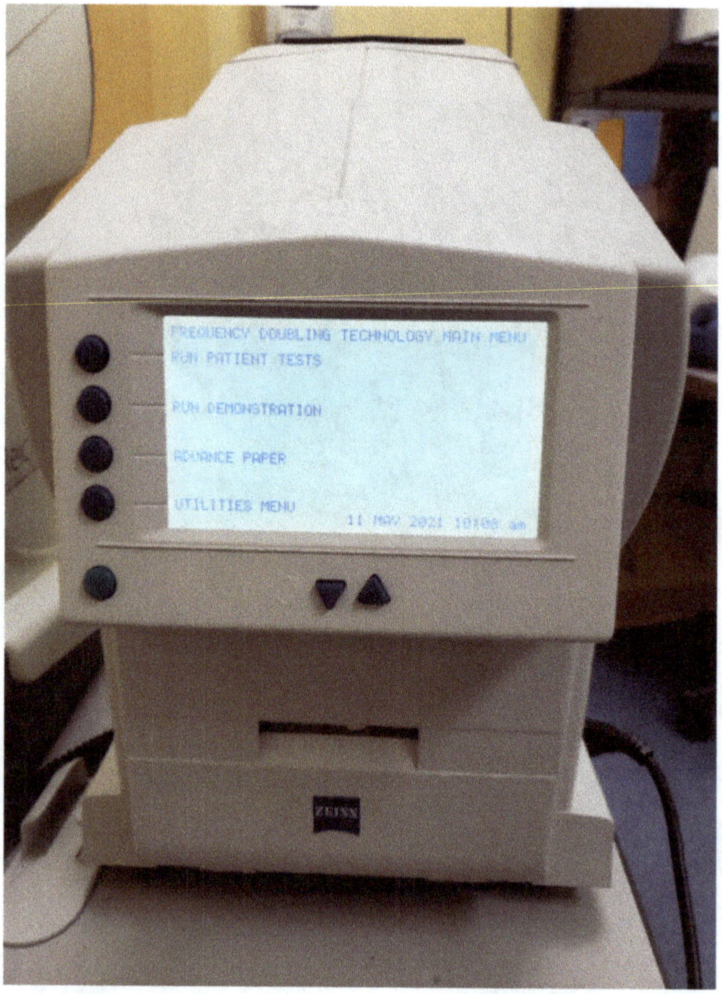

Equipment

1. Octopus 900 perimeter
2. Occluder or eye patch

Procedure

Step 1: Occlude one eye

Step 2: Place the calculated spectacle correction into the lens holder (spectacle correction should not be worn because they can cause false defects)

Step 3: Situate the child's head slowly within the dome where the chin is resting comfortably on the chin rest and the forehead is on the forehead rest

Step 4: Select the appropriate test. Follow the screen instructions to adjust and calibrate

Step 5: Start the test. Watch the on-screen display of the eye and remind the child to remain fixated on the central target.

Clinical Pearl: *If needed, adjust or turn off fixation control depending on child's fixation behavior, but it is recommended to leave it on medium setting.*

Step 6: When completed, switch the occluder to the other eye. Repeat for the other eye

WHITE SPHERE KINETIC PERIMETRY

Finally, we turn to a preferential looking method of perimetry called white sphere kinetic perimetry (WSKP). In WSKP the central and peripheral stimuli are 6-degree white spheres. The peripheral white sphere is mounted on the end of a long thin wand and is moved along one of the 4 arcs/arm from the periphery to the center of the arc perimeter; the child's reflexive orienting eye-head movement from fixation of the central stimulus toward the peripheral stimulus indicates its detection. WSKP has been used extensively to study normal maturation of visual field (Mohn & Van Hof-van Duin, 1986; Delaney et al., 2005) and to study various conditions that place children at risk of visual field loss, including cerebral visual impairment (Van Hof-van Duin et al., 1998), periventricular leukomalacia (Scher et al., 1989), intraventricular hemorrhage (Harvey et al., 1997), and history of antiepileptic medication (Agrawal et al., 2009). WSKP visual fields have also been used as an outcome measure in multicenter clinical trials of treatment for retinopathy of prematurity (Quinn et al., 1996, 2011).

WSKP is generally reserved for children that have multiple impairments that affect their cognitive and or motor abilities. The arc perimeter which the central fixation white sphere is mounted on consists of 2 hemi-spherical steel arcs attached to each other at 90 degrees and mounted on a custom tripod. This will in turn form four arcs/arms oriented on the 45, 135, 225, 315 degree meridians.

Advantages

- Highly successful for low functioning, multiply impaired children.
- A major advantage of using an arc perimeter is the ability to position wheelchair bound patients in between the arcs to perform the testing. This visual field test does not require the patient to engage with any triggers and does not require resting or stabilizing the head on a chin or forehead rest. Yet, this simple test can act as an effective tool to grossly map out a nonverbal, severely impaired child's functional field of view.

Disadvantages

- Difficult to administer, requires two examiners.
- Requires practice and training.

Equipment

1. Plain white spheres or Light-emitting-diode (LED)
2. Occluder or eye patch
3. Arc Perimeter

Procedure

Step 1: Occlude one eye either with an eye patch or occluder

Clinical Pearl: *If child refuses occlusion, perform the test binocularly to obtain a measurement of binocular functional field extent.*

Step 2: To successfully administer WSKP testing, two examiners are needed. One examiner is situated behind the arc perimeter, usually out of the field of view of the patient, and that same examiner is responsible for observing for any preferential looking behavior. The second examiner, situated behind the patient is presenting the peripheral target along the arcs

Step 3: The examiner presenting the peripheral target must exercise caution to move the target at a fixed rate - this can be achieved with practice, or by listening to an electronic metronome through an ear piece in order to sync movement speed to a constant audible rhythmic pattern. A movement speed of approximately 3 degrees per second is recommended. If movement speed of the peripheral target is too fast, it may cause an under estimation of the extent of the patient's visual field

Step 4: Recording and tabulation of the results require multiple steps. Where the tester notices a reflexive look corresponds to a point in the patient's visual field that can be quantified in degrees based off the marking on the arc/arm. Each data point representing a potential visual field extent is recorded on a data sheet where the data is extrapolated into a polar plot.

Clinical Pearl: *Some modifications and variations of WSKP exists. One modification is to make the central and the peripheral stimuli more salient. This is useful for severely impaired children who require a hyper-threshold stimulus to elicit the appropriate peripheral orienting responses. Kong Wand Perimetry is a variant of the WSKP where, instead of a plain white sphere for the central and peripheral target, an array of Super White LEDs housed within a 6-degree diffuse white hemisphere covering is used (Figure 6). The peripheral target is mounted on a 45-centimeter black steel wand and can be modulated temporally from non-flicker to 5 Hz. The central stimulus has identical properties. The transformation of the plain white sphere into a diffuse white light creates a stimulus that is more salient, and the flickering option enhances the effects further. When working with multiply impaired children that are seemingly difficult to engage, using a supra threshold stimulus like the target in Kong Wand Perimetry may yield success (Kong et al., 2009).*

FUTURE DIRECTIONS

Visual fields are constantly evolving. With today's technology, we can see visual fields re-adapted with virtual reality perimetry systems such as the VisuALL S system perimetry by Keeler (Olleyes, 2020). Objective visual field testing (requiring no patient input/response) is also a possibility now with the objectiveFIELD analyzer by Konan Medical (Konan Medical, 2021). Objective visual testing relies on the patient's pupillary responses and can be a solution to meeting the needs of a more objective means of visual field testing particularly important for pediatric patients.

Figure 6. Demonstration of a modified WSKP method called Kong Wand Perimetry. Employs an arc perimeter with 4 arms/arc labelled "A" "B" "C" "D". Central ("E") and peripheral ("F") stimulus is a 6-degree sized LED-based target that can switch from non-flicker to a flicker of 5 hz. Small hash marks along the arcs (white arrow) indicates a measure of visual field extent in degrees

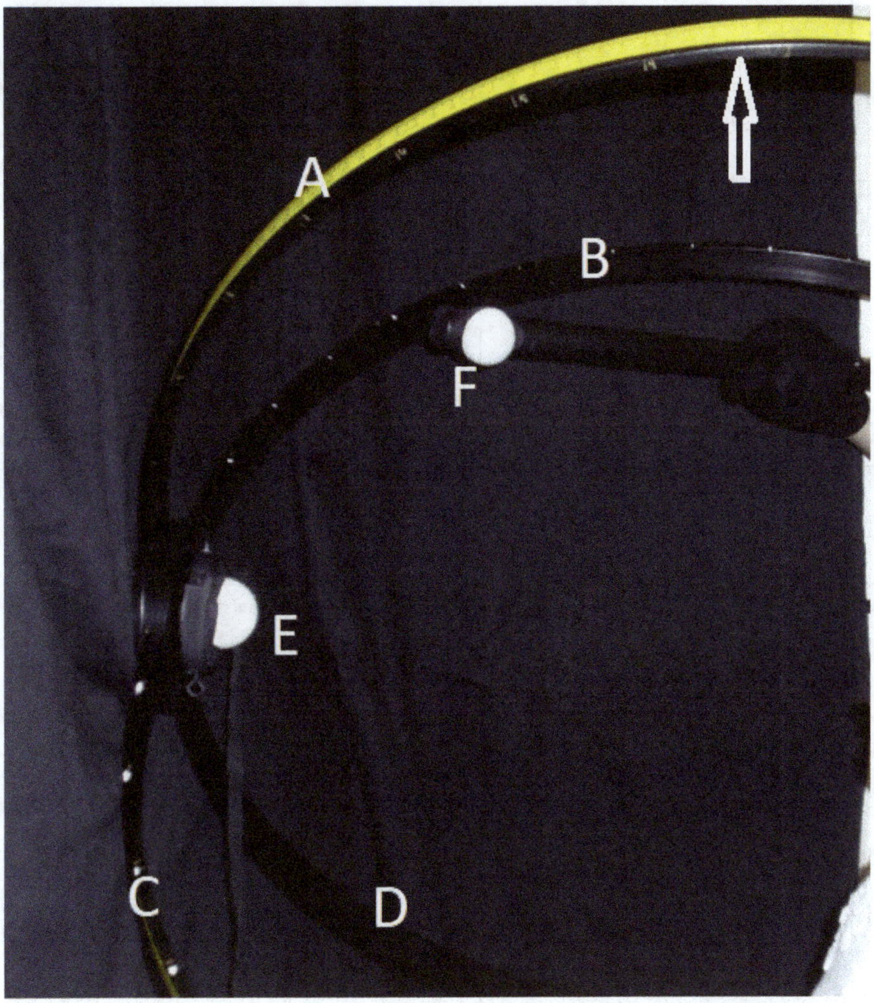

CONCLUSION

When working with young children, unpredictability will be certain and sometimes no test will be tolerated by the child. Through the many methods of visual field testing described in this chapter, it is most important to be able to select the testing method that best fits the child's cognitive and motor abilities. Variations of some of the techniques explained serve as examples of modifications that the clinician can make to the testing as long as the goals of visual field measurement are met and the data from the testing is enough to construct a functional analysis of the patient's monocular or binocular visual field extent.

Table 1. Summary and clinical pearls of various visual field tests

Visual Field Test	Depth of Visual Field Analysis	Cognition Level for patient to complete testing	Clinical Pearls	Modifications or alternative ways of testing
Confrontation Visual Field Test	• Gross or Functional	• Low	• Easy to administer • Low Cost • Can perform on any patient as part of entrance exam	• Use of larger more salient targets • Can use patient's reflexive looking to identify awareness of peripheral stimulus • Can do binocular field if patient refuses monocular testing
Finger Counting Field Test	• Gross or Functional	• Moderate	• Easy to administer • Low Cost • Can perform on any patient as part of entrance exam	• Use finger motion instead of counting fingers • Can do binocular field if patient refuses monocular testing
Goldmann Perimetry	• Gross or Functional and Threshold	• Low to moderate	• Difficult to administer • Requires practice and training • Results can be very consistent and will give a more in-depth analysis on patient's visual field and any associated visual pathway disorder	• Can use patient's reflexive looking to identify awareness of peripheral stimulus • Can do binocular field if patient refuses monocular testing
Frequency Doubling Technology Perimetry	• Threshold	• High	• Easy to administer, but only for high functioning patients	• None
Automated Static Perimetry: Humphrey perimetry & Octopus perimetry	• Threshold	• High	• Moderately easy to administer but only for high functioning patients • Results can be very consistent and will give a more in-depth analysis on patient's visual field and any associated visual pathway disorder	• None
White Sphere Kinetic Perimetry	• Gross or Functional	• Low	• Difficult to administer • Requires practice and training. • Setup is difficult as it requires 2 examiners (one behind the arc perimeter and one behind the patient) • Highly successful for low functioning – multiply impaired patient's that need a visual field analysis	• Use of larger more salient targets • Can do binocular field if patient refuses monocular testing

When working with the pediatric population, the unpredictability of the child's attention span, stamina, and overall behavior/cooperation must always be considered. This is especially true in the case of visual field analysis. Repeating entire tests in the case of the automated perimeters, for example, or retesting certain quadrants multiple times in the case of WSKP, is necessary to establish confidence that the results obtained are unaffected by the child's behavior. In some cases, repeating the test on a different day may be necessary.

Always keep an open mind and remain versatile. If testing is not initially successful or the patient does not seem to be engaged, try changing to a more interesting or salient target. As mentioned above this can be as simple as going from a 3mm white sphere to a larger 1-inch sized colorful finger puppet in the case of confrontation field testing.

A final pearl to end this chapter with is to use the power of observation. The clinician can make an overall sense of the child's visual field functionality by observing the child's movements from the waiting area to the exam room and noting the child's ability to locate objects or people in his/her surroundings. These observations of the child's spatial awareness will shed light on the intactness and functionality of the child's visual field.

REFERENCES

Agrawal, S., Mayer, D. L., Hansen, R. M., & Fulton, A. B. (2009). Visual fields in young children treated with Vigabatrin. *Optometry and Vision Science*, *86*(6), 767–773. doi:10.1097/OPX.0b013e3181a7b3fc PMID:19417698

Anderson, A.J., & Johnson, C.A. (2003). Frequency-doubling technology perimetry. *Ophthalmology Clinics of North America, 16*(2), 213-25.

Anderson, D. R. (1987). *Perimetry With and Without Automation* (2nd ed.). CV Mosby Company.

Carlson, N. B., & Kurtz, D. (2016). *Clinical Procedures for Ocular Examination* (4th ed.). McGraw-Hill.

Chou, S. Y., & Digre, K. M. (1999). Neuro-ophthalmic complications of raised intracranial pressure, hydrocephalus, and shunt malfunction. *Neurosurgery Clinics of North America, 10*(4), 587–608. doi:10.1016/S1042-3680(18)30160-8 PMID:10529972

Delaney, S. M., Dobson, V., & Mohan, K. M. (2005). Measured visual field extent varies with peripheral stimulus flicker rate in very young children. *Optometry and Vision Science, 82*(9), 800–886. doi:10.1097/01.opx.0000178059.39998.bd PMID:16189489

Gilbert, C., Rahi, J. S., & Quinn, G. E. (2003). *The Epidemiology of Eye Disease* (2nd ed.). Arnold.

Harvey, E. M., Dobson, V., Luna, B., & Scher, M. S. (1997). Grating acuity and visual-field development in children with intraventricular hemorrhage. *Developmental Medicine and Child Neurology, 39*(5), 305–312. doi:10.1111/j.1469-8749.1997.tb07436.x PMID:9236696

Heijl, A., Lindgren, G., & Olsson, J. (1987). A package for the statistical analysis of computerized visual fields. *Documenta Ophthalmologica, 49*, 153–168. doi:10.1007/978-94-009-3325-5_23

Heijl, A., & Patella, V. M. (2002). *The Field Analyzer Primer: Essential Perimetry* (3rd ed.). Carl Zeiss Meditec.

Kim, S. K., Wang, K. C., Hwang, Y. S., Kim, K. J., Chae, J. H., Kim, I. O., & Cho, B. K. (2008). Epilepsy surgery in children: Outcomes and Complications. *Journal of Neurosurgery. Pediatrics, 1*(4), 277–283. doi:10.3171/PED/2008/1/4/277 PMID:18377302

Kocabeyoglu, S., Uzum, S., Mocan, M. C., Bozkurt, B., Irkec, M., & Orhan, M. (2013). Comparison of visual field test results obtained through Humphrey Matrix Frequency doubling technology perimetry versus standard automated perimetry in healthy children. *Indian Journal of Ophthalmology, 61*(10), 276–279. PMID:24145558

Konan Medical. (2021). *objectiveFIELDTM Objective Field Analyzer (OFATM)*. Retrieved October 17, 2021, from https://www.konanmedical.com/objectivefield

Kong, J., Johnson, C., Kran, B., Wright, D., & Mayer, L. (2009). *Assessment of Visual Fields in Deafblind Children* [Poster presentation]. American Academy of Optometry. https://www.aaopt.org/detail/knowledge-base-article/assessment-visual-fields-deafblind-children

Mayer, D. L., & Fulton, A. B. (2004). *Pediatric Ophthalmology & Strabismus*. Elsevier Science Limited.

Mohn, G., & Van Hof-van Duin, J. (1986). Development of the binocular and monocular visual fields of human infants during the first year of life. *Clinical Vision Sciences*, *1*, 51–64.

Molia, L., Winterkorn, J. M., & Schneider, S. J. (1996). Hemianopic visual field defects in children with intracranial shunts: Report of two cases. *Neurosurgery*, *39*, 599–603. PMID:8875494

Olleyes. (2020). *Olleyes Virtual Visual Field Products*. Retrieved October 17, 2021, from https://olleyes.com/

Patel, D. E., Cumberland, P. M., Walters, B. C., Russell-Eggitt, I., & Rahi, J. S.OPTIC Study Group. (2015). Study of Optimal Perimetric Testing in Children (OPTIC): Feasibility, Reliability and Repeatability of Perimetry in Children. *PLoS One*, *10*(6), e0130895. doi:10.1371/journal.pone.0130895 PMID:26091102

Quinn, G. E., Dobson, V., Hardy, R. J., Tung, B., Palmer, M. D., & Good, W. V. (2011). Visual field extent at 6 years of age in children who had high-risk prethreshold retinopathy of prematurity. *Archives of Ophthalmology*, *129*(2), 127–132. doi:10.1001/archophthalmol.2010.360 PMID:21320954

Quinn, G. E., Dobson, V., Hardy, R. J., Tung, B., Phelps, D. L., & Palmer, M. D. (1996). Visual fields measured with double-arc perimetry in eyes with threshold retinopathy of prematurity from the Cryotherapy for Retinopathy of Prematurity Trial. *Ophthalmology*, *103*(9), 1432–1427. doi:10.1016/S0161-6420(96)30487-9 PMID:8841302

Racette, L., Fischer, M., Bebie, H., Hollo, G., Johnson, C. A., & Matsumoto, C. (2016). *Visual Field Digest: A guide to perimetry and the Octopus perimeter* (6th ed.). Haag-Streit AG.

Rahi, J. S., & Gilbert, C. E. (2005). *Pediatric Ophthalmology and Strabismus* (3rd ed.). Elsevier Saunders.

Scher, M. S., Dobson, V., Carpenter, N. A., & Guthrie, R. D. (1989). Visual and neurological outcome of infants with periventricular leukomalacia. *Developmental Medicine and Child Neurology*, *31*(3), 353–365. doi:10.1111/j.1469-8749.1989.tb04004.x PMID:2753239

Spry, P. G. D., Johnson, C. A., Anderson, A. J., Gunvant, P., Fingeret, M., Keltner, J. L., Wall, M., & Werner, J. S. (2008). *A Primer for Frequency Doubling Technology (FDT) Perimetry Using the Humphrey Matrix*. Carl Zeiss Meditec.

Suharwardy, J., & Elson, J. (1997). The clinical presentation of children with tumours affecting the anterior visual pathways. *Eye (London, England)*, *11*(6), 838–844. doi:10.1038/eye.1997.215 PMID:9537141

Van den Broek, E. G. C., Janssen, C. G. C., Van Ramshorst, T., & Deen, L. (2006). Visual impairments in people with severe and profound multiple disabilities; an inventory of visual functioning. *Journal of Intellectual Disability Research*, *50*(6), 470–475. doi:10.1111/j.1365-2788.2006.00804.x PMID:16672040

Van Hof-van Duin, J., Cioni, G., Bertuccelli, B., Fazzi, B., Romano, C., & Boldrini, A. (1998). Visual outcome at 5 years of newborn infants at risk of cerebral visual impairment. *Developmental Medicine and Child Neurology*, *40*, 302–309. PMID:9630257

Warburg, M. (1994). Visual impairment among people with developmental delay. *Journal of Intellectual Disability Research*, *38*(4), 423–432. doi:10.1111/j.1365-2788.1994.tb00421.x PMID:7949793

Wild, J. M., Ahn, H. S., Baulac, M., Bursztyn, J., Chiron, C., Gandolfo, E., Safran, A. B., Schiefer, U., & Perucca, E. (2007). Vigabatrin and epilepsy: Lessons learned. *Epilepsia*, *48*(7), 1318–1327. doi:10.1111/j.1528-1167.2007.01133.x PMID:17635558

Zeppieri, M., & Johnson, C. A. (2008). *Frequency Doubling Technology (FDT) Perimetry*. Imaging and Perimetry Society. Retrieved October 17, 2021, from http://webeye.ophth.uiowa.edu/ips/perimetryhistory/FDP/

KEY TERMS AND DEFINITIONS

Arc Perimeter: An alternative to the traditional dome perimeters such as the Humphrey or the Goldmann. The arc perimeter is made by joining 2 steel semi-circular arcs at a 90-degree array. This creates 4 arms at the 45, 135, 225, 315-degree meridians. The functional visual field test is carried out based off the 4 main meridians.

Binocular Field Extent: Visual field measured when both eyes are open.

Kinetic Perimetry: Perimetric test based on a moving peripheral stimulus.

Monocular Field Extent: Visual field measured when one eye is occluded.

Perimetry: A method of measuring a patient's visual field. Can be adapted to many different types of techniques.

Static Perimetry: Perimetric test based on fixed locations of peripheral stimuli being presented

Visual Field: How sensitive and to what extent a patient's spatial awareness is under conditions where the eye is fixated on a single area and there is no movement. Typically, more restricted nasally (55–60 degrees) than temporally (90–100 degrees).

Chapter 6
Pupil Examination in Children

Iason Mantagos
Boston Children's Hospital, USA

ABSTRACT

Pupillary evaluation is a crucial part of every pediatric eye exam. It provides information about the structure of the eye as well as the afferent and efferent function of the eyes. It remains a quick and efficient test in the ocular evaluation. This chapter reviews the relevant neuroanatomy and the different components of the pupillary exam. The light-reflex and swinging flashlight tests are reviewed, as well as how a reverse afferent pupillary defect is detected. Clinical examples and pearls are provided to help the reader better understand the different aspects of the exam.

INTRODUCTION

Pupil testing is a crucial component of every pediatric eye examination. The shape and movements of the pupils provide an enormous amount of diagnostic information. Unequal pupil size (anisocoria) or a relative afferent pupillary defect (RAPD) may indicate a serious intracranial pathology or a benign physiological condition. An RAPD may be produced by retinal disorders (including but not limited to retinal detachment, and retinal vascular disease such as central retinal artery occlusion), unilateral or asymmetric optic nerve pathology, as well as chiasmal compression and optic tract lesions due to an uneven number of optic fibers undergoing hemidecussation at the chiasm (Balcer, 2019). An RAPD will NOT be produced by refractive error, media opacities including cataracts, lesions posterior to the lateral geniculate body and non-physiologic visual loss.

BACKGROUND

Relevant Neuroanatomy

Pupillary responses depend on the afferent and efferent neurologic pathways of the eyes, which will be reviewed in detail in this chapter.

DOI: 10.4018/978-1-7998-8044-8.ch006

After light enters the eye, passing through cornea, anterior chamber, and lens it will eventually reach the retina, where it will stimulate the photoreceptors which will convert light stimuli to neuronal impulses. The afferent path originates at the level of the retina and sends neuronal impulses to various central nervous system structures, including the primary visual cortex for further processing and image recognition and the pretectal nuclei of the brainstem for control of pupillary constriction via the visceral efferent fibers of the oculomotor nerve (Agur and Dalley, 2019).

The pupillary-light reflex arc is polysynaptic and its afferent path is cranial nerve II and the efferent path is cranial nerve III (Figure 1). The afferent pathway starts at the level of the retina, ganglion cells project to the pretectal nuclei bilaterally in the midbrain. As nerve fibers pass through the chiasm hemidecussation of the nasal fibers occurs. The ganglion cell nerve fibers of the pupillary pathway exit the optic tract just anterior to the lateral geniculate nucleus at the brachium of the superior colliculus. The pretectal nuclei project crossed fibers via the posterior commissure, and uncrossed fibers to the Edinger-Westphal nucleus of cranial nerve III. The efferent path of the pupillary light reflex is the parasympathetic pathway which will be described in the following paragraphs.

The iris has both sympathetic and parasympathetic innervation. The size of the pupil depends on the balance between the sympathetic innervation to the dilator muscle of the iris and the parasympathetic innervation to the sphincter muscles of the iris.

Sympathetic innervation starts at the hypothalamus (McDougal and Gamlin, 2015). First-order neurons descend through the brain stem to the spinal cord in the intermediolateral column where they synapse in the ciliospinal nucleus of Budge-Waller, between the 7th cervical and the 2nd thoracic vertebrae. From there, the postsynaptic second-order fibers exit the spinal cord and ascend to terminate at the superior cervical ganglion at the level of the angle of the jaw and the carotid artery bifurcation. From the superior cervical ganglion, the postganglionic third-order fibers surround the internal carotid artery and enter the cavernous sinus. They briefly join cranial nerve VI, then join the nasociliary branch of the ophthalmic division of cranial nerve V, passing through the ciliary ganglion (without synapsing at the ciliary ganglion), before finally reaching the iris dilator muscle via the long ciliary nerves.

Parasympathetic innervation of the iris sphincter muscles originates at the Edinger-Westphal nucleus (McDougal and Gamlin, 2015). The preganglionic parasympathetic fibers travel within cranial nerve III, after the cranial nerve III bifurcation in the cavernous sinus the parasympathetic fibers travel in the inferior division of cranial nerve III until they reach and synapse at the ciliary ganglion. From there, the postsynaptic fibers will reach the iris sphincter via the short posterior ciliary nerves.

Clinically in the absence of ocular pathology, stimulation of one eye with light results in bilateral pupillary constriction. This occurs because of the double decussation of the fibers involved in the light reflex pathway, first at the chiasm and second at the posterior commissure where the pretectal nuclei project crossed fibers to the Edinger Westphal nucleus.

In addition to the pupillary-light reflex pathway, there is the near-reflex pathway which is responsible for pupillary constriction during accommodation (Kardon, 2008). Even though the neuroanatomic pathway responsible for the near-reflex is not as well defined, its efferent path is also through cranial nerve III with fibers originating in the rostral Edinger-Westphal nucleus.

Figure 1. Sympathetic and parasympathetic innervations of the eye

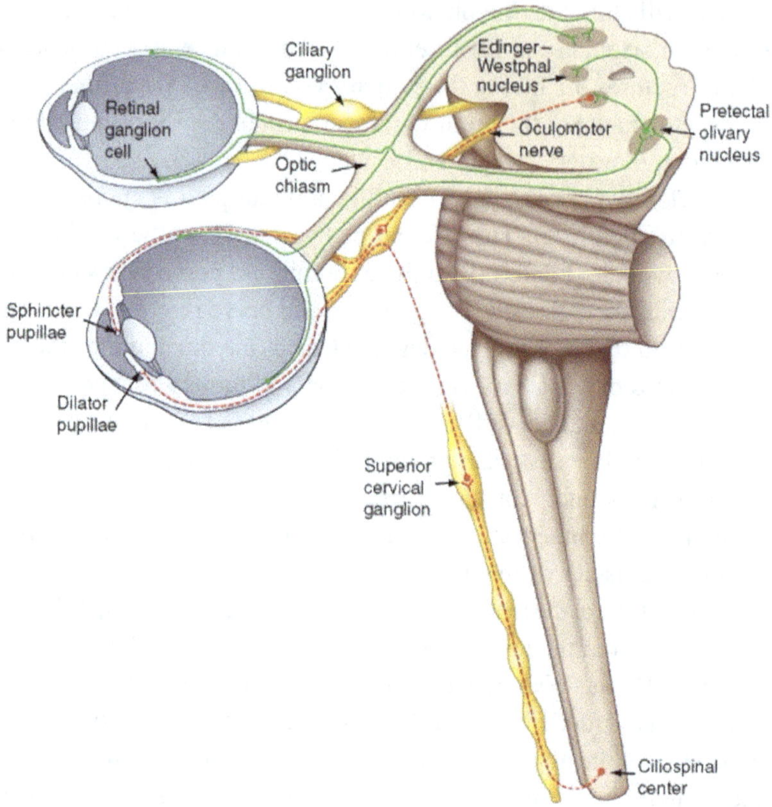

NORMAL PUPILLARY RESPONSES

In the absence of pathology, both pupils will constrict when light is shined to either eye. This occurs as a result of the double decussation of nerve fibers described in the previous paragraph.

CLINICAL EXAMINATION

Evaluating pupillary reactions to light is a simple way of checking the integrity of the visual pathway. Clinical examination of the pupils consists of (Lessell and Kim, 2008):

1. Observation
2. Light-reflex test, where one evaluates the direct and consensual pupillary responses
3. Swinging flashlight test (also known as the Marcus Gunn test), where we are observing for differences in pupil reactions between the two eyes
4. Near-reflex test, where we evaluate pupillary responses during accommodation

Equipment (Figure 2 shows a transilluminator, a near visual acuity card with pupil gauge and child fixation target)

1. Transilluminator
2. Pupil gauge
3. Neutral density filter bar

Figure 2. Left: transillumination Center: Near visual acuity with pupil gauge Right: Fixation target

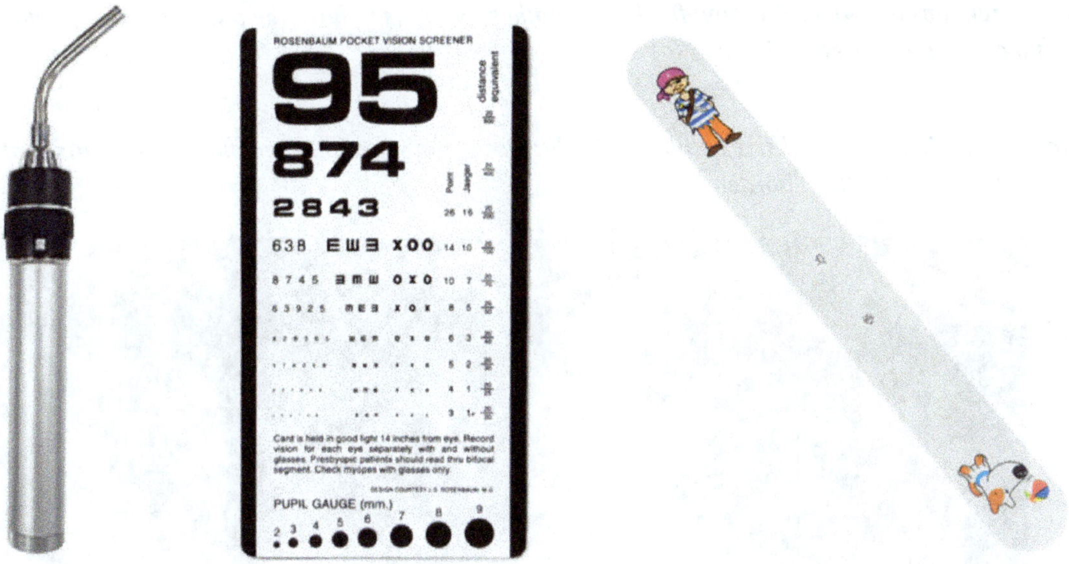

Procedure

Clinical examination of the pupils consists of:

Step 1: Observation

Similar to other components of the physical exam, observation of the pupils under normal lighting is the first step. One notes the size of each pupil, any difference in the size of each pupil, as well as the contour of the pupil.

Clinical Pearl: *Distracting children by having them watch a movie at a distance is a great way to ensure adequate cooperation for an accurate exam. Visual acuity charts that will play cartoons and movies are essential for providers that routinely examine children.*

Irregularities of the contour of the pupil should be further investigated with slit-lamp examination. In children, irregularities of the pupillary contour can be congenital or acquired. Congenital defects of the iris include aniridia, coloboma and corectopia, while acquired defects can be traumatic iris tears or posterior synechiae secondary to inflammation among other causes. Figure 3 shows an inferior nasal iris coloboma and a posterior synechiae secondary to uveitis.

If anisocoria is noted, which is unequal size of the pupils, the diameter of each pupil should be recorded in millimeters both under regular lighting and under dim lighting. Using a pupil gauge allows accurate recording of the size of each pupil, it is best done by placing the pupil gauge next to the pupil being measured. If the difference in the pupil size is greater in a brightly lit room, then the more dilated pupil is likely to be the pathologic pupil; whereas if the anisocoria is more notable in a dimly lit room then the pathologic pupil is the smaller one.

Clinical Pearl: *In children who are frightful and close their eyes as you approach them, one can evaluate the pupil size and look for asymmetry by using the retinoscope. Slightly dim the room lights and sit far enough from the child so that you can illuminate both pupils simultaneously with the retinoscope. For a child that remains uncooperative and frightful, another option is to have the parents take a photograph of the face using their smart phone.*

Figure 3. Left: Inferior-nasal iris coloboma Right: Posterior synechiae secondary to uveitis (note the irregularity of the pupillary border)

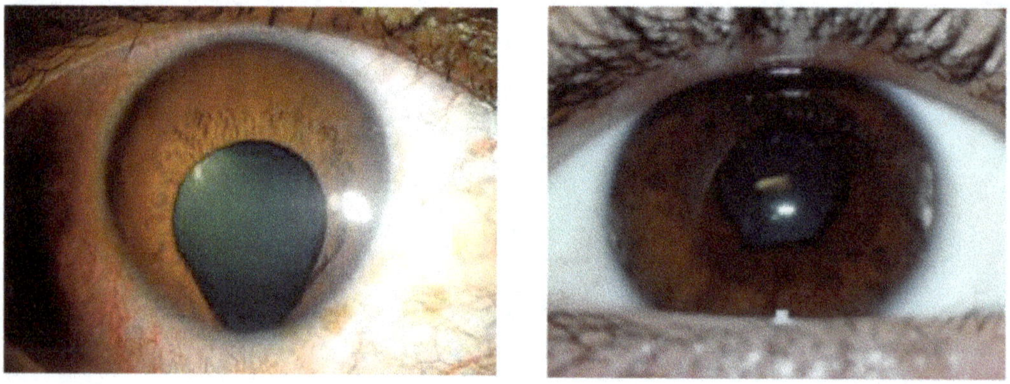

For anisocoria that is greater in the dark, one should consider further pharmacologic testing for Horner's syndrome to differentiate it from physiologic anisocoria, which can be present in up to 20% of the population (Lam and Thompson, 1987). In physiologic anisocoria a 1 to 1.5mm difference in pupil size can be observed. While pharmacologic testing for Horner's syndrome is beyond the scope of this chapter, associated ocular signs that one should evaluate for include ipsilateral miosis, iris heterochromia (present in congenital Horner's syndrome with the involved eye having a lighter iris color) and dilation lag of the miotic pupil (Weinstein et al., 1980). Figure 4 shows congenital Horner's syndrome of the left eye with ipsilateral miosis, ptosis, and iris heterochromia.

Figure 4. Congenital Horner's syndrome of the left eye with ipsilateral miosis, ptosis and iris heterochromia

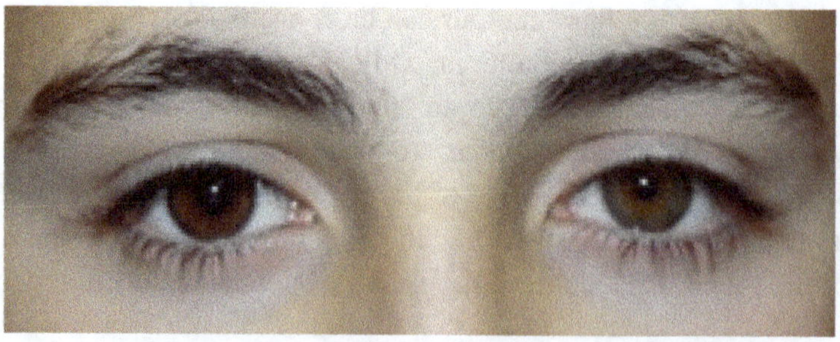

The differential diagnosis for anisocoria that is more notable in a lit room includes traumatic mydriasis from trauma to the iris sphincter muscle, Adie's tonic pupil, cranial nerve III palsy and pharmacologic dilation. When investigating the etiology of anisocoria it is important to review the medication history and to query specifically for the use of scopolamine patches and eyedrops. Associated signs of cranial nerve III palsy include ipsilateral ptosis, exotropia and hypotropia with limitation of elevation and adduction. Pharmacologic testing to differentiate between Adie's tonic pupil, cranial nerve III palsy and pharmacologic dilation can be done using dilute (0.125%) pilocarpine. Tonic pupils with denervation hypersensitivity will constrict with 0.125% pilocarpine, whereas dilated pupils due to cranial nerve III palsies and pupils that are pharmacologically dilated will not constrict. If after testing with dilute pilocarpine the pupil does not constrict, then the next step is to instill a drop of 1% pilocarpine and evaluate for pupillary constriction, a pharmacologically dilated pupil will not constrict but the pupil will constrict in the setting of cranial nerve III palsy.

Step 2: Light-Reflex Test - Figure 5 shows the light reflex test

1. Under dim illumination have the patient fixate at a distant target.
2. The transilluminator light (or a penlight) is shined to the right eye and the examiner records the pupillary response of the eye that is being illuminated; this includes the size of the pupil prior and after light was shone and the briskness of the response.
3. Repeat the same steps for the left eye.

Figure 5. Light-reflex test. Light shined to the right eye leads to pupillary constriction on the right (direct response) and the left (consensual response) eye

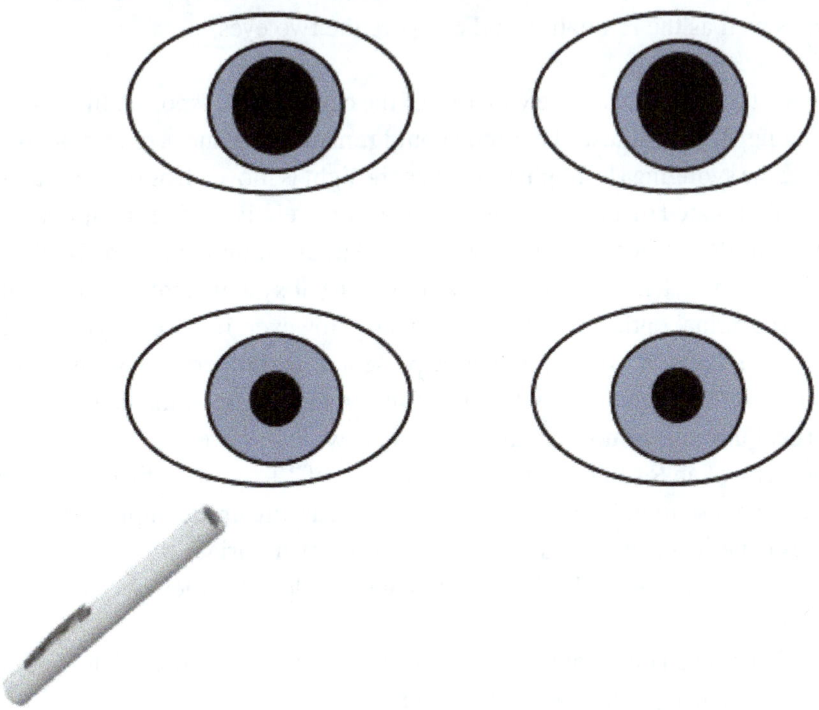

Evaluating how the eye responds when light is shone directly to it is called the direct response. The briskness of the response can be graded on a subjective 0 to 4+ scale.

The next step is to evaluate how the fellow eye responds at the same time, this is the consensual response.

4. Repeat steps 1 and 2, but this time observe how the left eye responds when light is shined to the right eye.
5. Repeat illuminating the left eye, but now observe and record how the right eye responds.

Clinical Pearl: *Approach with the light from beneath or from the side of the eye, instead of holding it directly in front of the child. This prevents the child from fixating at the light, accommodating and thus causing pupillary constriction from stimulation of the near-reflex.*

Step 3: Swinging Flashlight Test (Figure 6)

The swinging flashlight test follows the light-reflex test.

1. Continue having the child fixate at a distant target under dim illumination.
2. Shine a bright transilluminator light on to the right eye approximately one inch from the eye and slightly below the pupillary axis for about 3 seconds. Quickly move the light from one eye to the other while keeping the rhythm equal between the two eyes. For example, count 1, 2, 3 right eye, move the light directly across the bridge of the nose and count 1, 2, 3 left eye and repeat in a rhythmic fashion. Avoid using a wide beam of light that potentially illuminates the fellow eye at the same time.
3. Repeat the process for at least three to four cycles and observe the speed and the extent of the initial constriction as well as the re-dilation and compare the two eyes.

Compare the direct pupillary response with that of the consensual response. In the absence of pathology with the swinging flashlight test, the pupil should remain the same size or constrict slightly when illuminated. During the swinging flashlight test, when the light is moved from one eye to the other and the pupil dilates when illuminated that indicates the presence of a relative afferent pupillary defect (RAPD). A relative afferent pupillary defect is also known as a Marcus Gunn pupil. An RAPD is present when there is unilateral or asymmetric damage to the afferent visual system anterior to the lateral geniculate nucleus, including the retina, optic nerve and optic tracts. However, if there is symmetric damage to the anterior visual system then an RAPD might not be present (e.g., bilateral advanced glaucoma, bilateral optic neuropathy). In addition, patients with refractive errors, cataracts, media opacities (e.g., vitreous hemorrhage), cortical infracts, or non-organic vision loss will not have an RAPD.

Grading the severity of an RAPD can be done on a scale of 1+ to 4+, with 4+ being used when there is not even a direct response to light. A 4+ RAPD is known as amaurotic pupil. Grading on this scale is subjective, requires experience and has significant interobserver variability.

A more objective way of grading RAPD is with a neutral density filter bar (Bell et al., 1993):

1. After an RAPD has been confirmed as describe above, a neutral density filter bar is placed in front of the normal eye starting with the least dense filter.
2. Continue swinging the light from one eye to the other and observe the severity of the RAPD.

3. Move the neutral density filter bar to have a denser filter over the normal eye until you have eliminated the presence of the RAPD.
4. Record the filter that was required to eliminate the RAPD response.

Clinical Pearl: *Avoid prolonged illumination of one eye because it can produce a false RAPD.*

Figure 6. Swinging Flashlight Test. RAPD is present on the right A. Pupils under normal conditions B. Slight symmetrical pupillary constriction when light shined to the right eye C. Both pupils constrict further when light shined to the left eye D. Pupillary dilation when light moved and shined to the right eye again

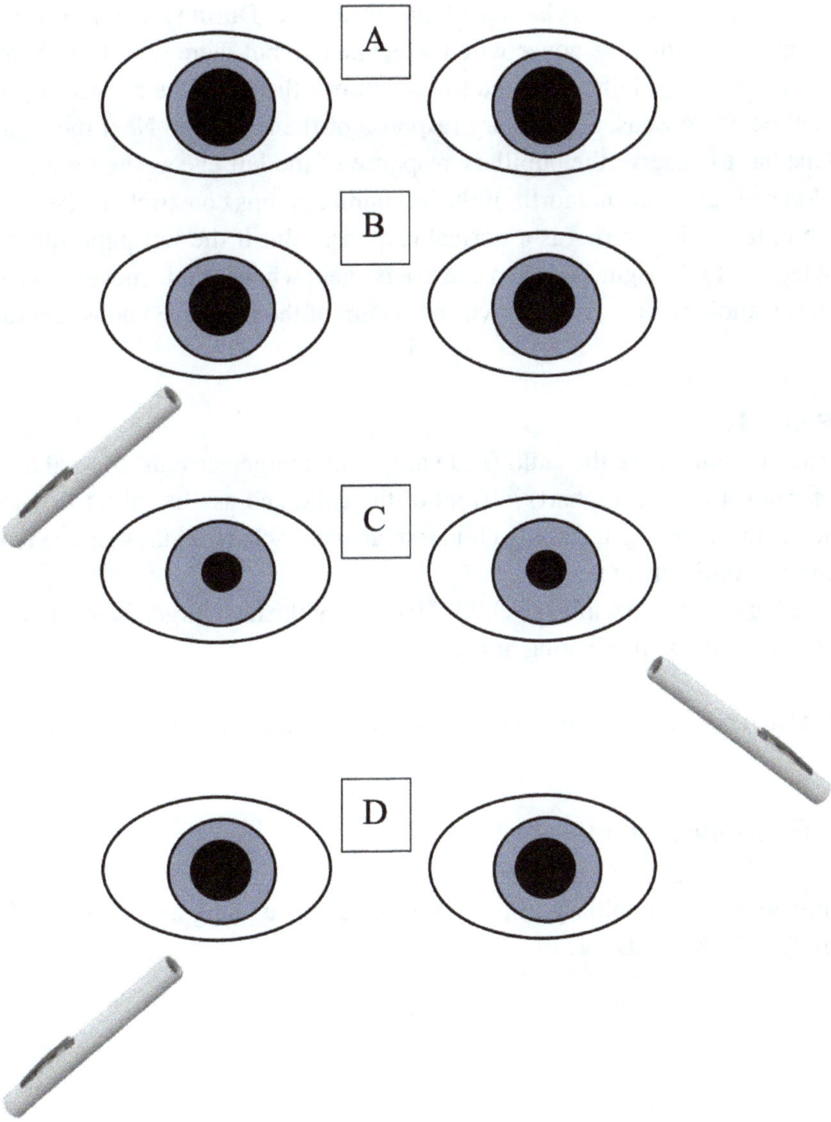

Evaluating for a Reverse Relative Afferent Pupillary Defect

The presence of an RAPD can still be determined in the setting of a pupil that is pharmacologically dilated or constricted, or in the setting of pupillary anomalies that prevent normal pupillary reaction (e.g., posterior synechiae). This is not an uncommon scenario, where patients with unilateral pathology are pharmacologically dilated but continue to require monitoring of their afferent visual system. Common examples include patients with hyphema or eyes after eye surgery, where pharmacologic dilation is common. In this setting, the suspected pathologic eye might not have direct nor consensual pupillary responses, but if one observes the fellow eye during the swinging flashlight test one can determine if a relative afferent pupillary defect is present.

Clinical Example:

The right eye has a hyphema and is pharmacologically dilated. During the light-reflex test, when light is shined to the right eye a direct response will not be elicited, but there will be a consensual pupillary response of the left eye; when light is shined to the left eye there will be a direct response of the left eye, but there will be no consensual pupillary response of the right eye. Next the swinging flashlight is performed. One has to observe the pupillary response of the left eye as the light is moved from the right eye to the left eye, and back and forth. If the left pupil remains constricted when the light is moved from the left eye to the right eye that is a normal response. But if the left pupil dilates as the light is moved from the left eye to the right, and then constricts again when light is moved back over the left eye then that indicates pathology in the afferent visual system of the right eye and is recorded as a positive reverse RAPD.

Step 4: Near-Reflex Test

1. Under normal lighting, have the child fixate at a distant target such as a visual acuity chart.
2. Bring a near target (toy, near chart) in front of the child and ask her/him to switch fixation from the distance to the near target. Asking child to read a near chart ensures she/he is accommodating and fixating appropriately at near.
3. Note the pupillary response while the child is fixating at the near target. Normal response is a slight pupillary constriction while fixating at near.

Clinical Pearl: *One can simultaneously test the near-reflex and evaluate accommodation by dynamic retinoscopy.*

Recording of Pupillary Testing

It is very common for normal pupillary responses to be recorded using the acronym PERRLA.

The acronym PERRLA stands for:

P = Pupils
E = Equal
R = Round
R = Reactive (reactive to light with next letter)
L = Light

A = Accommodation (reactive to accommodation)

If the near-reflex was not tested, then one should record the response as PERRL.

However, in patients with pupillary abnormalities more detailed recording of the responses should be made, include the size of the pupil in brightly and dimly lit conditions, briskness of reactivity, presence and severity of an RAPD.

An example of detailed pupillary responses follows:

Table 1. Documentation of pupillary exam

	Pupil Size		Briskness of reaction to light	RAPD
	Dark	Light		
OD	6 mm	3 mm	3+	
OS	6 mm	3 mm	1+	2+

CONCLUSION

In conclusion, pupillary evaluation is a crucial part of every pediatric eye exam as it can detect ocular and neurologic disease. Pupil testing is a quick, sensitive and low-cost test that provides valuable insight into possible pathology of at the anterior visual pathways, midbrain and autonomic nervous system. However, there can be a significant learning curve in mastering the different aspects of the exam and subtle defects can be missed. Grading RAPD is also highly subjective and there can be significant interobserver variability.

ACKNOWLEDGMENT

The author would like to thank Tak-Man Kimberly Fung, OD for her illustration contributions to this chapter.

REFERENCES

Agur, A. M., & Dalley, A. F. (2019). *Moore's essential clinical anatomy* (6th ed.). Wolters Kluwer.

Balcer, L. J. (2019). Pupillary disorders. In G. T. Liu, G. T. Volpe, & S. L. Galetta (Eds.), *Neuro-ophthalmology diagnosis and management* (3rd ed., pp. 417–421). Elsevier Inc.

Bell, R. A., Waggoner, P. M., Boyd, W. M., Akers, R. E., & Yee, C. E. (1993). Clinical grading of relative afferent pupillary defects. *Archives of Ophthalmology, 111*(7), 938–942. doi:10.1001/archopht.1993.01090070056019 PMID:8328935

Kardon, R. (2008). The pupils and accommodation. In D. M. Albert & J. W. Miller (Eds.), *Albert & Jakobiec's. Principles and practice of ophthalmology* (pp. 4029–4048). Elsevier Inc. doi:10.1016/B978-1-4160-0016-7.50296-4

Lam, B. L., Thompson, H. S., & Corbett, J. J. (1987). The prevalence of simple anisocoria. *American Journal of Ophthalmology, 104*(1), 69–73. doi:10.1016/0002-9394(87)90296-0 PMID:3605282

Lessell, S., & Kim, J. W. (2008). Clinical examination. In D. M. Albert & J. W. Miller (Eds.), *Albert & Jakobiec's. Principles and practice of ophthalmology* (pp. 3813–3816). Elsevier Inc. doi:10.1016/B978-1-4160-0016-7.50281-2

McDougal, D. H., & Gamlin, P. D. (2015). Autonomic control of the eye. *Comprehensive Physiology, 5*(1), 439–473. PMID:25589275

Weinstein, J. M., Zweifel, T. J., & Thompson, H. S. (1980). Congenital Horner's syndrome. *Archives of Ophthalmology, 98*(6), 1074–1078. doi:10.1001/archopht.1980.01020031064011 PMID:7387512

KEYWORDS AND DEFINITIONS

Amaurotic Pupil: A light without light perception, the involved pupil does not react to light (direct response), but will constrict when light is shined to the fellow normal eye (consensual response).

Horner Syndrome: Disruption of the sympathetic innervation of the eye, classically characterized by ipsilateral miosis, ptosis and anhidrosis (lack of sweating).

Light-Reflex Test: A test used to evaluate direct and consensual pupillary responses.

Marcus Gunn Pupil: A pupil that exhibits a relative afferent pupillary defect.

Neutral Density Filter Bar: An optical filter that reduces the intensity of light used to quantify the extent of a relative afferent pupillary defect.

Posterior Synechiae: Adhesions at the pupillary margin between the posterior iris and the anterior lens surface.

Pupil: Circular opening in the center of the iris.

Relative Afferent Pupillary Defect: Defect of the afferent visual pathway of one eye relative to the other eye.

Swinging Flashlight Test: A test used to evaluate for differences in pupil reactions between the two eyes and for the presence of a relative afferent pupillary defect.

Chapter 7
Ocular Motility Testing in Children

M. H. Esther Han
https://orcid.org/0000-0002-8114-0472
SUNY College of Optometry, USA

ABSTRACT

The purpose of this chapter is to provide the main indications, background, and procedures when assessing eye movement function in the pediatric patient. The assessment of extraocular motility function includes version and ductions using the H pattern test in order to determine the presence of underaction or overactions of the extraocular muscles (EOM). EOM testing detects abnormalities in the structural and neurological integrity caused by an acquired or congenital disease of the central nervous system. Deficits in eye movement function can also contribute to poor academic performance which requires a developmental approach to the assessment of saccadic and pursuit eye movements to determine if a referral for optometric vision therapy is indicated. For the older child who is reading to learn, an assessment of reading eye movements using objective tests, such as the Visagraph and/or the ReadAlyzer, will guide the direction of the management plan.

INTRODUCTION

Eye movement testing in the pediatric population assesses a child's visual system on several levels and should be evaluated during the primary care examination. First, the structural and neurological integrity is assessed to rule-out the presence of an acquired or congenital disease of the central nervous system requiring a neurological evaluation (London, 2020; Scheiman & Wick, 2020). Second, visual function and developmental status is assessed to determine the presence of learning related vision problems that may impact academic performance (Birnbaum, 1983; Maples, 2017; Rouse, 2006; Taub 2012).

There is a high prevalence of ocular motility function deficits in children with special needs (Taub, 2012). This can range from congenital or acquired strabismus due to cranial nerve palsies or due to delays in visual development. In addition, growing public health interest in sports-related concussions require clinicians to understand that ocular motility deficits are common visual sequela seen in particularly the

DOI: 10.4018/978-1-7998-8044-8.ch007

adolescent population (Graham et al., 2014; Master et al., 2016; Galloway et al., 2017). Although poor reading ability is the main indication for testing in the pediatric population, some additional commonly reported vision symptoms associated with ocular motility deficits include:

- Loss of place, omission of words when reading.
- Poor efficiency with reading and other academic assignments resulting in poor reading comprehension.
- Difficulty fixating, locating, or tracking objects.
- Poor attention and easily distractible with sustained visual activities.
- Vague asthenopic symptoms around the head or eyes.
- Poor coordination of body and eyes.
- Vertigo, dizziness, motion sickness.

This chapter will be divided into two parts: Part I: Structural & Neurological Status and Part II: Visual Function and Developmental Status. Specific clinical procedures to accurately assess versional or conjugate ocular motility function in the pediatric patient will be presented.

PART I: STRUCTURAL AND NEUROLOGICAL STATUS

Versions and Ductions

Versions and ductions assess the structural and neurological integrity by detecting the presence of a congenital or an acquired disease of the central nervous system which may require further neurological evaluation. There are six extraocular muscles in each eye: superior rectus (SR), inferior rectus (IR), lateral rectus (LR), medial rectus (MR), superior oblique (SO), and inferior oblique (IO) (Ciuffreda & Tannen, 1995; Wong, 2008). See Table 1 for the primary, secondary, and tertiary actions as well as the cranial nerve innervation for each muscle. In addition, a mneumonic "RAD SIN" aids in remembering the functions of the muscles. "RAD" refers to the rectus muscles adducting while "SIN" refers to the superior muscles intorting. The actions of each muscle for eye movements depend upon the actual position of the eye (Ciuffreda & Tannen, 1995; Wong 2008).

Versions and ductions testing would rule-out the presence of extraocular muscle underactions or overactions. Cranial nerve palsies may lead to muscle paresis or paralysis. A paralysis occurs when there is complete nerve damage resulting to no movement in the direction of the diagnostic action field. A paresis occurs when there is partial nerve damage resulting in varying degrees of muscle restriction. When differentiating a palsy of recent onset, the secondary deviation (when the deviated affected eye is fixating) is typically larger than the primary deviation (when the unaffected eye is fixating) (Griffin & Borsting, 2010). When a cranial nerve palsy is suspected, the goal is to determine if there is a congenital or a recently acquired cranial nerve palsy. For example, in a child manifesting a constant esotropia in one eye, a sixth nerve palsy can be seen if the lateral rectus of the affected eye does not abduct. If this same child also reported a recent onset diplopia and a recent onset esotropia, a consult is urgently required to determine the presence of an active neurological disease process. The most common cause of acute cranial nerve palsies was found to be neoplasms. About 20% in children (0-14 years) and in 31% in adolescents (15-19 years) (Park et al., 2019).

Table 1. Extraocular muscle cranial nerve innervations and actions

EXTRAOCULAR MUSCLES	CRANIAL NERVE INNERVATION	MUSCLE ACTIONS		
		Primary	**Secondary**	**Tertiary**
Superior Rectus	III (Oculomotor)	Elevation	Intorsion	Adduction
Inferior Rectus	III (Oculomotor)	Depression	Extorsion	Adduction
Lateral Rectus	VI (Abducens)	Abduction		
Medial Rectus	III (Oculomotor)	Adduction		
Superior Oblique	IV (Trochlear)	Intorsion	Depression	Abduction
Inferior Oblique	III (Oculomotor)	Extorsion	Elevation	Abduction
MNEUMONIC: Rad Sin				
"R"ectus "ad"duct, Obliques abduct				
"S"uperior "in"tort, Inferior Extort				

(Ciuffreda & Tannen, 1995; Wong 2008)

The following is a summary of the characteristics of each cranial nerve palsy affecting ocular motility:

- Cranial Nerve IV Palsy: Most pediatric fourth nerve palsies are congenital (Holmes et al., 1999; Priya et al. 2021).
    - Primary gaze: A fourth nerve palsy would manifest a hyper deviation of the affected eye in primary position. With a careful case history with the older child, a small excyclodeviation and small eso deviation may be noted subjectively (Griffin & Borsting, 2010).
    - Diplopia and gaze: This patient may report vertical diplopia that worsens in inferior gaze and with convergence.
    - Motility finding: An underaction of the superior oblique muscle would be noted.
    - Compensatory head tilt: A compensatory head tilt would also be observed as this is the ocular position which minimizes diplopia. If there was a right superior oblique muscle weakness from a right fourth nerve palsy, the child may be noted to have a left head tilt, a left head turn, with chin depression (Griffin & Borsting, 2010). The child would be attempting to look towards superior right gaze.
- Cranial Nerve VI Palsy: The most common etiology of a pediatric sixth nerve palsy is trauma (Priya et al., 2021).
    - Primary gaze: A sixth nerve palsy would manifest as an esotropia of the affected eye in primary position.
    - Diplopia and gaze: If diplopia is reported, the patient would report horizontal diplopia worse in the direction of the affected eye (Griffin & Borsting, 2010).
    - Motility finding: There would be an underaction of the lateral rectus of the affected eye or a gaze restriction in the direction of the affected eye.
- Cranial Nerve III Palsy: Congenital cases make up most pediatric third nerve palsies (Holmes et al., 1999; Priya et al. 2021). Congenital cases exhibit aberrant regeneration, also known as misdirection syndrome, resulting in some of the following characteristics: jaw-wink reflex, widening of the eyelids upon depression, adduction and eye retraction upon elevation, and some pupillary involvement (miotic pupils) (Griffin & Borsting, 2010).

- Primary gaze: Third nerve palsy would manifest the classic "down and out" position in which the affected eye would be exotropic (due to medial rectus weakness) and hypotropic (due to a weakness in the inferior rectus and inferior oblique muscles) in primary gaze (Griffin & Borsting, 2010).
- Diplopia and gaze: A patient may not report diplopia as the eyelid of the affected eye may be ptotic due to weakness of the levator palpebrae muscle.
- Ocular and motility findings: Given the innervational pathway of the nerve, a fixed dilated pupil may be noted. In addition to the weaknesses of the medial rectus, inferior rectus, and inferior oblique muscles, there will be limited depression noted during abduction due to the inferior rectus weakness. With the older child, a careful evaluation may elicit the abduction and intorsion of the eye upon depression.

Indication for Versions and Ductions

The evaluation of versions should be a part of every pediatric examination to ensure the neurological and structural integrity of the extraocular muscles and the associated cranial nerve innervations. Ductions are performed when an abnormality (underaction, overaction, gaze restriction) is noted during versional testing. A paretic versus a paralytic muscle can be concluded with duction testing. Then the affected extraocular muscle can be better isolated when re-assessed monocularly.

Equipment for Versions and Ductions

For both versions and ductions, any object that is visually interesting and appropriate for the age of the child can be used as a tracking target. In younger children, more stimulating targets may be effective visually. Auditory stimulating targets can also work. Any one of the following can be used:

Figure 1. Examples of fixation cubes

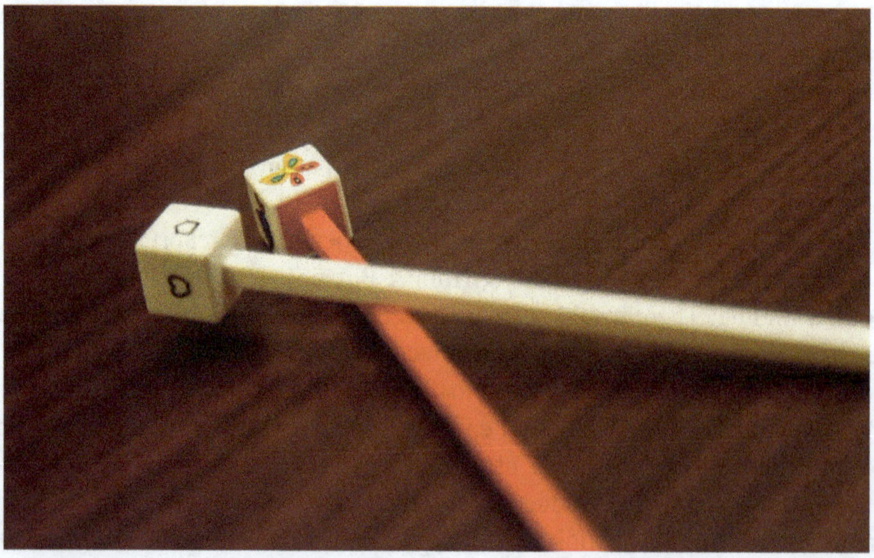

1. Fixation Stick with pictures (See Figure 1)
2. Pen Tip
3. Penlight or Transilluminator
4. Wolff Wand (See Figure 2)

Figure 2. Wolff Wands

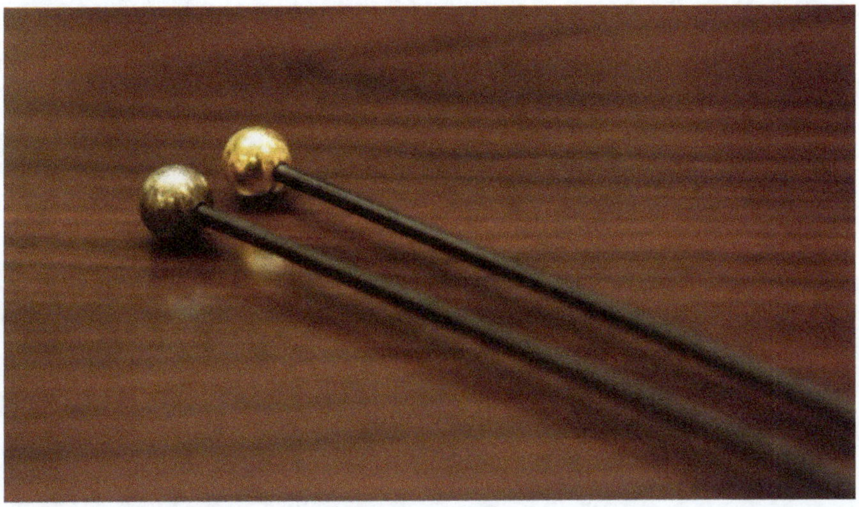

Procedure for Versions

Extraocular eye muscles are clinically examined by direct observation of eye movements in the six diagnostic action fields as indicated in Figure 3 and Figure 4. Versions are tested binocularly as follows:

Figure 3. Extraocular motility testing: six diagnostic action fields and H pattern

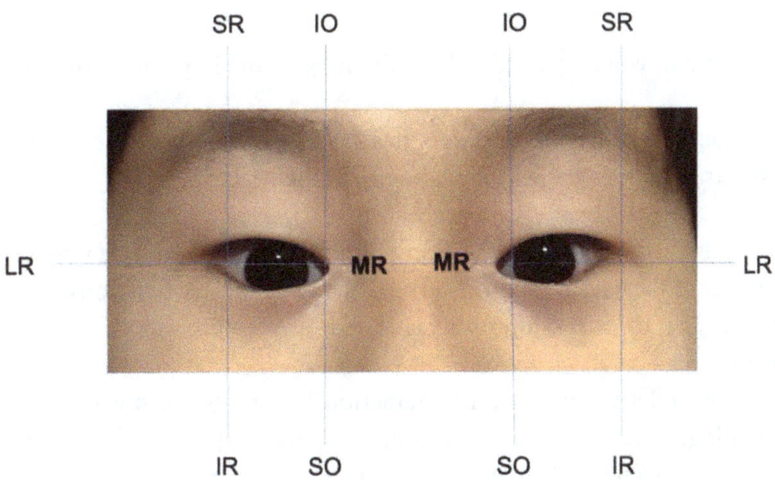

Figure 4. Six cardinal positions of gaze
Source: (Wong, 2007) (© 2007, Oxford University Press. Used with Permission.). "Used with permission of Oxford, from Wong, A.M. (2007). Eye movement disorders. Oxford University Press; permission conveyed through Copyright Clearance Center, Inc."

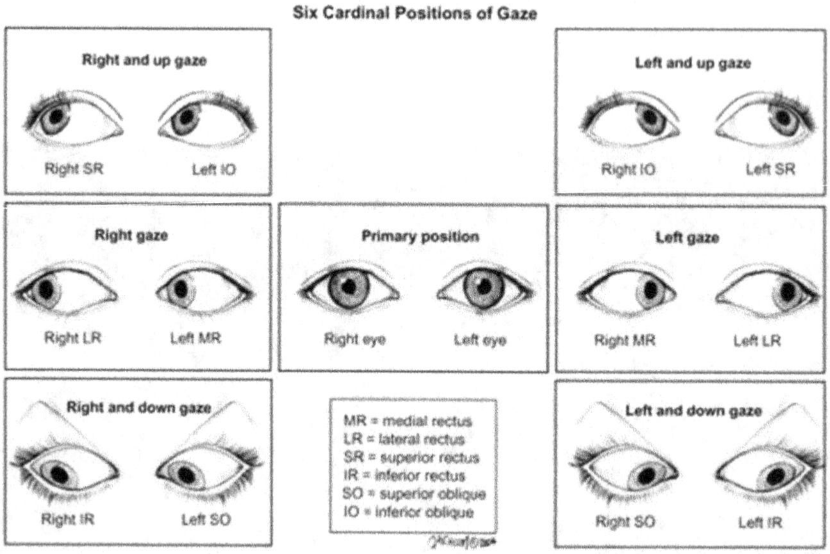

Step 1: Patient wears habitual correction

Step 2: Use an appropriate fixation target based on the patient's maturity level (20/80 stimulus size) (Griffin & Borsting, 2010; Schlange & Maino, 2001). The more developmentally delayed, a larger target should be used. A light can be used to simultaneously observe the Hirschberg reflexes

Step 3: Hold the target about 16 inches away (40 cm)

Step 4: Have the child follow the fixation target with minimal head movement as it moves in an H pattern as demonstrated in Figure 4 and Figure 5 below to evaluate the position of each eye in the six diagnostic positions. Try to stay at each position for a few seconds to ensure ocular alignment. To get a good view of both eyes in down gaze, remember to lift the upper eyelids as demonstrated in Figure 5.

- For the younger patient, you may need to have them touch the target to ensure he or she is fixating accurately.
- Alternatively, a younger and smaller child's head can be moved in different positions while the eyes are looking straight ahead at an interesting fixation target.

Step 5: Ask and/or observe if they experience any double vision by noting whether the patient can maintain fixation or if the eyes begin to alternate at any of the six positions

Step 6: Note any ocular pain by observing for tearing, excessive blinking or flinching at any of the six diagnostic positions

Step 7: Evaluate if there is a relative overaction, underaction, or paralysis of any of the extraocular muscles in any of the six diagnostic positions. For example, in Figure 4, when the patient is looking in left and up gaze and there is a possible overaction of the right inferior oblique muscle, more of the iris would be seen under the right upper eyelid as compared to the left eye. This type of comparison would be done for each of the six diagnostic positions

Step 8: Record: The presence of any specific underacting or overacting muscles, gaze restriction or deficit (elevation, depression, abduction, adduction), ocular pain, and diplopia.

- Grading System for versions/ductions:
  - Overactions are recorded with a "+" and underactions with a "-".
  - The grading ranges from 0 to 4 with each number representing a 25% change. Mentally divide the area between the midline and the canthus into three sections, each representing 25% (London, 2020).
  - For example: Left lateral rectus underaction, *Grade 4- (Eye cannot pass the midline). Negative pain or diplopia.*
- For normal versions/ductions: Record if extraocular motility (EOM) is full and smooth. Some abbreviations used for normal cases are: "FROM" (full range of motion) or SAFE (smooth, accurate, full, and extensive).

Figure 5. Extraocular motility testing in a pediatric patient: H pattern

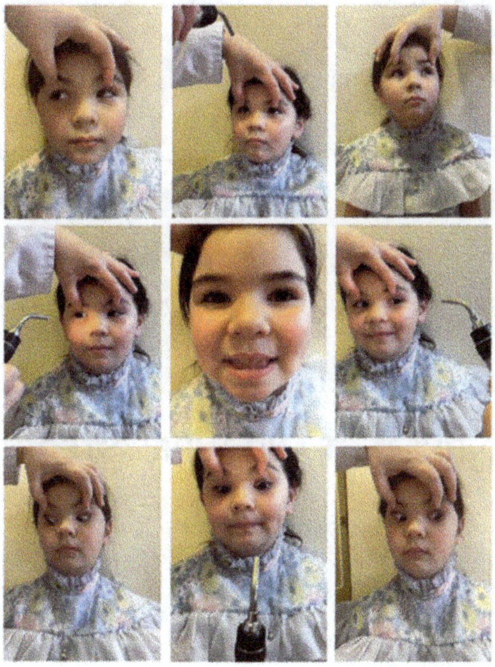

Procedure for Ductions

If an abnormality is noted during version testing, then ductions should be performed monocularly to confirm the presence of an isolated extraocular muscle weakness and to differentiate the paretic versus the paralytic muscle.

Step 1: The fixation target is moved into the six diagnostic positions in the H-pattern with one eye being occluded. As seen in Figure 3, the function of each muscle is tested as the target is moved in the following positions:

1. When the eye turns in (nasally) and horizontally, the function of the medial rectus muscle is being tested.
2. When the eye turns out (temporally) and horizontally, the function of the lateral rectus muscle is being tested.
3. When the eye turns down and out (temporally), the inferior rectus is being tested.
4. When the eye turns up and out (temporally), the superior rectus is being tested.
5. When the eye turns eye up and in (nasally), the inferior oblique muscle is being tested.
6. When the eye turns down and in (nasally) the superior oblique muscle is being tested.

Step 2: Interpretation:

1. If no abnormalities are noted during ductions but noted during versions, a paretic muscle weakness is present.
2. If limitations are noted during both version and duction testing, there is likely a paralytic muscle.
3. For these cases, a mechanical restriction of the muscle may exist and a referral for further investigation is needed.

Step 3: Use the same recording and grading systems described above for version testing.

Clinical Pearl: *When deficiencies in elevation, depression, and adduction are noted during extraocular motility, start to suspect a third nerve palsy. Carefully evaluate for a ptosis and pupillary abnormalities (Griffin & Borsting, 2010).*

Clinical Pearl: *Congenital cranial nerve palsy cases will not report symptoms such as diplopia unless it is a decompensated case.*

BIELSCHOWSKY HEAD-TILT TEST AND THREE-STEP TEST

These tests are used mainly to confirm the extraocular muscle responsible for a manifest vertical deviation usually related to a superior oblique weakness due to a Cranial Nerve IV Palsy (Miller et al., 2008).

Indication

The Bielschowsky Head Tilt Test is used to confirm whether the superior oblique muscle is responsible for a measured hyper deviation. The Three-Step test is also known as the Parks-Three-Step Test and is used to isolate a single paretic muscle in the presence of a vertical deviation. These tests are performed when a motility abnormality is noted during version and duction testing.

Equipment

The equipment is the same as described under the version and duction section above.

Procedure

The Bielschowsky Head Tilt Test is the third step of the Three-Step Test. The result can be positive or negative. A positive result is recorded when the hypertropia increase when the head is tilted in the direction of the affected eye. For example, a right hypertropia will increase as the head is tilted to the right. This suggests that the right hypertropia is due to an underacting right superior oblique muscle.

Three-Step Test

The Three-Step Test involves evaluating a vertical deviation under three conditions:

Step 1: Which eye has the hyper deviation in primary position?
Step 2: Which eye has the greater hyper deviation in right or left gaze (approximately 30 degrees away) (Griffin & Borsting, 2010)?
Step 3: Which eye has the greater hyper deviation in right or left head tilt (approximately 40 degrees toward the right or left shoulder)? During this step, the evaluating clinician should also match the head tilt of the patient when objectively measuring the hyper deviation
Step 4: Which eye has the greater hyper deviation in upgaze or downgaze? This step can be performed when the results of the Three-Step Test are questionable.

- For example, if there is a question between the right superior oblique and the left superior rectus muscle of the other eye. If the hyper worsens in downgaze, this identifies a superior oblique muscle weakness since it normally acts as a depressor. If the hyper worsens in upgaze, this suggests a superior rectus muscle weakness since it acts as an elevator.

There are 8 possible combinations that potentially can identify the paretic muscle causing the vertical deviation. Since the most common etiology for a recent onset vertical deviation would be due to a superior oblique muscle weakness. The following are the combinations to be aware of when administering the Three-Step Test:

- Right Superior Oblique:
  - Right hyper in primary gaze
  - Left gaze shows a greater hyper
  - Right head tilt shows a greater hyper
- Left Superior Oblique:
  - Left hyper in primary gaze
  - Right gaze shows a greater hyper
  - Left head tilt shows a greater hyper

Clinical Pearl: *One advantage of the Bielschowsky Head Tilt Test will point to an underlying superior oblique muscle weakness even in a long-standing case when spread of comitancy has occurred (Griffin & Borsting, 2010).*

Clinical Pearl: *Another advantage of the Bielschowsky Head Tilt Test is in the presence of a bilateral fourth nerve palsy which can occur in congenital cases (Miller et al., 2008). In these cases, a positive result will be seen on both right and left head tilts in which a right hyper deviation will increase on right head tilt and a left hyper deviation will also increase on left head tilt (Griffin & Borsting, 2010).*

Clinical Pearl: *During the Three-Step Test, asking for subjective responses even in older children during step three may result in unreliable responses as the head tilt itself creates a hyper deviation.*

Clinical Pearl: *Due to the spread of comitancy in long-standing vertical deviations, the Three-Step Test is recommended to be administered in recent onset acquired cases (Miller et al., 2008; Griffin & Borsting, 2010).*

PART II: VISUAL FUNCTION AND DEVELOPMENTAL STATUS

The muscles in each eye work together to produce eye movements such as pursuits, saccades, and vergences which can be evaluated and compared to known age expected norms (Ciuffreda & Tannen, 1995; Miller et al., 2008; Wong, 2008). Pursuit eye movements are smooth and slow conjugate movements which track moving targets. Saccades are fast rapid conjugate eye movements associated with abrupt changes in fixation from one target to another. Vergence movements are disconjugate or non-conjugate eye movements and involve a convergence or divergence of the lines of sight to fixate an object at near or in the distance.

PURSUITS

Pursuit eye movements are slow (up to 30-40 degrees/second), smooth, continuous, and conjugate eye movements used when the eyes follow an object of interest (Ciuffreda & Tannen, 1995; Griffin & Grisham, 2010; London, 2020; Barrett, 2014). A pursuit eye movement is initiated by target motion and is described by its gain (eye velocity/target velocity) and latency (Ciuffreda & Tannen, 1995; Barrett, 2014). A gain of 1.0 indicates that the target and the eye move at the same velocity. The latency for a pursuit eye movement is typically 100-150 ms. Visual pathways responsible for pursuit movements include cortical and brainstem input (Ciuffreda & Tannen, 1995; Pola & Schnell, 2020).

In infants, pursuit eye movements are clinically measurable by two to three months of age but are asymmetrical. Pursuit eye movement ability is present in patients as young as one month (London, 2020; Barrett, 2014). Temporal to nasal target motion is relatively accurate but nasal to temporal target movement is jerky. It becomes more symmetrical after 4 to 6 weeks of age (London, 2020). Monocular pursuits are also more accurate than binocular pursuits in infants between 1 and 5 months of age. Adult level accuracy of pursuits is seen after 5 months of age (Pola & Schnell, 2020).

Birnbaum (1993) described that pursuit eye movements are "influenced not only by neuromuscular integrity, but also by attention, spatial judgements, and motor organization, performance is related to age and developmental level." Therefore, the ability, quality, and accuracy of pursuit eye movements point to the child's visual developmental status. Excessive tension or effort suggests that the pursuit movement is not automatic, and the child will not have the ability to simultaneously process other information. This inability can contribute to learning related vision problems for the school age child. Although pursuit movements do not have a direct role in reading like saccadic movements, it is believed that the high level of oculomotor control and visual attention required to produce good eye movements are important markers of academic success.

The extraocular motility and smooth pursuit testing are typically performed simultaneously by simple subjective observation using a moving fixation target or a more structured approach developed by the Northeastern State University College of Optometry (NSUCO). During a primary care evaluation, ocular motility and pursuits are typically performed binocularly (versions) but if needed, can be performed monocularly (ductions) as described earlier.

Indications

Specifically, the evaluation of the ability, quality, and accuracy of pursuit eye movements provides insight into a child's visual developmental status. Deficiencies contribute to functional/developmental vision problems which inhibit academic performance. It can be evaluated using the Direct Observation method or the NSUCO protocol.

Equipment

The equipment is the same as described under the version and duction section above.

Procedure

Pursuits Direct Observation

Step 1: Patient wears their habitual spectacle correction

Step 2: Use an appropriate fixation target based on the patient's maturity level (20/80 stimulus size) (Griffin & Borsting, 2010; Schlange & Maino, 2001). The more developmentally delayed, a larger target should be used

Step 3: Hold the target at 16 inches away (40 cm)

Step 4: Evaluate smooth pursuits by having the patient follow the target as it is moved across their full range of horizontal and vertical eye movements, creating an H pattern movement with the target.

- For young children, instruct the child to follow just with their eyes only and not to move their body or their head.
- See Table 2 for descriptions of age-expected observations during pursuit eye movement testing. Specifically, note the following:
  1. Quality of eye movements, i.e., smooth versus jerky
  2. Accuracy
  3. Qualitative differences between the two eyes

4. Head movements
5. Motor-overflow (tongue, head, neck, or body movement)
6. Presence of a midline jump or difficulty crossing the midline
7. Unusual head and body postures i.e., tilts, turns

- If a child has gross head movements during testing, hold on to the head gently while moving the target. Alternatively, the child's head can be gently rotated while keeping the target still.

Step 5: Recording the pursuit movements using one of two systems:

1. Qualitative Descriptions
    a. Full and smooth
    b. Jerky movements with loss of fixation
    c. Needs repeated verbal instruction
2. Numerical Grading System for Pursuits: Any score less than 3+ is documented as poor performance (Griffin & Borsting, 2010; London, 2020; Schlange & Maino, 2001).
    a. 4+: Smooth and accurate
    b. 3+: One fixation loss
    c. 2+: Two fixation losses
    d. 1+: More than 2 fixation losses, inability to do the task

Table 2. Pursuits: age expected observations

Age	Expected Observations
4-5 years	• Head and body movement may be present but can be inhibited when instructed to not move the head • Overflow (motor, verbal, gustatory) may be present.
6-7 years	• Horizontal pursuits are smooth and well-sustained with minimal head movement • Overflow should not be present • Midline jumps should not be consistently present
9 years	• Horizontal pursuits are smooth and well-sustained with minimal head movement • Overflow should not be present • Midline jumps should not be consistently present
10 years	• Automaticity should be present • Pursuit testing can be done in the presence of a cognitive demand (e.g. conversing with clinician) without affecting pursuit movement performance

(Birnbaum, 1993)

NSUCO Direct Observation of Pursuits

This is a more structured recording system when testing pursuit eye movements. The normative values exist for males and female children aged 5 to 14 years. It can be performed both monocularly and binocularly as needed.

Procedure

Step 1: Patient is standing with feet shoulder width apart
Step 2: A single target is held at the patient's midline and is moved in a circle about 20 cm in diameter

Step 3: Two rotations are made in both the clockwise and counterclockwise directions

Step 4: The maximum distance the target should be held is 40 cm away or at a minimum distance of the Harmon working distance (distance from the child's elbow to the middle knuckle) (Maples, 2017)

Step 5: Make observations of:

- Ability: Number of rotations completed
- Accuracy: Number of refixations
- Degree of head movement: No movement to gross movement
- Degree of body movement: No movement to gross movement

Step 6: Record observations:

- A score ranging from 1 to 5 is given for each of the categories (See Table 3)
- Determine if the patient's performance is age appropriate by comparing the patient's score to the minimal acceptable score by age and gender as described in Table 4 for males and females
- The minimal score refers to performance greater than one standard deviation from the mean (Maples & Ficklin, 1988)

Table 3. NSUCO scoring criteria: Direct observation of pursuits

ABILITY *Can the patient keep his attention under control to complete 2 rotations in each direction?*			**ACCURACY** *Can the patient accurately and consistently fixate so that no noticeable refixation is needed?*	
1	Cannot complete ½ rotation in either the clockwise or counterclockwise direction		1	No attempt to follow the target or requires greater than 10 refixations
2	Complete ½ rotation in either direction		2	Refixations 5-10 times
3	Completes 1 rotation in either direction but not 2 rotations		3	Refixations 3-4 times
4	Completes 2 rotations in one direction but less than 2 rotations in the other direction		4	Refixations 2 or less
5	Completed 2 rotations in each direction		5	No refixations
HEAD MOVEMENT *Can the patient accomplish the pursuit without moving his or her head?*			**BODY MOVEMENT** *Can the patient accomplish the pursuit without moving his or her body?*	
1	Large movement of the head or body at any time		1	Large movement of the head or body at any time
2	Moderate movement of the head or body at any time		2	Moderate movement of the head or body at any time
3	Slight movement of the head or body (>50% of time)		3	Slight movement of the head or body (>50% of time)
4	Slight movement of the head or body (<50% of time)		4	Slight movement of the head or body (<50% of time)
5	No movement of head or body		5	No movement of head or body

(Maples, 2017; Taub, 2012; Maples & Ficklin, 1988)

Table 4. NSUCO pursuit test minimal acceptable score by age and gender

	ABILITY		ACCURACY		HEAD MOVMENT		BODY MOVEMENT	
AGE	Male	Female	Male	Female	Male	Female	Male	Female
5	4	5	2	3	2	3	3	4
6	4	5	2	3	2	3	3	4
7	5	5	3	3	3	3	3	4
8	5	5	3	3	3	3	4	4
9	5	5	3	4	3	3	4	4
10	5	5	4	4	4	4	4	5
11	5	5	4	4	4	4	4	5
12	5	5	4	4	4	4	5	5
13	5	5	4	4	4	4	5	5
14 or >	5	5	5	4	4	4	5	5

(Scheiman & Wick, 2020; Maples et al., 1992)

Clinical Pearl: *Be aware that a common error made during pursuit testing is moving the target at an inappropriate speed or in a non-smooth manner (London, 2020).*

Clinical Pearl: *The advantage of direct observation pursuit testing is that its fast, easy, and an inexpensive way to assess eye movements with minimal patient cooperation.*

Clinical Pearl: *The disadvantage of direct observation pursuit testing is that it is very subjective and inter-clinician reliability is very low. It is also dependent on the examiner's clinical experience particularly when examining pediatric patients. It is an acquired skill that requires an astute observer especially when there are subtle eye movement restrictions.*

Clinical Pearl: *In very young children, the ability to monocularly fixate and accurately follow a small target can offer a quick and gross qualitative assessment of visual acuity.*

Clinical Pearl: *The advantage of using the NSUCO Direct Observation of Pursuit method is that it has been well-studied and demonstrates good reliability between and within clinicians, good test-re-test reliability, and good validity (Maples, 2017; Taub, 2012; Maples & Ficklin, 1988).*

SACCADES – LARGE GROSS SACCADIC MOVEMENTS

Saccades are conjugate eye movements that re-directs fixation from one object of interest to another in a rapid stepwise manner (Ciuffreda & Tannen, 1995; London, 2020). When target movement is greater than 30-40 degrees per second, saccades are used rather than pursuit movements to maintain fixation on the target. Saccades are the fastest of all eye movements with velocities as high as 700 degrees per second (Barrett, 2014). About 85% of saccadic eye movements are less than 15 degrees in amplitude (Ciuffreda & Tannen, 1995; London, 2020).

Saccades, like pursuit eye movements, require both cortical and brainstem input. Different areas of the brain are responsible for horizontal eye movements than for vertical and torsional eye movements (London, 2020). Unlike with pursuits, the velocity and the amplitude of the saccadic eye movement is adult-like at an early age and is due to the maturity of the brainstem components (Pola & Schnell, 2020). While brainstem processes develop over weeks to months during development, the cortical processes can continue to change over several years of development. This makes it important for the clinician to have standardized testing and expected age norms when evaluating older children.

Saccadic eye movement testing also probes for adequate visual spatial organization which is noted when a child easily switches fixation from one target to another. In addition, testing assesses a patient's visual attention ability by observing the distractibility level in the presence of extraneous peripheral stimuli. Children with learning disabilities and poor readers generally score lower on the NSUCO test of pursuits and saccades than normal children who are good readers (Birnbaum, 1993; Maples, 2017).

Indications

Testing saccades is indicated to assess whether deficiencies are contributing to the presence of functional/developmental vision problems such as learning related vision problems, particularly with respect to reading. Pediatric testing of saccades can be divided into the evaluation of larger gross saccades and the evaluation of fine saccades required in reading (London, 2020).

Tests of larger gross saccades include the Direct Observation method and the NSUCO protocol. The NSUCO method has a normative scale for children ages 5 to 15 years.

Equipment

Direct Observation and NSUCO Direct Observation of Saccades

Two objects that are different but visually interesting and appropriate for the age of the patient as described under the version and duction section. Younger patients require more stimulating targets; visually as well as auditory stimulating targets will work.

Any one of the following can be used:

- 2 Fixation Sticks (See Figure 1)
- 2 Pen Tips with different colors
- Wolff Wands (small gold and silver spheres fixed to metal rods) (See Figure 2)

Procedure

Direct Observation Saccades

Saccadic movement test can be performed by simply presenting two different targets and observing the patient's eye movements as they fixate from one target to another. During a primary care evaluation, saccades are typically performed binocularly but if needed, can be performed monocularly.

Step 1: Patient wears their habitual spectacle correction

Step 2: The testing distance can be 40 to 50 cm from the patient

Step 3: Present two age-appropriate targets separated enough so the patient does not need to move their head or body to fixate from one target to another. Maximum target separation should be about 20-40 cm apart (20-40 degrees) (Maples, 2017; London, 2020; Schlange & Maino, 2001)

Step 4: Ask the child to look from one target to the other target as you call out that target. For example: *"When I say "red" look at the red target and keep looking at that target until I say "blue", then look at the blue target"*. Say the targets both rhythmically and non-rhythmically with a pause of 1-2 seconds in between

Step 5: Test the horizontal, vertical, and diagonal directions. Near-far along the z-axis can also be tested. About five cycles are completed in each direction depending on patient maturity and cooperation.

Step 6: Make observations of the following:

- Percent undershooting (hypometric) or overshooting (hypermetric) movements
- Fixation losses and the presence of corrective saccades
- Head posture (tilt or turns)
- Qualitative differences between the two eyes
- Difficulties within specific directions (diagonal, vertical, horizontal)
- Ability to match the beat (rhythmic timing)
- Head and or body movements
- Presence of a midline jump or difficulty crossing the midline
- Tensing of neck/facial muscles

Step 7: Record the following:

- Age expected norms: *By 8-9 years*: Accurate and well-sustained movements with minimal head and minimal overflow; 10% undershoot is normal (Birnbaum, 1993).
- Qualitative Description:
  - 15% undershoot, smooth, accurate, rhythmic match, OU, OD, OS
  - Midline jump with loss of fixation, with head movement
  - Needs repeated verbal instruction
  - Grading System Saccades: Any grade less than 3+ is documented as poor performance (See Table 5)

Table 5. Saccadic eye movement grading systems

Grade	Southern California College of Optometry (SCCO)	Saccades Grading System
4+	Smooth and accurate	Accurate
3+	Slight undershoot	One inaccuracy
2+	Gross under/overshooting	Two inaccuracies
1+	Inability to do the task	More than 2 inaccuracies

(Griffin & Borsting, 2010; London, 2020; Schlange & Maino, 2001)

NSUCO Direct Observation of Saccades

This is a more structured recording system when testing saccadic eye movements. The normative values exist for males and female patients aged 5 to 14 years. It can be performed both monocularly and binocularly as needed.

Step 1: Patient is standing with feet shoulder width apart

Step 2: Targets are held 10 cm on each side of the patient's midline. The maximum distance the target should be held is 40 cm away or at a minimum distance of the Harmon working distance (distance from the child's elbow to the middle knuckle).

Step 3: Do not make any instructions regarding head movement. Test only HORIZONTAL saccades. Perform five cycles. Say to the child, "*When I say red, look at the red target. When I say green, look at the green target. Don't look until I tell you to.*"

Step 4: Make observations of the following:

- Ability: Number of cycles
- Accuracy: Amount of over or undershooting
- Degree of head movement: No movement to gross movement
- Degree of body movement: No movement to gross movement

Step 5: Record the following:

- A score ranging from 1 to 5 is given for each of the categories (See Table 6)
- Determine if the patient's performance is age appropriate by comparing the patient's score to the minimal acceptable score by age and gender as described in Table 7 for males and females
- The minimal score refers to performance greater than one standard deviation from the mean (Maples & Ficklin, 1988)

Clinical Pearl: *If the case history is positive for reading difficulty (i.e., loss of place and/or skipping words when reading), then a 10-15 cm (10-15 degree) target separation is used to better assess the quality of reading related saccades. In reading most saccades are about 1-3 degrees to each word so separating the targets about 10-15 degrees simulates the return sweep to the beginning of the next line (Ritter & Steiner, 2021).*

Clinical Pearl: *If difficulty is noted during saccadic eye movement testing, longer pauses can be given between targets and/or the target separation can be decreased to make the activity easier.*

Clinical Pearl: *Direct observation saccades are based upon the clinician's subjective interpretation and the inexperience clinician may not have enough experience to use a particular rating system effectively. Good saccadic performance does not directly correlate with reading eye movements (Scheiman & Wick, 2020).*

Clinical Pearl: *Saccades are easily performed with minimal equipment, particularly for the young preschool or early school age patients and children with developmental delays.*

Table 6. NSUCO scoring criteria: direct observation of saccades

	ABILITY *Can the patient keep his attention under control to complete 5 round trips in each direction?*		**ACCURACY** *Can the patient accurately and consistently fixate so that no noticeable correction is needed?*
1	Completes less than 2 round trips	1	Large over- or undershooting is noted 1 or more times
2	Completes 2 round trips	2	Moderate over- or undershooting is noted 1 or more times
3	Completes 3 round trips	3	Constant slight over- or undershooting noted (>50% of time)
4	Completes 4 round trips	4	Intermittent slight over- or undershooting noted (<50% of time)
5	Completes 5 round trips	5	No over or undershooting noted
	HEAD MOVEMENT ***Can the patient accomplish the saccade without moving his or her head?***		**BODY MOVEMENT** ***Can the patient accomplish the saccade without moving his or her body?***
1	Large movement of the head or body at any time	1	Large movement of the head or body at any time
2	Moderate movement of the head or body at any time	2	Moderate movement of the head or body at any time
3	Slight movement of the head or body (>50% of time)	3	Slight movement of the head or body (>50% of time)
4	Slight movement of the head or body (<50% of time)	4	Slight movement of the head or body (<50% of time)
5	No movement of head or body	5	No movement of head or body

(Maples, 2017; Taub, 2012; Maples & Ficklin, 1988)

Table 7. NSUCO saccade test minimal acceptable score by age and gender

	ABILITY		ACCURACY		HEAD MOVMENT		BODY MOVEMENT	
AGE	**Male**	**Female**	**Male**	**Female**	**Male**	**Female**	**Male**	**Female**
5	5	5	3	3	2	2	3	4
6	5	5	3	3	2	3	3	4
7	5	5	3	3	3	3	3	4
8	5	5	3	3	3	3	4	4
9	5	5	3	3	3	3	4	4
10	5	5	3	3	3	4	4	4
11	5	5	3	3	3	4	4	5
12	5	5	3	3	3	4	4	5
13	5	5	3	3	3	4	5	5
14 or >	5	5	4	3	3	4	5	5

(Scheiman & Wick, 2020; Maples et al., 1992)

Clinical Pearl: *The NSUCO method is a more structured method and norms exist for children ages 5 to 14 years.*

Clinical Pearl: *As with pursuit testing, the NSUCO Direct Observation of Saccades has also been shown to have good reliability between and within clinicians, good test-re-test reliability, and good validity (Maples, 2017; Taub, 2020, Maples & Ficklin, 1988).*

SACCADES – FINE READING SACCADIC MOVEMENTS

Pediatric testing of saccades can be divided into the evaluation of larger gross saccades described above and the evaluation of finer smaller reading saccadic movements (London, 2020). Optometric evaluation of these reading eye movements can be done with the Developmental Eye Movement (DEM) Test and the Readalyzer/Visagraph Test.

Developmental Eye Movement (DEM) Test

The DEM test provides an objective measurement of a patient's tracking ability and may provide insight into visual information processing during reading tasks. A psycho-physical and verbal-visual evaluation of fine saccades required in reading eye movements. Observations made during testing can also provide insight into the patient's visual memory, speed of speech, attention, and spatial awareness.

The DEM evaluates fine saccades required in reading eye movements that was developed by Richman and Garzia in 1987 (Griffin & Borsting, 2010). It is specifically a visual-verbal test which assesses oculomotor skills and rapid automatized naming (RAN). RAN is a visual-verbal skill that involves rapid naming of a series of visual targets. It is important to rule out the presence of RAN deficits when evaluating for saccadic deficits as patients with reading disabilities also demonstrate poor RAN abilities (Tassinari & DeLand, 2005).

The DEM attempts to separate eye movement speed from RAN abilities so the clinician can assess whether the patient has age-appropriate saccades, age-appropriate RAN, or deficits in one or both. The *Vertical Score* represents the patient's RAN ability. The *Ratio Score* is the ratio of the Horizontal Time Score over the Vertical Time Score and represents the efficiency of saccadic eye movement speed in relationship to RAN ability. In general, a score below 15%ile (worse than one standard deviation below the mean) is considered clinically significant in the diagnosis of a saccadic deficit.

With the increased public health initiative by the Centers for Disease Control (CDC) of concussion awareness in youth sports, it is important to know when to evaluate for the presence of the visual sequela after a concussive event. The prevalence of saccadic deficits in concussions specifically in adolescents, ranging from 11 to 17 years, was found to be 29% (Master, et al., 2016). In this study, the DEM was utilized to diagnose the saccadic dysfunction using the criteria of one standard deviation below the mean for the Ratio Score and/or the Total Errors Score.

Indications

The DEM is typically administered to children of reading age with normative data ranging from age 6 to 13 years. It is indicated to be tested in patients with suspected learning related vision problems reporting the following vision symptoms:

- Excessive head movement when reading.
- Skipping lines or losing place while reading.
- Frequently loses place when copying.
- Omitting words or transposing words when reading.
- Requiring the use of a finger or marker to stay on line when reading.
- Reporting shifting of words on the page when reading.
- Re-reading lines unknowingly.
- Lacks comprehension when reading.

Equipment

1. Timer
2. DEM Test (See Figure 6)
3. Score Sheet

Procedure

Step 1: The patient should be wearing their habitual near prescription

Step 2: Perform at the habitual near distance or Harmon working distance (distance from the child's elbow to the middle knuckle)

Step 3: Administer the Pretest to determine if the child can name the ten numbers correctly. Otherwise, the patient is untestable. This subtest is not timed but should be correctly done in 12 seconds or less. Finger pointing is ONLY permitted during this section

Step 4: If the Pretest is completed successfully, administer Test A.

- Time the child while reading the 40 vertically aligned numbers from top to bottom starting with the left column and continue to the top of the right column.
- Also note the errors. The types of errors are substitution (s), addition (a), transposition (t), and omission (o) errors. These errors are used to calculate the adjusted time if indicated.

Step 5: Repeat Step 4 for Test B asking the patient to read in a similar fashion. The times for Test A and Test B are added to get the Vertical Time.

Step 6: Administer Test C. Ask the patient to read 16 lines of 80 numbers horizontally like reading a book and time the patient. Record the time to complete this subtest and note the errors.

Step 7: Score the DEM (The formulas are listed on the scoresheet.)

- Four scores are obtained from this test are the Vertical Time, Horizontal Time, Ratio, and Total Errors
- Vertical Time (V): Total of Test A and Test B times. An adjusted vertical time may need to be calculated. The formula is on the scoresheet but typically is not done for the Vertical Time since there are so few errors
- Horizontal Time (H): If there are omission (o) or addition (a) errors, then the adjusted time needs to be calculated using the formula below but is also on the Score Sheet

Adjusted Horizontal Time = Test C Time x (80/80 – o + a)

- Ratio (R): Ratio = Horizontal Time/Vertical Time
- Errors (E): Total Errors = s + o + a + t

Step 8: Recording: Calculate z-scores based upon the mean and standard deviation (SD) by referring to the DEM age-related normative data and then determine the patient's percentile ranks.

Figure 6. DEM test

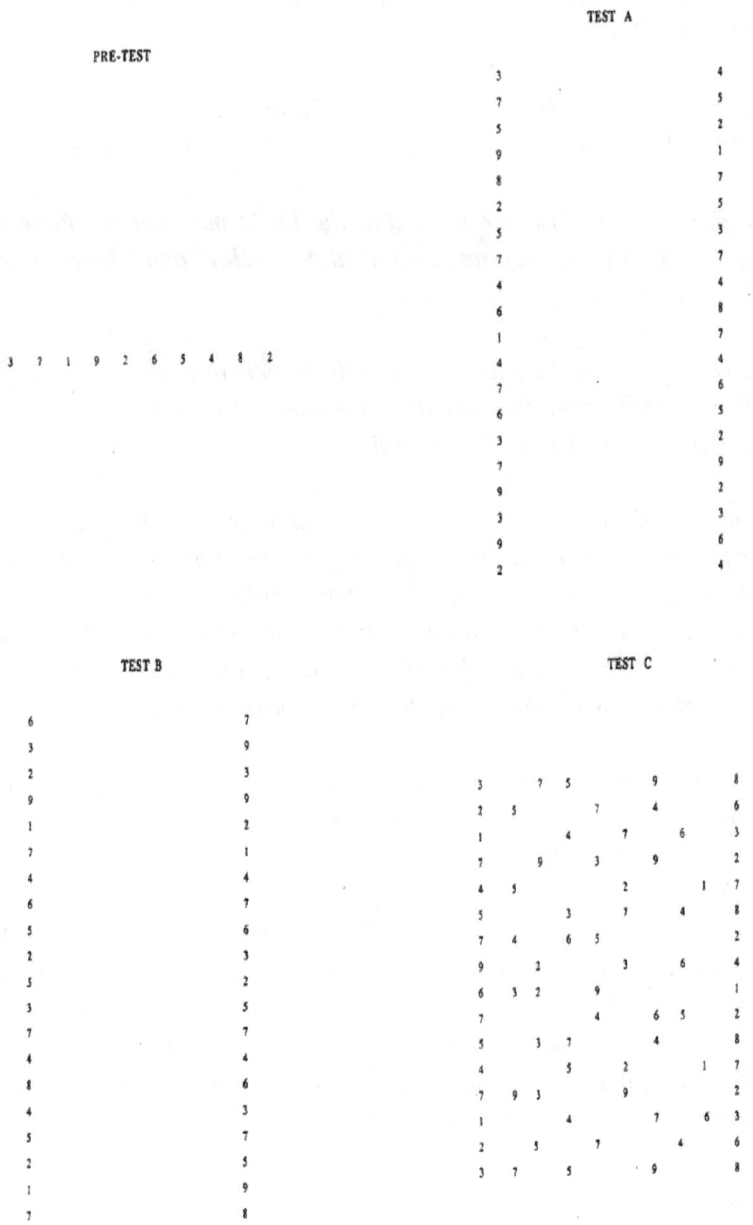

- **Interpretation:**
  - *Normal:* All scores are normal.
  - *Saccadic Deficit:* Adjusted Horizontal Score is high as compared to the Vertical Score thereby making the Ratio Score high also.
  - *RAN Deficit:* Both the Vertical and Horizontal Scores are high, but the Ratio Score is normal.
  - *RAN Deficit and Saccadic Deficit:* The Vertical and Horizontal Scores are high, but the Horizontal Score is higher making the Ratio Score high as well.
  - *Error Score:* Used independently to assess the eye movement accuracy.

Clinical Pearl: *The DEM has a high intra-subject test-retest and inter-examiner reliability (Birnbaum, 1993; Tassinari & DeLand, 2005).*

Clinical Pearl: *Tassinari and DeLand (2005) demonstrated a statistically significant relationship between poor DEM performance (Ratio and the Vertical Scores) and symptomatic patients.*

Clinical Pearl: *Ayton, et al. (2009) determined that the DEM may not correlate with saccadic eye movements and symptomatology, but they did conclude that the Horizontal Score is well-correlated with reading performance and visual processing speed.*

Clinical Pearl: *The DEM can also be used to assess the effects of attention on the DEM Error Score on Test C. Coulter et al. (2000) found that attention not fatigue may affect accuracy over time in those patients performing poorly on the DEM with excessive errors in the second half of Test C.*

Clinical Pearl: *Poor English fluency can adversely affect scores on this test. However, if the clinician can administer the test in Spanish, norms have been determined for children ages 6 to 11 years (Fernandez-Velazquez & Fernandez-Fidalgo, 1995). Some differences were reported for 6-year-olds, Spanish speakers were found to be significantly slower in the Vertical and Horizontal Scores, but the Ratio score was not found to be different. The DEM test appeared to be reliable, and its results could be used efficiently and reliably when evaluating Spanish speaking children.*

Clinical Pearl: *Children with severe speech deficits may have significant difficulty with the DEM test. This test should not be administered to children with special needs with developmental delays due to the high cognitive demands (Maples, 2017).*

Clinical Pearl: *The King-Devick (KD) (See Figure 7) is another fine saccadic eye movement test currently utilized as a sideline test to determine if an athlete can return to play (Ayton, et al, 2009; Tjark, et al., 2013). KD test is now administered through a standard sized iPad device only. A non-electronic version of the KD test is no longer available and the evidence-based studies are based upon the electronic version of the test. For reading, it is called the K-D Test Pro Reading. For post-concussions, it is called the K-D Test Pro Baseline or K-D Test Pro Monitoring.*

Figure 7. King-Devick test

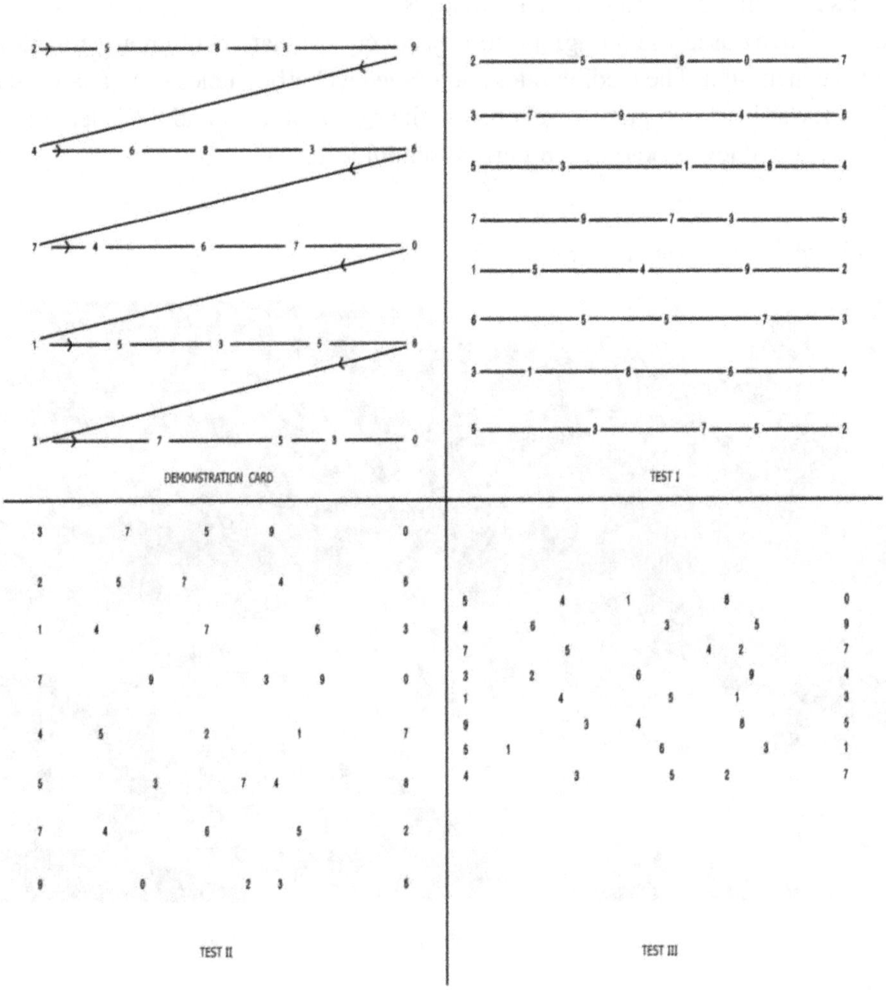

VISAGRAPH AND READALYZER

The Visagraph and ReadAlyzer (Figure 8) are two electrooculographic instruments which use goggles with infrared limbal sensing eye movement recorders to specifically analyze eye movements during reading (Scheiman & Wick, 2020; Taub, 2012). Normative data exists for elementary school children through adulthood.

The Visagraph and the ReadAlyzer minimize the clinician's subjective interpretation of the child's saccadic eye movements. Grade appropriate cognitive reading material is used to better correlate findings to reported reading difficulties. For example, does the child have an oculomotor dysfunction or a language-based reading dysfunction, or both? This system provides objective reading eye movement analysis using age and grade normative data. The child is instructed to answer 10 true-false questions after reading a paragraph, resulting in a high likelihood that the individual demonstrates true reading eye movements during the test. Clinically, it should be noted that the eye movement analyses are valid when the comprehension level is at least 70% or better. Further explanation of the test is provided in the

Procedures section. Specific summary reports and eye movement recordings are available to monitor progress and/or share with inter-professional providers.

Tannen, et al. (2015) used the Visagraph to objectively evaluate oculomotor function in children diagnosed with a concussion. The reading rates and grade level efficiencies were analyzed and 68% had a reading efficiency at least two grade levels below their current level and 82% demonstrated reading speeds at least two grade levels below their current school level.

Figure 8. ReadAlyzerTM unit, goggles, story book

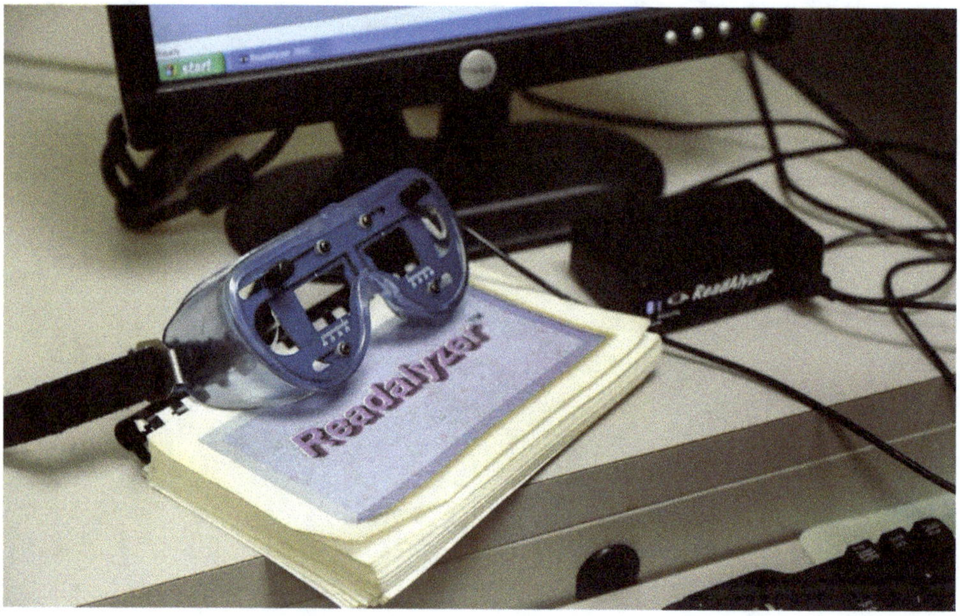

Indications

The Visagraph/ReadAlyzer testing is indicated with older children to obtain an objective assessment and recording of fine reading saccadic eye movements. It can help the clinician determine if the child has a reading/language deficit, a saccadic deficit, or whether there are deficits in both areas.

Equipment

- Visagaph IIITM Software, Visagraph IIITM Goggles, and Visagraph Test Booklet. There is also the Visagraph USB. Support can be found at the following website: www.readingplus.com/support/visagraph-support/
- ReadAlyzerTM Software, infrared goggles, and English Story Book with either 50- or 100-word passages (See Figure 9). Additional ReadAlyzer Long Stories which are reading passages with an average length of 800 words. Currently, the ReadAlyzer 2K is available with wireless goggles.

Procedure

There is not a universally accepted standard protocol to administer the Visagraph/ReadAlyzer. In general, it is important for the child to be comfortable with the test set up in order to perform multiple trials.

Step 1: Child wears habitual prescription for reading under the googles
Step 2: Have the child hold the reading material at eye level. Instruct the child to look at the fixation dot at the top of the page. When a beep is heard, the child is instructed to read the text quietly and thoroughly since there will be true/false questions to answer after the reading
Step 3: Have the child read two or more paragraphs. The reading material can be either at the child's current reading level, or one grade below the child's current reading level. The first trial is a practice trial. The second trial is included in the analysis if comprehension is at least 70% (Tannen & Ciuffreda,1997). If 70% is not achieved after three trials, then the reading level is reduced by one grade level. Reading at the reduced grade level provides a more accurate evaluation of only the reading eye movements without fluency and reading comprehension impacting the analysis results.
Step 4: Interpretation: Use the Grade Level Efficiency (GLE) findings to determine whether the patient has an oculomotor based or language-based problem (Tannen & Ciuffreda,1997).

- *Category I:* Oculomotor efficiency-based problem exists when the GLE is two grade levels below after reading text one grade below their current grade level. In addition, the GLE does NOT improve by at least three grade levels when tested with reduced grade level text.
- *Category II:* Language-based reading problem exists when the GLE while is found to be at least two grade levels below their current grade level even while reading text slightly below their current grade. Improved GLE is noted by at least three grade levels when tested with reduced grade level text.

Clinical Pearl: *The patient should hold the book at the eye level to read while wearing goggles. If they are keeping the book down and they are also looking in down gaze, then accurate saccadic and fixational eye movements are not measured. When the child is viewing in down gaze, the upper eye lids will cover the eyes thereby preventing the sensors from being able to record the eye movements.*

Clinical Pearl: *These units are more expensive than the visual-verbal test or direct observation methods of saccadic testing.*

Clinical Pearl: *A standard protocol that is universally accepted with good repeatability has not yet been established. However, it is agreed that multiple trials should be administered with at least one practice trial be administered before the baseline measurements are taken.*

Clinical Pearl: *For young children, more than one baseline test session may be required to establish a stable and repeatable baseline. Since this is not practical in the pediatric population, it is suggested that the child reads a paragraph silently for the first trial and the next trial the child reads aloud (London, 2020).*

Clinical Pearl: *First and second graders with reading disabilities will be hard to evaluate as the text will be very difficult.*

Clinical Pearl: *Testing is not indicated with uncooperative or hyperactive patients since steady goggle positioning is important to get the best recordings.*

Clinical Pearl: *It is also not indicated for patients whose first language is not English. The Visagraph III is available in English and German only. But the ReadAlyzer is available in Spanish, Dutch, Italian, Norwegian, and Arabic.*

CONCLUSION

This chapter provides the clinician with the tools required to evaluate the pediatric patient from infancy through school-age. Primarily, the structural and neurological integrity of the visual system is examined in the early years to diagnose common visual conditions that require further management and treatment such as amblyopia and strabismus. In addition, it is important to be aware of how to diagnose acquired or congenital diseases of the central nervous system requiring further neurological consultation.

For the school-age child the integrity of visual function as related to their developmental status is evaluated to ensure that there are no learning related vision dysfunctions. In this chapter much of the testing emphasized saccadic eye movements particularly large gross saccadic eye movements versus fine reading saccadic eye movements. The case history and age of the child will drive which of the tests will be administered. In addition, depending on the severity of the symptoms and the diagnoses, a referral is typically made for extensive testing and treatment with a clinician with advanced competency training in pediatric optometry and/or optometric vision therapy. In such cases, interprofessional management (teachers, pediatricians, occupational therapy, and physical therapy providers) will become an important part of the care of the pediatric patient with ocular motility deficits.

REFERENCES

Ayton, L. N., Abel, L. A., Fricke, T. R., & McBrien, N. A. (2009). Developmental eye movement test: What is it really measuring? *Optometry and Vision Science*, *86*(6), 722–730. doi:10.1097/OPX.0b013e3181a6a4b3 PMID:19417709

Barrett, B. T. (2014). Assessment of binocular vision and accommodation. In D. B. Elliot (Ed.), *Clinical procedures in primary eye care* (4th ed., pp. 147–208). Elsevier Saunders.

Birnbaum, M. H. (1993). *Optometric management of nearpoint vision disorders*. Butterworth Heinemann.

Caloroso, E. E., & Rouse, M. W. (1993). *Clinical management of strabismus*. Butterworth-Heinemann.

Ciuffreda, K. J., & Tannen, B. (1995). *Eye movement basics for the clinician*. Mobsy.

Ciuffreda, M. A., Ciuffreda, K. J., & Santos, D. (2003). Visagraph baseline analysis and procedural guidelines. *Journal of Behavioral Optometry*, *14*(3), 60–64.

Colby, D., Laukkanen, H. R., & Yolton, R. L. (1998). Use of the Taylor Visagraph II system to evaluate eye movements made during reading. *Journal of the American Optometric Association, 69*(1), 22–32. PMID:9479933

Coulter, R. A., & Shallo-Hoffman, J. (2000). The presumed influence of attention on accuracy in the Developmental Eye Movement (DEM) Test. *Optometry and Vision Science, 77*(8), 428–432. doi:10.1097/00006324-200008000-00010 PMID:10966069

Fernandez-Velazquez, F. J., & Fernandez-Fidalgo, M. J. (1995). Do DEM test scores change with respect to the language? Norms for Spanish-speaking population. *Optometry and Vision Science, 72*(12), 902–906. doi:10.1097/00006324-199512000-00009 PMID:8749338

Galetta, K. M., Brandes, L. E., Maki, K., Dziemianowicz, M. S., Laudano, E., Allen, M., Lawler, K., Sennett, B., Wiebe, D., Devick, S., Messner, L., Galetta, S. L., & Balcer, L. J. (2011). The King-Devick test and sports-related concussion: Study of a rapid visual screening tool in a collegiate cohort. *Journal of the Neurological Sciences, 309*(1-2), 34–39. doi:10.1016/j.jns.2011.07.039 PMID:21849171

Gallaway, M., Scheiman, M., & Mitchell, G. L. (2017). Vision therapy for post-concussion vision disorders. *Optometry and Vision Science, 94*(1), 68–73. doi:10.1097/OPX.0000000000000935 PMID:27505624

Graham, R., Rivara, F. P., Ford, M. A., & Spicer, C. M. (2014). *Sports-related concussions in youth: Improving the science, changing the culture*. The National Academies Press.

Griffin, J. R., & Borsting, E. J. (2010). *Binocular anomalies: theory, testing, and therapy* (5th ed., Vol. 1). Optometric Extension Program Foundation, Inc.

Holmes, J. M., Mutyala, S., Maus, T. L., Grill, R., Hodge, D. O., & Gray, D. T. (1999). Pediatric third, fourth, and sixth nerve palsies: A population-based study. *American Journal of Ophthalmology, 127*(4), 388–392. doi:10.1016/S0002-9394(98)00424-3 PMID:10218690

London, R. (2020). Evaluation of ocular motor function. In P. H. Schnell, M. B. Taub, & R. H. Duckman (Eds.), *Visual development, diagnosis, and treatment of the pediatric patient* (2nd ed., pp. 336–353). Wolters Kluwer.

Maples, W. C. (2017). Oculomotor dysfunctions: Classification of saccadic and pursuit deficiencies. In L. J. Press (Ed.), *Applied concepts in vision therapy* (pp. 262–292). Ridgevue Publishing.

Maples, W. C., Atchley, J., & Ficklin, T. (1992). Northeastern State University College of Optometry's oculomotor norms. *Journal of Behavioral Optometry, 3*(6), 143–150.

Maples, W. C., & Ficklin, T. W. (1988). Interrater and test-retest reliability of pursuits and saccades. *Journal of the American Optometric Association, 59*(7), 549–552. PMID:3403903

Master, C. L., Scheiman, M., Gallaway, M., Goodman, A., Robinson, R. L., Master, S. R., & Grady, M. F. (2016). Vision diagnoses are common after concussion in adolescents. *Clinical Pediatrics, 55*(3), 260–267. doi:10.1177/0009922815594367 PMID:26156977

Miller, N. R., Newman, N. J., Biousse, V., & Kerrison, J. B. (2008). *Walsh and Hoyt's Clinical neuro-ophthalmology: The essentials* (2nd ed.). Wolters Kluwer.

Park, K. A., Oh, S. Y., Min, J. H., Kim, B. J., & Kim, Y. (2019). Acquired onset of third, fourth, and sixth cranial nerve palsies in children and adolescents. *Eye (London, England), 33*(6), 965–973. doi:10.103841433-019-0353-y PMID:30760897

Pola, J. R., & Schnell, P. H. (2020). Eye movements. In P. H. Schnell, M. B. Taub, & R. H. Duckman (Eds.), *Visual development, diagnosis, and treatment of the pediatric patient* (2nd ed., pp. 79–99). Wolters Kluwer.

Ritter, S., & Steiner, A. (2021). *Anomalies of visual sensorimotor function lab manual* (17th ed.). SUNY College of Optometry.

Rouse, M. W. (2006). Optometric assessment: visual efficiency problems. In M. M. Scheiman & M. W. Rouse (Eds.), *Optometric management of learning-related vision problems* (2nd ed., pp. 335–367). Mosby Elsevier.

Scheiman, M., & Wick, B. (Eds.). (2020). *Clinical management of binocular vision: Heterophoric, accommodative, and eye movement disorders* (5th ed.). Wolters Kluwer.

Schlange, D. G., & Maino, D. M. (2001). Clinical behavioral objectives: Assessment techniques for special populations. In D. M. Maino (Ed.), *Diagnosis and management of special populations* (pp. 151–188). Mosby-Year Book, Inc.

Tannen, B., & Ciuffreda, K. J. (1997). A proposed addition to the standard protocol for the Visagraph II™ eye movement recording system. *Journal of Behavioral Optometry, 18*(6), 143–147.

Tannen, B., Darner, R., Ciuffreda, K. J., Shelley-Tremblay, J., & Rogers, J. (2015). Vision and reading deficits in post-concussion patients: A retrospective analysis. *Vision Development and Rehabilitation, 1*(3), 206–213.

Tassinari, J. T., & DeLand, P. (2005). Developmental eye movement test: Reliability and symptomology. *Optometry (St. Louis, Mo.), 76*(7), 387–399. doi:10.1016/j.optm.2005.05.006 PMID:16038866

Taub, M. B. (2012). Comprehensive examination procedures. In M. B. Taub, M. Bartuccio, & D. M. Maino (Eds.), *Vision diagnosis and care of the patient with special needs* (pp. 155–183). Wolters Kluwer Health/Lippincott Williams & Wilkins.

Tjark, B. J., Dorman, J. C., Valentine, V. D., Munce, T. A., Thompson, P. A., Kindt, S. L., & Bergeron, M. F. (2013). Comparison and utility of King Devick and ImPACT® composite scores in adolescent concussion patients. *Journal of the Neurological Sciences, 334*(1-2), 148–153. doi:10.1016/j.jns.2013.08.015 PMID:24007870

Wong, A. M. (2007). *Eye movement disorders*. Oxford University Press.

KEY TERMS AND DEFINITIONS

Ductions: Monocular eye movements.

Gain: Refers to the ratio of the eye velocity to the target velocity.

Latency: Refers to the time the eye movement (pursuit or saccade) response occurs after target motion.

Pursuit: Slow, continuous, and conjugate (eyes moving in the same direction) eye movement used when the eyes follow an object that is moving slowly and smoothly.

Saccades: Rapid, step-like conjugate (eyes moving in the same direction) eye movements that redirects the line of sight from one position to another.

Vergence Eye Movements: Are non-conjugate eye movements in which the eyes are moving in opposite directions. These movements involve either a convergence or divergence of the line of sight of each eye to fixate an object at near or in the distance.

Versional Eye Movements: Are conjugate eye movements in which both eyes moving in the same direction. An example of versional eye movements is when both eyes are moving towards the right or the left at the same time.

Chapter 8
Refraction in the Pediatric Eye Examination

Marilyn Vricella
SUNY College of Optometry, USA

ABSTRACT

Accurate determination of refractive error is one of the most critical components of a pediatric eye examination. According to the National Eye Institute, refractive errors are the most common causes of correctable reduced vision in children. Children with uncorrected refractive error are more likely to have developmental delays, visual-related academic problems, and poor social skills or interactions. In addition to difficulty seeing, uncorrected refractive errors can contribute to developmental deficits of accommodation, binocular vision, and certain forms of strabismus, amblyopia, and perceptual function. The author provides the clinician an in-depth guide on how to determine the refractive error in pediatric patients. The chapter focuses on the specific techniques, advantages and disadvantages, equipment required, and step-by-step procedures for performing retinoscopy, objective refraction, and subjective refraction on children.

INTRODUCTION

Accurate determination of refractive error is one of the most critical components of a pediatric eye examination. Refractive errors of hyperopia, myopia and astigmatism are the most common types of vision problems in children (National Eye Institute, 2020). Although not as common, anisometropia is also a significant refractive error concern. In addition to difficulty seeing, uncorrected refractive errors can contribute to developmental deficits of accommodation, binocular vision, and certain forms of strabismus, amblyopia, and perceptual function. Therefore, an accurate determination of a child's refractive error is important.

Refraction is a procedure used to determine a patient's eyeglass prescription. In young children, this procedure can be somewhat tricky due to their inability to express themselves. For young and nonverbal children, clinicians tend to rely on objective findings instead of subjective findings to aid in the decision making of what to best prescribe. This chapter will focus on the specific techniques, advantages and

DOI: 10.4018/978-1-7998-8044-8.ch008

disadvantages, equipment required, and step-by-step procedures for performing retinoscopy, objective refraction, and subjective refraction on children.

BACKGROUND

Retinoscopy is an objective method to measure refractive error and is a valuable skill to the pediatric eye care provider. Retinoscopy can be performed on patients of all ages, is fast when performed by a practiced clinician, does not require any verbal responses and only minimal cooperation from the child, and can be performed with minimal equipment. For the younger child who lacks the maturity, understanding or ability to provide subjective responses, retinoscopy may be the sole method for measuring refractive error. For the older child who can perform a subjective refraction, retinoscopy provides a starting point that can be fine-tuned by a subjective refraction.

Principles and Methodology of Retinoscopy

Retinoscopy is performed with a retinoscope (Figure 1) and uses correcting lenses to quantify the refractive errors of hyperopia, myopia, and astigmatism in each eye. Specifically, retinoscopy uses lenses to bring the patient's far point to the peephole of the retinoscope where the eye of the examiner is positioned. Retinoscopy can be performed behind a phoropter (Figure 2), with lens racks (Figure 3), or with loose lenses (Figure 4). The age and maturity of the child will help decide how retinoscopy is performed.

Before beginning retinoscopy, the clinician should determine their working distance. This is the distance from the retinoscope to the phoropter. The working distance is typically 50 cm or 67 cm, which corresponds to a dioptric value of 2.00 D (one divided by 0.50 m) or 1.50 D (one divided by 0.67 m), respectively.

Figure 1. Retinoscope

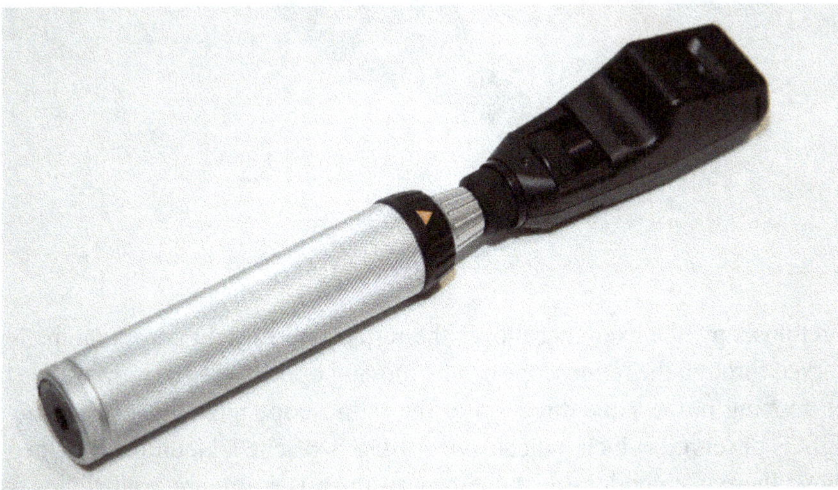

Figure 2. Phoropter

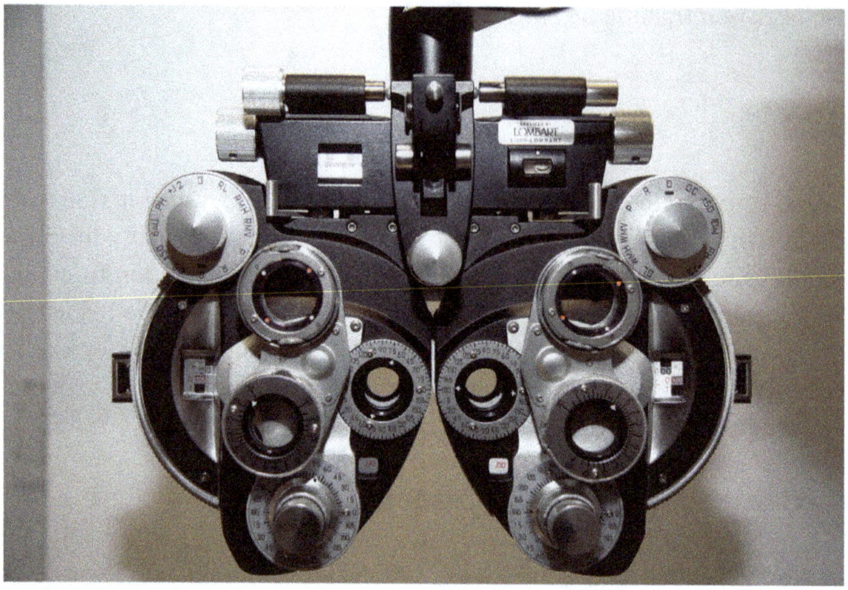

Figure 3. Lens racks

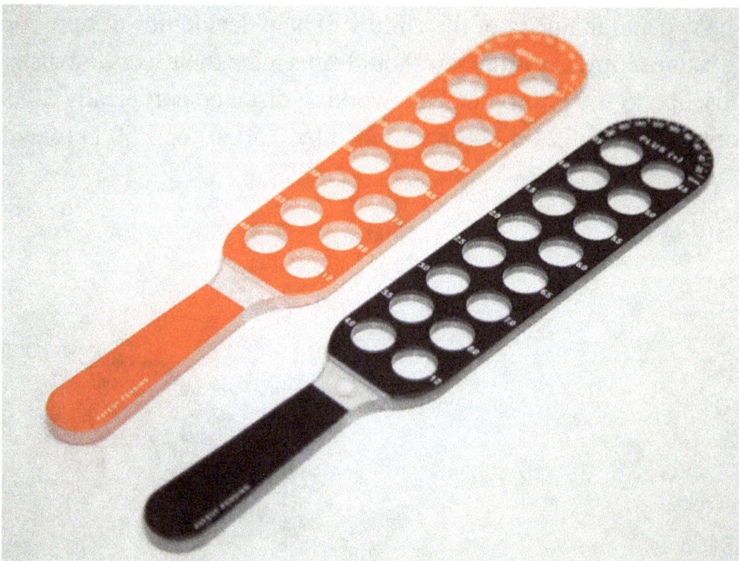

To perform retinoscopy, the examiner moves the retinoscope's light across the patient's pupil. The light reflex observed through the retinoscope can be moving opposite to the retinoscope movement (aka *against motion*), moving in the same direction of the retinoscope movement (aka *with motion*), or no movement of light is observed, which indicates *neutrality* is reached. Neutrality is when the reflex fills the entire pupil and there is no noticeable movement of the reflex. Figure 5 illustrates the principles of retinoscopy.

Figure 4. Loose lenses

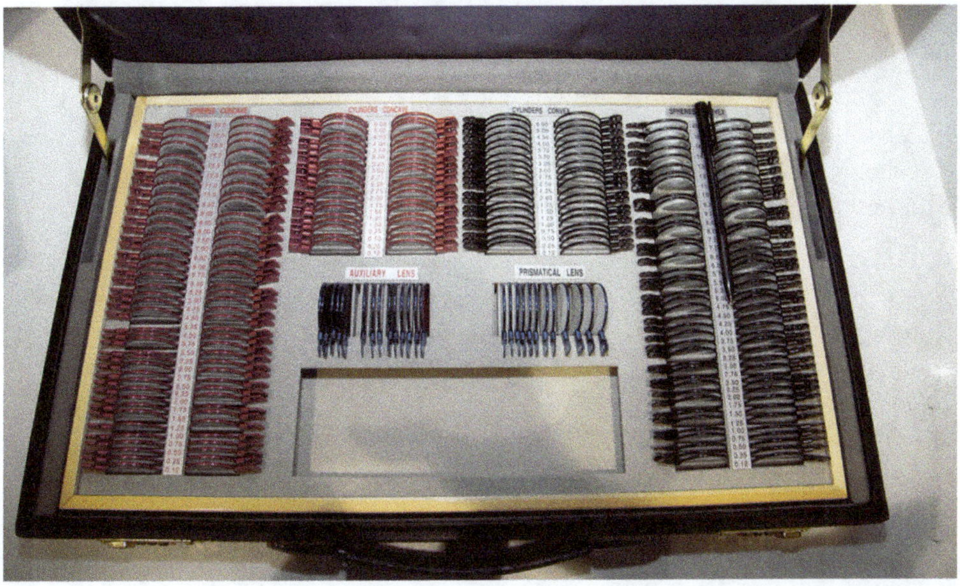

Figure 5. Principles of retinoscopy

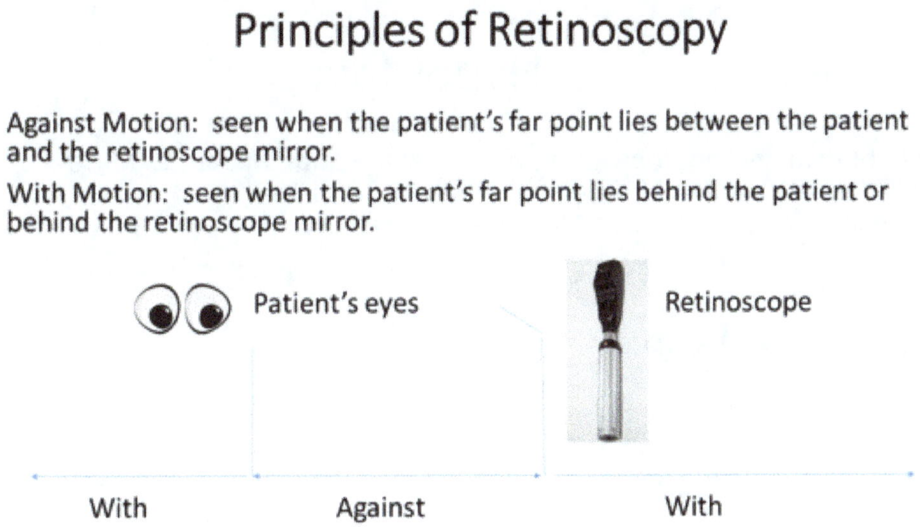

If the reflex is moving in the same direction of the retinoscope beam, then *plus* power lenses are introduced to neutralize the reflex. If the reflex is moving in the opposite direction of the retinoscope movement, *minus* power lenses are introduced to neutralize the reflex. Figure 6 illustrates the use of minus (or concave) lenses to neutralize the against motion observed in the case of a myopic refractive error. Figure 7 illustrates the use of plus (or convex) lenses to neutralize the with motion observed in the case of a hyperopic refractive error.

Figure 6. Myopia as seen during retinoscopy

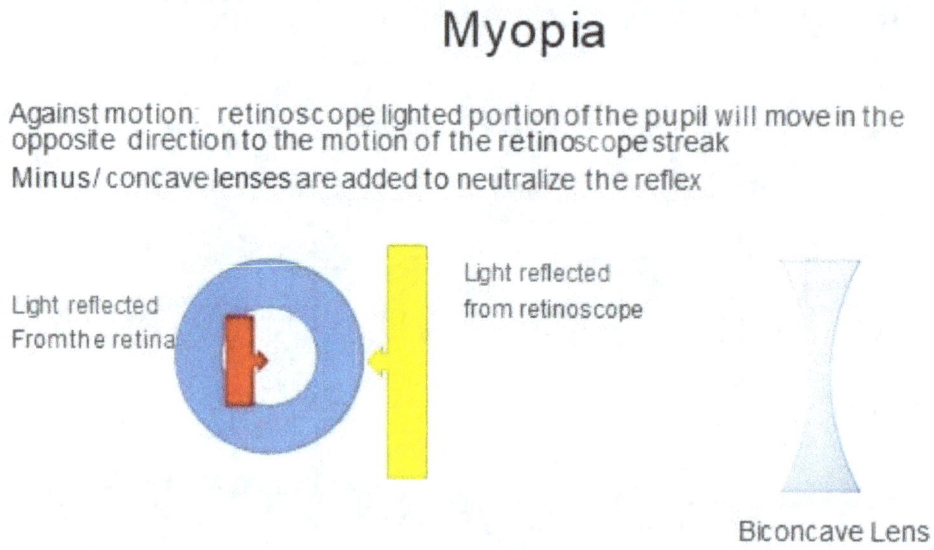

Figure 7. Hyperopia as seen during retinoscopy

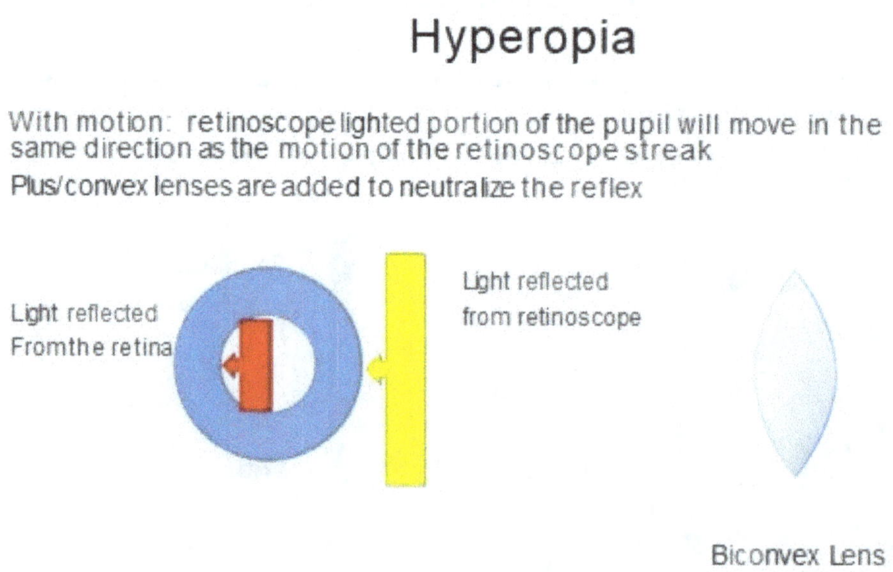

During retinoscopy, aside from the reflex movement, the clinician will also observe the quality of the reflex. The quality of the light reflex includes the speed, brilliance, and the width. If the speed is slow, brilliance is dull, and/or the width of the beam is thin, it means there is a relatively high uncorrected refractive error. Conversely, if the speed is fast, brilliance is bright, and/or the width of the beam is wide, there is a relatively low refractive error. When the reflex is at neutrality, the light will appear to fill up the entire pupil. Table 1 summarizes the various retinoscopy light reflex qualities and the refractive indications.

Table 1. Quality of retinoscopy light reflex and refractive indication

LIGHT REFLEX	QUALITY	REFRACTIVE INDICATION
Speed	Slow	Large refractive error, far point is far from the peephole of the retinoscope
	Fast	Small refractive error, far point is near the peephole of the retinoscope
Brilliance	Dull	Large refractive error, far point is far from the peephole of the retinoscope
	Brighter	Small refractive error, far point is near the peephole of the retinoscope
Width	Thin	Large refractive error, far point is far from the peephole of the retinoscope
	Wide	Small refractive error, far point is near the peephole of the retinoscope

When performing retinoscopy, the clinician will determine if the eye is spherical or if it is astigmatic. A spherical eye has the same reflex motion, brightness and speed in all meridians and is neutralized with the same lens in both principal meridians. If the reflex quality changes as the retinoscope beam is rotated, the eye has astigmatism. To determine the principal meridians, the retinoscope streak is rotated until it aligns with the pupil reflex such that the reflex moves in unison with the retinoscope streak; the two principal meridians are 90 degrees away from each other.

Once the two principal meridians are located, the clinician should first neutralize the meridian with the more *with motion* (i.e., the more hyperopic, or least myopic meridian). To find the more hyperopic (or less myopic) meridian, the clinician rotates the beam of the retinoscope light until it coincides with the slower *with motion* meridian. The more hyperopic meridian is neutralized first. If both meridians are against motion, then the meridian with the least (fastest) against motion is neutralized first. If the reflex is "against motion" i.e., the reflex is moving in the opposite direction of the retinoscope beam, then minus power lenses should be added to neutralize the reflex. If the reflex is "with motion" i.e., the reflex is moving in the same direction of the retinoscope beam then plus power lenses should be added to neutralize the reflex.

When using a streak retinoscope, the orientation of the beam is always perpendicular to the meridian being examined. If all meridians are neutralized with the same lens, the refractive error is spherical. When two different lenses are required to neutralize the reflexes, it is an eye with astigmatic refractive error. Most astigmatism has the principal meridians 90 degrees apart and is referred to as regular astigmatism. Less common is irregular astigmatism, when the two principal meridians are not 90 degrees apart. For example, Figure 8 shows a retinoscope light beam oriented vertically. In this position, the 180th meridian is being measured. Similarly, when the retinoscope light beam is oriented horizontally, the 90th meridian is being measure. In other words, the meridian that is being neutralized is always 90 degrees away from the retinoscope's light beam orientation.

The power of the lenses required to neutralize the retinoscopic reflex is the gross refractive error. The child's actual refractive error is the net of the power of the neutralizing lens **minus** the dioptric value of the clinician's working distance. For example, a clinician performs retinoscopy at 50 cm, and has the following results:

Figure 8. Illustrates a vertical beam of light from the retinoscope in the child's right eye
Photo courtesy of SUNY College of Optometry

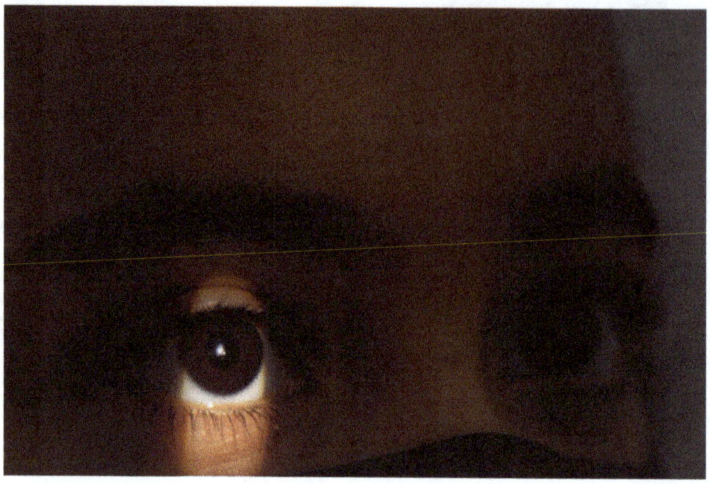

For the right eye:

- Lens to neutralize the 90-degree meridian: +4.00 D
- Lens to neutralize the 180-degree meridian: +4.00 D
- The child's net refractive error in the 90-degree meridian is +4.00 D - 2.00 D = +2.00 D
- The child's net refractive error in the 180-degree meridian is +4.00 D - 2.00D = +2.00 D
- The child's actual refractive error for the right eye is +2.00 D sphere

For the left eye:

- Lens to neutralize the 90-degree meridian: -1.75 D
- Lens to neutralize the 180-degree meridian: -1.00 D
- The child's net refractive error in the 90-degree meridian is -1.75 D - 2.00 D = -3.75 D
- The child's net refractive error in the 180-degree meridian is -1.00 D - 2.00D = -3.00 D
- The child's actual refractive error for the left eye is -3.00 – 0.75 x 180

Clinical Pearl: *When performing retinoscopy if the quality of the reflex is difficult to judge because the against motion reflexes are usually dimmer than the with motion reflexes, introduce large dioptric "jumps" of minus lenses (e.g. -3.00 D steps) until with motion is observed and then decrease the minus lens power until neutrality is reached. If the reflex becomes dimmer with large minus lens jumps, then try adding a high plus lens and observe if the reflex is brighter. The process of using high plus or minus lens jumps when the reflex is dull helps to ensure large refractive errors are not missed.*

Clinical Pearl: *Retinoscopes come with two light sources, a streak or a spot. The most widely used is the streak retinoscope which reflects a rectangular beam from a line source, while the spot retinoscope reflects a round light from a circular source (Rutner and Bartolone, 2020). The benefit of the spot retinoscope is that the clinician can identify the astigmatism axis without having to change the orientation of the light source. Additionally, with the spot retinoscope light, the clinician is able to quickly observe changes in the pupillary light reflex, enabling easier detection of fluctuations in accommodation during the procedure. However, the streak retinoscope allows for easier determination of astigmatism axis.*

OBJECTIVE REFRACTION

This section covers the three most popular clinical methods of objective refraction: dry retinoscopy (aka static retinoscopy), cycloplegic retinoscopy, and Mohindra retinoscopy.

Dry retinoscopy is an objective refraction technique performed without cycloplegic ophthalmic drops. An objective test does not require verbal feedback from the patient. However, to obtain an accurate retinoscopy finding, accommodation should be relaxed. Uncontrolled or fluctuating accommodation can lead to inaccurate measurements, usually resulting in less plus/more minus power. In addition, when accommodation is not controlled, astigmatism can be overestimated, underestimated or astigmatism that is not existent may be found. The best way to ensure accommodation is relaxed and controlled during retinoscopy is to provide the child with an interesting and engaging distance target to view. For a young child, the use of a short video with sound and animation projected at distance allows for increased attention and a relaxed state of accommodation.

Dry retinoscopy can be performed using a phoropter, or in free space using loose lenses or lens racks. Using lens bars or loose lenses are preferred when performing retinoscopy on an infant, young child or any child who is unable to sit behind a phoropter. The advantage of free space retinoscopy is that it can be performed while the infant or child is sitting on the parent's lap or while seated in a stroller in a comfortable position.

It is important to control accommodation in young children to obtain an accurate refraction. Even when providing a distance target, a young child's refractive error may fluctuate due to a child's shifting fixation, large ability to accommodate and/or short attention span. If the child has fluctuations in accommodation, the clinician may notice that the child's pupil size changes during retinoscopy. A cycloplegic retinoscopy will allow the clinician to obtain an objective refractive error, control accommodation and dilate the pupil, preparing the patient for an ophthalmoscopic examination.

Cycloplegic retinoscopy is recommended to obtain an accurate refraction in children under 12 years of age (McCullough, et al., 2017). A cycloplegic refraction is especially necessary for all children with strabismus, amblyopia, and anisometropia (AOA, 2017). At times, due to the difficulty in fully suppressing the ciliary body function, cycloplegic findings may not always be consistent or complete and a repeated cycloplegic examination may be needed to obtain an accurate result.

Cyclopentolate ophthalmic solution is the drug of choice for cycloplegic refraction due to its rapid onset of action, minimal side effects, and minimal residual accommodation (Rutner and Bartolone, 2020). Cycloplegic refraction may be performed after 10-15 minutes of instillation in individuals with light irides and after 30 to 40 minutes in individuals with dark irides (Wickum & Amos, 2008). Cyclopentolate is available in 0.5%, 1% and 2% concentration; however, the 2% is rarely used because of its increased risk for significant side effects (Rutner and Bartolone, 2020). Psychiatric reactions and behavioral disturbances have been associated with the use of cyclopentolate, especially with the higher 2% concentration (Bausch & Lomb, 2021). Tropicamide ophthalmic solution is less frequently used as a cycloplegic agent and should be considered when cyclopentolate is contraindicated or not available. Tropicamide 1% has been shown to be an effective measure of refractive error in non-strabismic infants (AOA, 2017). Tropicamide is available in 0.5% and 1% concentrations.

The 0.5% cyclopentolate concentration can be used in most infants less than 12 months of age and 1.0% cyclopentolate can be used in older children (AOA, 2017). Infants, young children, children with spastic paralysis, or brain damage have a higher reported susceptibility to cyclopentolate (Baush & Lomb, 2021). In children with Down Syndrome, cyclopentolate should be used with caution (Bausch & Lomb,

2021). Since increased susceptibility to side effects from cyclopentolate have been reported in infants, young children and children with spastic paralysis or brain damage, the use of concentrations higher than 0.5% is not recommended (Frazier and Jaanus, 2008). Tropicamide 0.5% can be used in most infants up to 1 year old, and 1% may be used thereafter. A topical anesthetic (0.5% proparacaine) may be instilled initially to improve the corneal penetration and effectiveness of the cycloplegic drop, and to avoid the stinging sensation caused by subsequent drops. It is recommended to use punctal occlusion (using digital pressure to compress the lacrimal sac) for 2 to 3 minutes after instillation, especially in young children and infants to reduce systemic absorption (Bausch & Lomb, 2021).

Mohindra retinoscopy is an objective dry retinoscopy method of determining refractive error without the use of cycloplegic drops. Because Mohindra retinoscopy is performed with the child fixating at a near target (the light of the retinoscope held 50 cm from the child), it is a useful refraction technique in infants and young children or any patient who is not interested in fixating a distant target (Rutner and Bartolone, 2020). Mohindra retinoscopy is particularly useful in instances where there are exam time constraints, for follow up visits when a refraction is indicated, in children who are extremely anxious about drops, when parents decline drops use, and for children who have systemic risk of adverse reactions from cycloplegic agents. Several studies have confirmed Mohindra retinoscopy findings are closely correlated with cycloplegic refraction in children, but without the need to use cycloplegic drops (Kauser et al., 2020; Borghi and Rouse, 1985; Natarajan et al., 2016). To calculate the final refractive error, an adjustment factor of -1.25 D is added to the neutralizing lens. For example, if neutrality is achieved with +2.00-1.00x180, the final refractive error is +0.75-1.00x180. And since tonic accommodation is greater in young children, using a lower adjustment factor of -0.75 D in children under 2 years and -1.00 D in children greater than 2 years provides for an even closer agreement between Mohindra retinoscopy and cycloplegic retinoscopy (Saunders and Westall, 1992). For example, for a 4-year-old, if neutrality is achieved with +2.00-1.00x180, the final refractive error is +1.00-1.00x180.

Dry Retinoscopy with Phoropter

Equipment: (Figure 9 shows the equipment used for retinoscopy with phoropter)

1. Retinoscope
2. Phoropter
3. Distance fixation target (such as a 20/400 letter/picture with red/green overlay as shown in Figure 10)

Procedure

Step 1: Clean the phoropter and set all lenses to zero power

Step 2: Position the phoropter such that the child's eyes are aligned through the ocular

Step 3: Set the pupillary distance and adjust the vertical alignment

Step 4: Instruct the child to look at a distance target provided at child's eye level and to let the doctor know if at any time the target is blocked

Step 5: Perform retinoscopy on the left eye. Add lenses to the left eye until a fast against motion is observed. This "fogging" technique is to help minimize accommodation

Step 6: Perform retinoscopy on the right eye. Determine the most hyperopic principal meridian. Add spherical lenses until a neutral reflex is observed

Step 7: If astigmatism is present, neutralize the second principal meridian by turning the cylinder axis dial to align with the retinoscope light beam (this will be 90 degrees away from the most hyperopic principal meridian in step 6)

Step 8. Repeat steps 6 and 7 for the left eye

Figure 9. Equipment for retinoscopy with phoropter
Photo courtesy of SUNY College of Optometry.

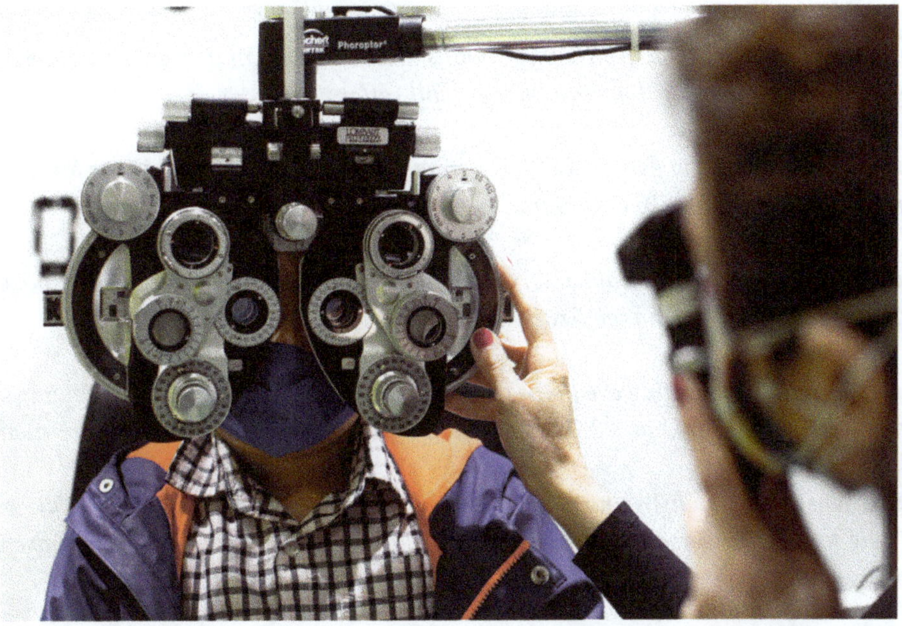

Figure 10. Large letter with red-green overlay as a distance fixation target during retinoscopy

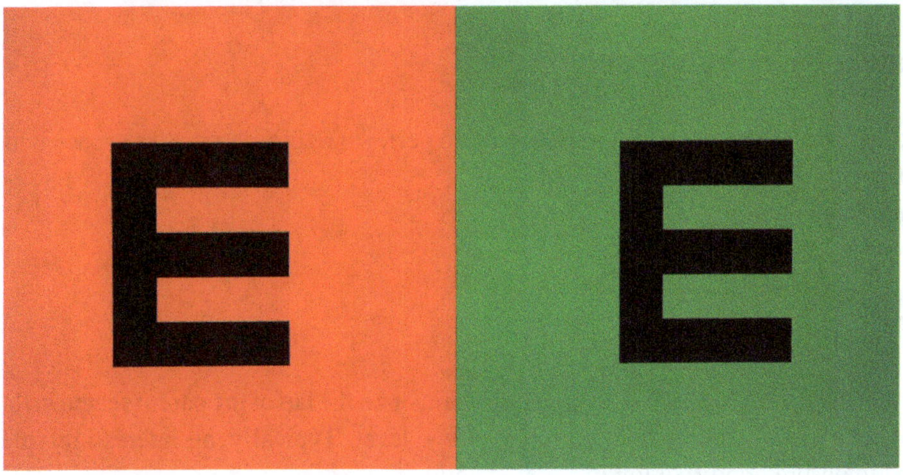

Clinical Pearl: *For a clinician's whose working distance is 67 cm, the "R" lens in the phoropter can be dialed in before beginning retinoscopy. The "R" lens is equivalent to +1.50 D. The benefit of using this lens is that after performing retinoscopy, the R lens can be removed, and the child's final prescription is the power of the lenses that are in the phoropter as the R lens already compensates for the working distance.*

Clinical Pearl: *Retinoscopy is best performed in dim light conditions to maximize pupil size. However, for young children who are afraid of the dark, retinoscopy can be performed with room lights on.*

Clinical Pearl: *Since children tend to have large pupils, it is important that when performing retinoscopy, the clinician focuses on the central portion of the pupil reflex.*

Clinical Pearl: *If the eye has an extremely high refractive error and the clinician is far away from neutral, this can misleadingly look like a "neutral" reflex.*

Clinical Pearl: *For an eye that is strabismic, occlude the fixating eye and perform retinoscopy slightly off the visual axis to allow for distance fixation.*

Clinical Pearl: *Fogging the fixating eye helps to ensure more accurate retinoscopy findings. The fogged eye is typically left with +1.50 D or +2.00 D additional plus power over the actual refractive error.*

Clinical Pearl: *When performing retinoscopy on the child's right eye, the clinician should be positioned to the child's right and vice versa for the left eye. The clinician looks through the retinoscope aperture with the right eye and directs the beam of light toward the child's right pupil.*

Clinical Pearl: *Advantages of using the phoropter for retinoscopy includes ease of adding "fogging" lenses to the fixating eye to control accommodation, and the ability to quickly make small lens power changes (such as 0.25 D) and axis changes (as small as one degree).*

Dry Retinoscopy in Free Space

Equipment: (Figure 11 shows the equipment used to perform retinoscopy in free space with lens racks)

1. Retinoscope
2. Distance fixation target
3. Loose lenses or lens racks

Procedure

Step 1: Position the child comfortably in the exam chair, or on the lap of the parent seated in the exam chair

Step 2: Provide a large distance fixation target at eye level. Typically, an interesting video is recommended to ensure good fixation in a young child.

Step 3: Instruct the child to look at the distance target. The clinician should make sure not to block the child's view of the fixation target

Step 4: "Fog" both eyes to relax accommodation. This can be accomplished with lenses in a pediatric trial frame. Select the lens power that provides a fast *against* motion in each eye

Step 6: Perform retinoscopy on the right eye. Determine the most hyperopic principal meridian. Add spherical lenses until a neutral reflex is observed

Step 7: If astigmatism is present, neutralize the second principal meridian (this will be 90 degrees away from the most hyperopic principal meridian in step 6) by holding spherical lenses until a neutral reflex is observed. Be sure to align the retinoscope light beam with the retinoscopic reflex

Step 8. Repeat steps 6 and 7 for the left eye

Figure 11. Equipment used to perform retinoscopy in free space with lens racks
Photo courtesy of SUNY College of Optometry

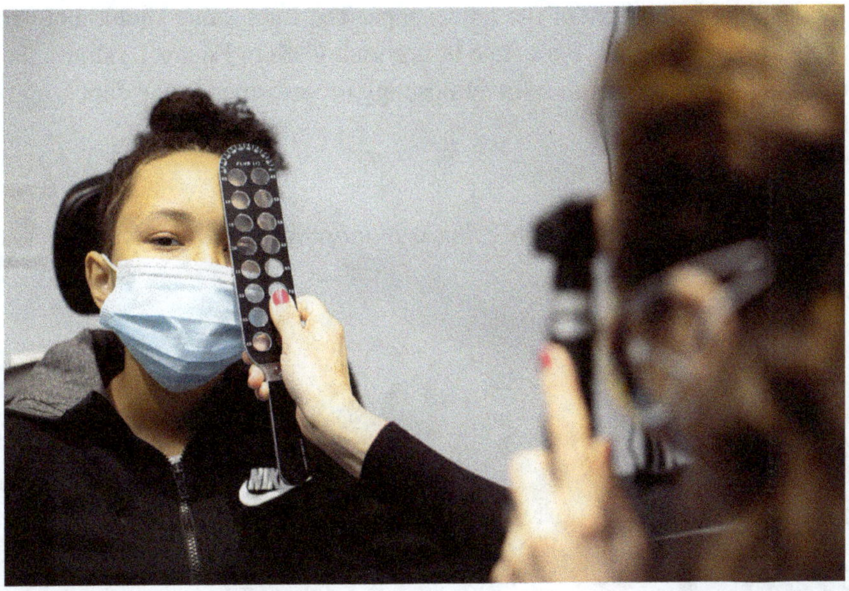

Clinical Pearl: *Retinoscopy in young children can be difficult. Singing popular tunes and asking the child to sing along can reduce some fear. Asking the parent to hug the child can also provide better fixation.*

Clinical Pearl: *Perform retinoscopy with the child in the stroller. Some children are more cooperative if they are allowed to remain seated in something familiar and comfortable.*

Clinical Pearl: *Ask another person to assist with holding the child's attention at a distance by presenting interesting hand-held toys that light up and make noise.*

Clinical Pearl: *It can be more challenging to control accommodation when performing retinoscopy in free space. Using premade "fogging" spectacles of +1.50 D sphere OU or +2.00 D sphere OU can be worn comfortably by the child during retinoscopy to control accommodation.*

Clinical Pearl: *Purchase lens racks with a printed axis compass to assist with astigmatism axis determination (Good-lite, 2021).*

Clinical Pearl: *Assessing pupil size changes during dry retinoscopy provides information on accommodation stability.*

Clinical Pearl: *Retinoscopy allows the clinician to view the clarity of media which can provide clues on ocular health.*

Mohindra Retinoscopy

Mohindra retinoscopy is performed monocularly and in a dark room under a non-accommodative state. The target for this method is the light of the retinoscope. The light target should not stimulate accommodation and represents the patient's dark state of accommodation. Figure 12 shows the procedure for performing Mohindra retinoscopy. Mohindra retinoscopy is performed in the dark with the retinoscope as the only light source.

Figure 12. The procedure for performing Mohindra retinoscopy. Note the room lights are left on for photography purposes
Photo courtesy of SUNY College of Optometry.

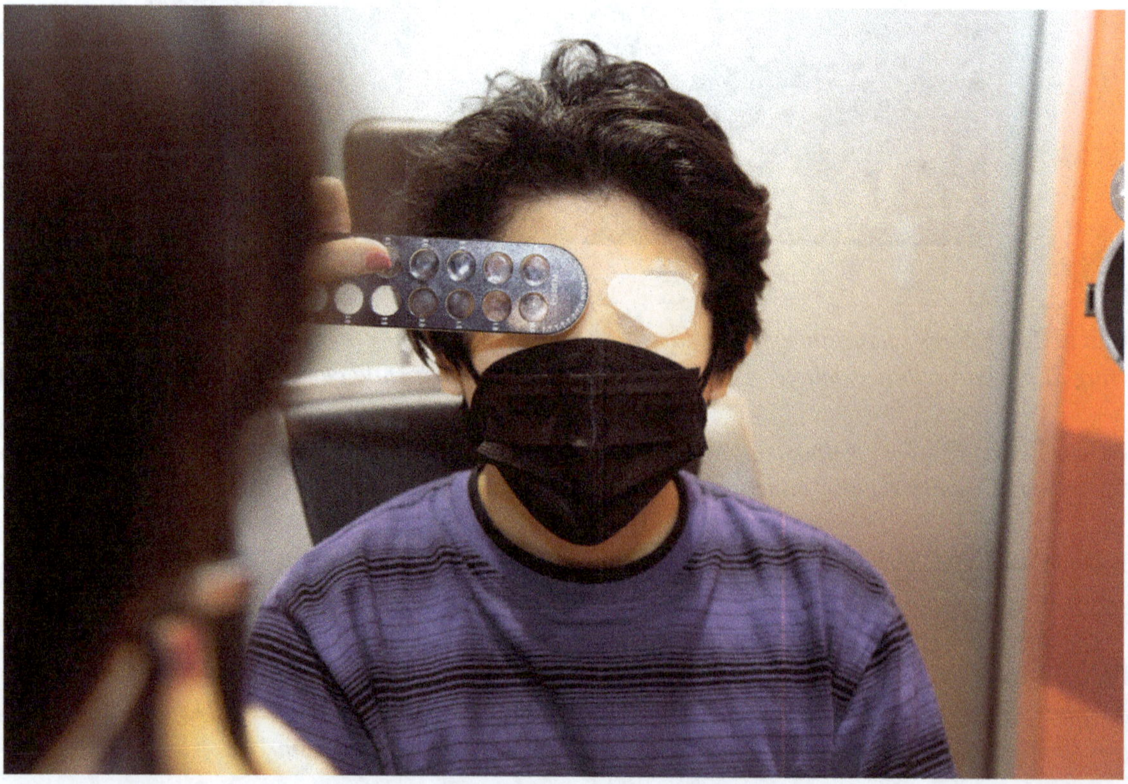

Equipment:

1. Retinoscope
2. Eye patch (Figure 13 shows a plastic eye patch; Figure 14 shows adhesive eye patches)
3. Loose lenses or lens rack

Figure 13. A black eye patch with elastic strap

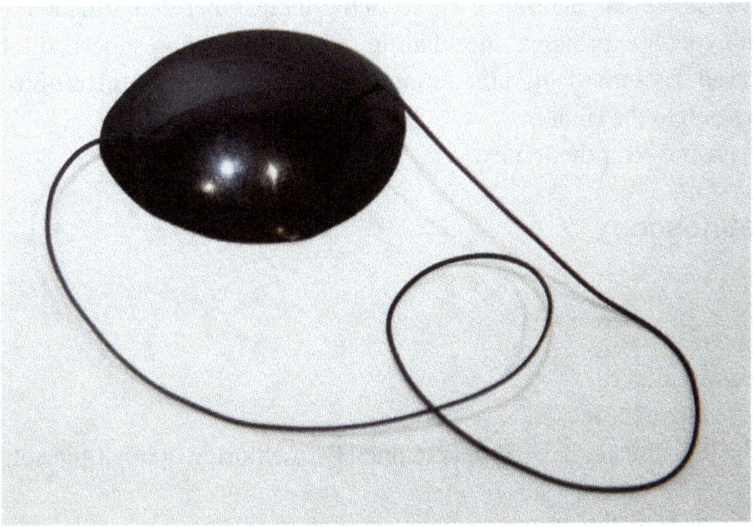

Figure 14. Adhesive eye patches

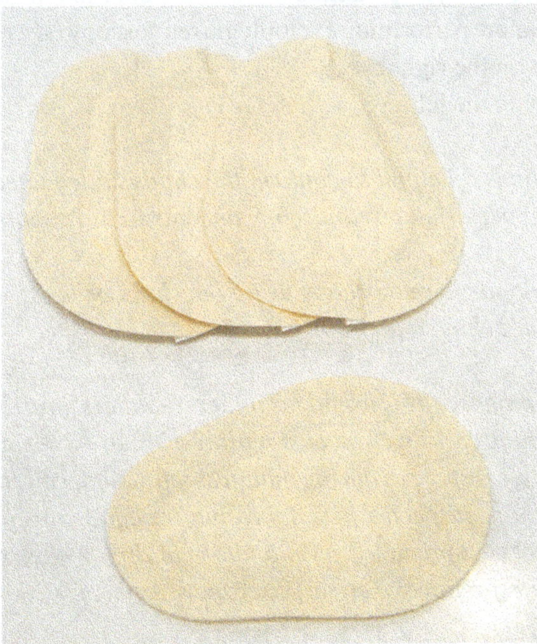

Procedure

Step 1: Occlude the left eye.
Step 2: Hold the retinoscope at 50 cm from the patient's right eye
Step 3: Direct the attention of the child to fixate at the retinoscope light
Step 4: Perform retinoscopy on the right eye. Determine the most hyperopic principal meridian. Add spherical lenses until a neutral reflex is observed
Step 5: If astigmatism is present, neutralize the second principal meridian (this will be 90 degrees away from the most hyperopic principal meridian in step 4) by holding spherical lenses until a neutral reflex is observed. Be sure to align the retinoscope light beam with the retinoscopic reflex
Step 6: Switch the patch to the right eye.
Step 7. Repeat steps 4 and 5 for the left eye

Cycloplegic Retinoscopy

Equipment:

1. Retinoscope
2. Distance target or video
3. Phoropter, loose lenses or lens rack
4. 0.5% or 1% Cyclopentolate, 0.5% Proparacaine Hydrochloride ophthalmic solution

Procedure

Step 1: If a topical anesthetic eye drop will be used, administer first
Step 2: Instill 2 drops 0.5% or 1% cyclopentolate ophthalmic solution in each eye 5 minutes apart
Step 3: Wait 10- 30 minutes before performing cycloplegic retinoscopy (see page 7 Objective Refraction).
Step 4: Perform retinoscopy on the right eye
Step 5: Perform retinoscopy on the left eye

Clinical Pearl: *The author finds it helpful to confirm the child is adequately cyclopleged by looking at the quality of the reflex when performing retinoscopy and ensure it is not fluctuating.*

Clinical Pearl: *Perform cycloplegic retinoscopy using lens bars or loose lenses for infants and young children who are unable to sit behind a phoropter.*

Clinical Pearl: *Cycloplegic retinoscopy is useful for infants, toddlers, preschoolers, non-communicative or uncooperative patients, children with suspected malingering or hysterical amblyopia, children with variable/inconsistent subjective responses during manifest refraction, children with strabismus, children with suspected latent hyperopia, suspected psuedomyopia/traumatic myopia, amblyopia, those whose visual acuity does not correct to a predicted level and/or children whose symptoms seem unrelated to the nature or degree of manifest refractive error (Wickum & Amos, 2008).*

Clinical Pearl: *When instilling drops into a child's eyes is difficult, it is best to minimize the number of drops to increase the likelihood of successful administration. In this case do not use a topical anesthetic prior to use of cycloplegic agent.*

Clinical Pearl: *When instilling eye drops in a child is challenging, some practitioners find the use of spray drops to instill a cycloplegic agent helpful. Spray administration of drops works well for toddlers who are apprehensive of drops.*

OBJECTIVE REFRACTION WITH HANDHELD AUTOREFRACTION

A handheld autorefractor is a portable method of determining the refractive error of the eye without the need for subjective input from the child. Handheld autorefractors are easier to use in young children than tabletop models. Adequate positioning and fixation are needed for accurate handheld autorefractors readings. Thus, autorefractors is a good tool for school-aged children but does not replace retinoscopy in infants and young children. Step-by-step procedures on how to use the more popular autorefractors are provided in this section.

Clinical Pearl: *Auto refraction can underestimate hyperopia and overestimate myopia due to proximal accommodation if cycloplegia is not used.*

Retinomax

The Retinomax is a portable, wireless, handheld autorefractor (Figure 15). There is a melody that is played in child mode to assist in keeping the child's attention (Righton, 2018). The Multi-Ethnic Pediatric Eye Disease Study (MEPEDS) evaluated the testability of the Retinomax auto refractor after cycloplegia in children 6 to 72 months old and found that 89% of children were testable when the procedure was performed by an optometrist or ophthalmologist with a subspecialty training in pediatrics (Borchert, 2008).

Advantages

The new auto quick measurement allows the instrument to enter Quick mode if no measurement is taken within six seconds. A measurement is then taken in 0.07 seconds. The Retinomax series of handheld autorefractors also provide keratometry readings.

Disadvantages

It requires stable fixation and a stable instrument. It must be held against the child's forehead. It is difficult to use with excessive blinking.

Figure 15. Retinomax handheld autorefractor in use
Photo courtesy of SUNY College of Optometry

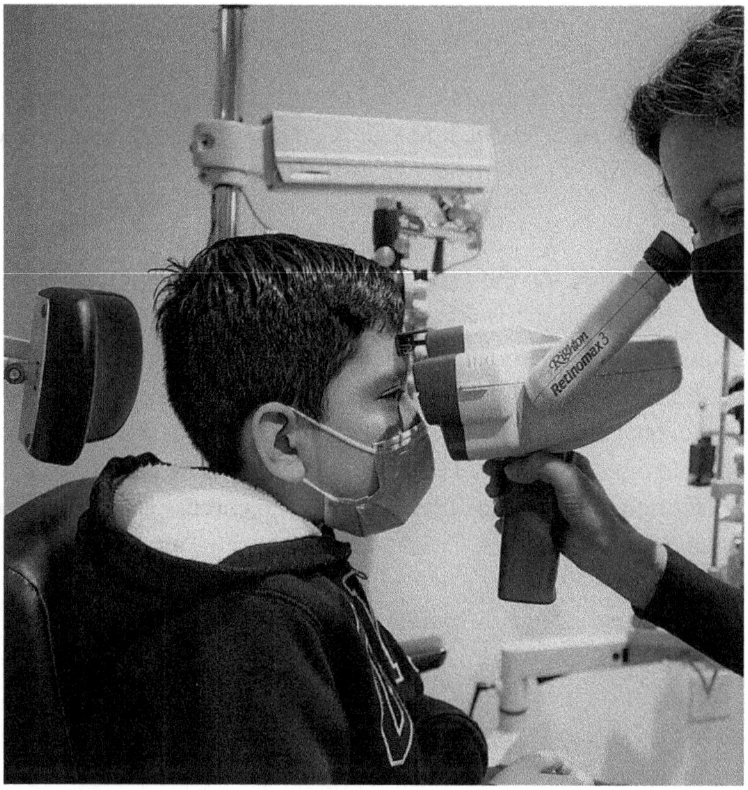

Procedure

Step 1: Clean the forehead rest
Step 2: Select the "regular mode"
Step 3: Clinician adjusts the eye piece for clarity
Step 4: Position the Retinomax in front of the child's right eye and stabilize the forehead rest on the child's forehead
Step 5: Instruct the child to fixate on the center target and not to blink during the procedure.
Step 6: Align the pupil with the middle of the screen. The circle of 4 white dots should be aligned and clear and the examiner should ensure the mire ring (circle of dots) is in the center of the pupil.
Step 7: Readings are automatically taken, and results are viewed on the screen or can be printed
Step 8: Repeat steps 5-7 for the left eye.

For a more comprehensive review of the instrument, please see the manufacturer's instructions.

Welch Allyn Sure Sight

The Welch Allyn Sure Sight (Skanaeateles Falls, NY) is a "child friendly" portable handheld auto refractor (Figure 16). The instrument is small, and the measurements are taken at a 14-inch distance from the child, which is less threatening to a child. The measurements are quick, and the lights and sound are attention grabbing to a young child.

Advantages

Welch Allyn Sure Sight has a calibration setting for both children and adults. Readings come with a reliability number and the distance between the child and the machine is less threatening.

Disadvantages

Welch Allyn Sure Sight recorded myopia more often when used on non-cyclopleged children (Iuorno, et al., 2004).

Figure 16. Welch Allyn Sure Sight set up
Photo courtesy of SUNY College of Optometry

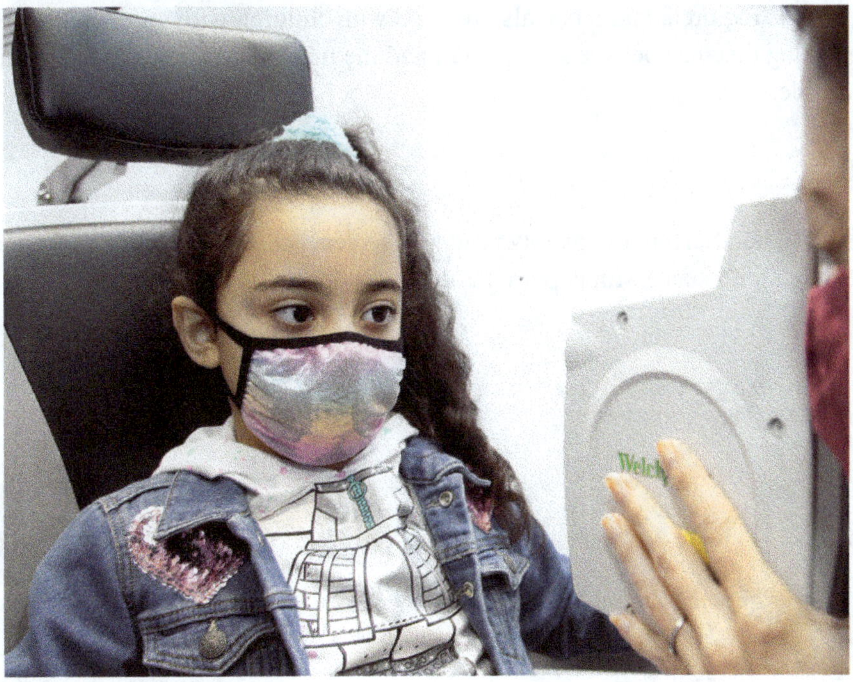

Procedure

Step 1: Hold the Welch Allyn Sure Sight 14 inches (~36 cm) in front of the child's right eye
Step 2: Select the child mode setting
Step 3: Press the Go button to initiate measurements
Step 4: Look through the view port and align the cross hair with the patient's pupil
Step 5: Instruct the child to fixate on the red central light (amongst the green peripheral blinking lights)

Step 6: Readings are automatically taken
Step 7: A "tah dah" sound played when testing is complete
Step 8: Repeat steps 4-7 for the left eye

For a more comprehensive review of the instrument, please see the manufacturer's instructions.

Welch Allyn Spot

The Welch Allyn Spot Vision Screener (Skanaeateles Falls, NY) is a handheld, portable auto refractor that offers fast binocular screening with a one-second capture time and a non-threatening 3-foot working distance (Figure 17). It is powered for mass screening events and can be used in children as young as 6 months old.

Advantages

The Welch Allyn Spot Vision Screener is easy to use with minimal user training required. Minimal patient cooperation is required, and it can also be used with children with special needs. It is quick and has a non-threatening distance between the patient and the machine. Wireless printing and Wi-Fi connectivity is available.

Disadvantages

Welch Allyn Spot Vision Screener is mainly used as a screener tool. Some children cannot hold steady fixation long enough for a successful capture to occur.

Figure 17. Welch Allyn Spot vision screener set up
Photo courtesy of SUNY College of Optometry

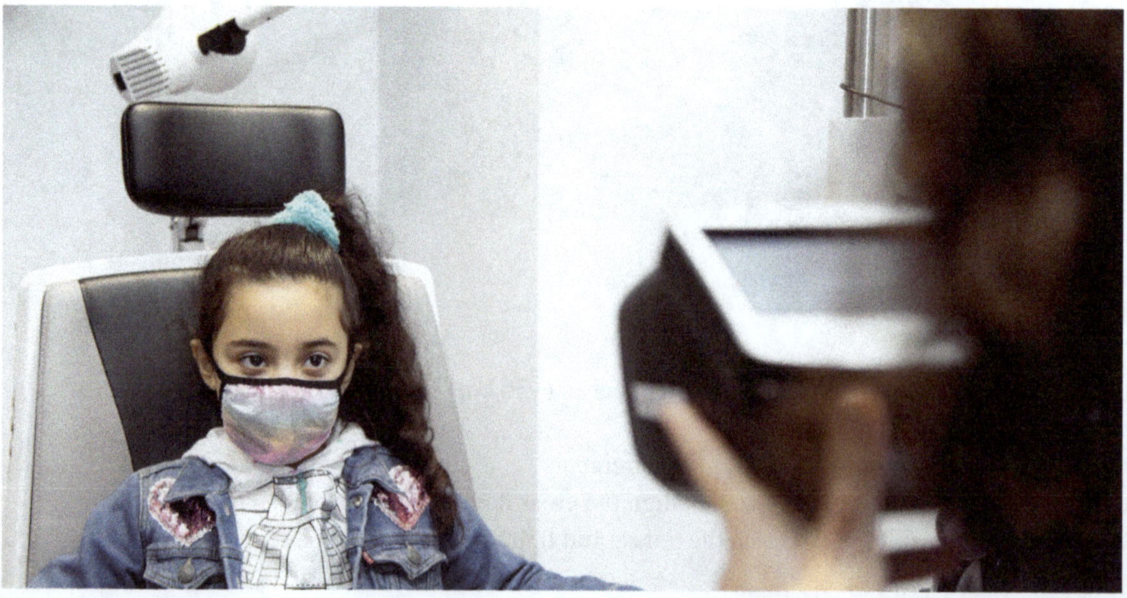

Procedure

Step 1: Hold Welch Allyn Spot Vision Screener one meter (3 feet) at eye level from child's eyes
Step 2: Select the age range of the child
Step 3: Press the Start button
Step 4: Move the instrument vertically to align with the child's eyes and move closer or further away from the child until the images of child's eyes are clear on the screen. The screen prompts if the instrument is too close or too far from the child
Step 5: When measurements are automatically taken, a spinning wheel appears on the screen. Hold the instrument steady until the readings are complete

For a more comprehensive review of the instrument, please see the manufacturer's instructions.

PlusOptix

The PlusOptix Binocular Auto Refractor (Nuremberg, Germany) is a handheld binocular autorefractor that provides values for refractive error, pupil diameters, pupil distance as well as gaze asymmetry (Figure 18). There are three different models, two of which are portable and one that is stationary.

Figure 18. PlusOptix

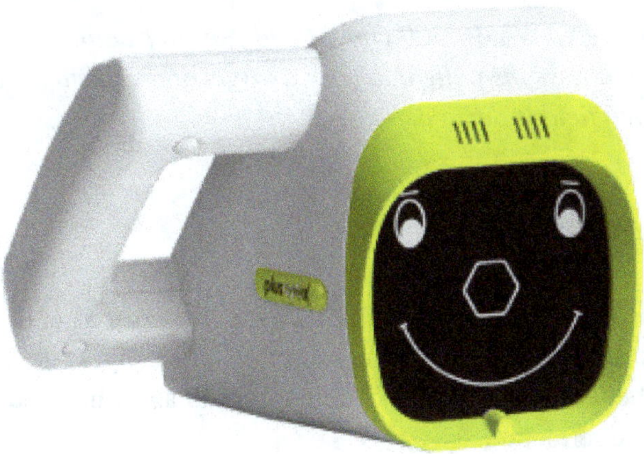

Advantages

The PlusOptix uses an infrared light to limit glare. It features an internal patient database and a CSV interface so it can be integrated into EMR systems. Results can be recorded either electronically or in paper charts.

Disadvantages

Some children cannot hold steady fixation long enough for a successful capture to occur. Pupil diameter must be between 3 mm and 8 mm.

Procedure

Step 1: Hold the PlusOptix hand-held instrument in front of the child's right eye and 1 meter (3.3 feet) away from the child in a room without any direct sunlight
Step 2: Select mode of choice: monocular right eye/left eye or binocular
Step 3: Press the Go button
Step 4: Instruct the child to look at the nose of the smiley face. There is also a warble sound to direct the child's attention
Step 5: Move the instrument vertically until the child's eyes are viewable in the monitor, and move the instrument closer or further from the child until the image of the eyes are clear in the monitor
Step 6: Readings are automatically taken
Step 7: Repeat steps 4-5 for the left eye (if the monocular mode was selected)

For a more comprehensive review of the instrument, please see the manufacturer's instructions.

Clinical Pearl: *The Grand Seiko WAM-5500 Open Field Auto refractor (Hiroshima, Japan) is a non-portable auto refractor that allows the patient to view a target at any distance and can be considered in older children when an open field is desired.*

SUBJECTIVE REFRACTION

Subjective refraction is further refinement of a child's refractive error after dry retinoscopy. Since subjective refraction requires the ability of a child to report visual changes, the child's maturity level and ability to focus is often a better determinant than chronological age when deciding whether a child can provide a reliable subjective refraction.

Subjective refraction can be performed using a phoropter or in free space with a trial frame. For older children, the subjective refraction can be performed using a phoropter with the dry retinoscopy findings in place. For younger children or any child who is unable to sit behind the phoropter (e.g., very young, very fidgety, in a wheelchair) subjective refraction can be carried out with the use of a trial frame and loose lenses. For those who are not able to give reliable subjective responses, the retinoscopy findings are placed in a trial frame and visual acuities are measured to see if there is any increase in vision. This allows the clinician to have a quantitative measure and is necessary in the management of amblyopia and in those who require follow up for visual acuity monitoring. The younger the child, the more the clinician will rely on an accurate retinoscopy finding to reach a final spectacle prescription. With both methods of subjective refraction, the goal is to provide a prescription that provides the child with the best visual acuity.

Subjective refraction consists of three parts: monocular (best sphere, cylinder axis refinement, cylinder power refinement), binocular balance (to equalize the accommodation stimulus between the two eyes), and binocular sphere refinement (to determine the best sphere binocularly). There are two main methods to perform binocular balance: The Prism Dissociation method and the Successive Alternate Occlusion method.

Clinical Pearl: *In the author's experience, with few exceptions, children age 6 and younger cannot complete a subjective refraction behind a phoropter because they lack the maturity, understanding, or ability to sit still.*

Clinical Pearl: *In the author's experience some 6 to 7 year olds and most children over the age of 7 can provide reliable subjective refraction responses.*

Subjective Refraction with Trial Frame

Equipment:

1. Pediatric trial frame (Figure 19)
2. Loose lenses
3. Hand-held JCC (Jackson Cross Cylinder)
4. Distance acuity chart
5. Occluder

Figure 19. Pediatric trial frames

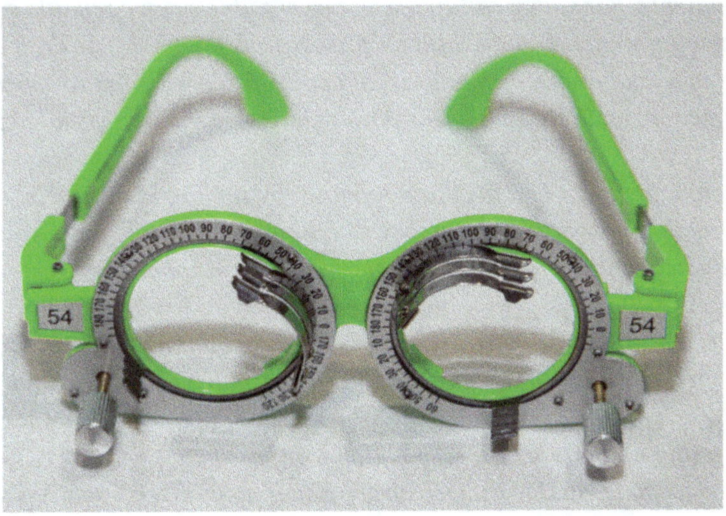

Procedure

Step 1: Place the dry retinoscopy findings in a trial frame

Step 2: Add half the power of the clinician's working distance lens (e.g., +0.75 D for a 67 cm working distance or a +1.00 D for a 50 cm working distance) to leave the eyes partially fogged before beginning the procedure

Step 3: Occlude the left eye

Step 4: Take distance visual acuity for right eye

Step 5: Adjust the sphere power using loose lenses in 0.25 D steps to obtain the best acuity with maximum plus

Step 6: If cylinder is present, refine the cylinder axis by holding the JCC with its **handle** parallel to the axis found on retinoscopy. The JCC is flipped to present position one, then flipped again for position two while keeping the handle parallel to the axis found on retinoscopy

Step 7: If cylinder is present, refine the cylinder power by holding the JCC with its **axes** parallel to the axis found on retinoscopy. The JCC is flipped to present position one, then flipped again for position two

Step 8: Remove the occluder from the left eye and place the occluder over the right eye

Step 9: Repeat steps 4-7 for the left eye

Step 10: Fog each eye by +1.00 D

Step 11: Display a single isolated line of letters (20/50 or 20/60)

Step 12: Perform binocular balance using the Successive Alternate Occlusion method. Alternately occlude one eye at a time and ask the child if the vision is clearer in one eye or the other

Step 13: If one eye is clearer, add +0.25 D to that eye and repeat step 12 until both eyes are equally blurred

Step 14: After the eyes are equally fogged, reduce the plus sphere binocularly in 0.25 D steps until the best VA is obtained. The least plus to obtain the best VA is the end point.

Clinical Pearl: *Trial frame refraction is usually done in adults with low vision and rarely performed in young pediatric patients. For young children who are not able to give reliable subjective responses, a complete trial frame refraction can be difficult to perform. For these cases, it is best to place the retinoscopy findings in a trial frame, measure visual acuity to see what improvement there is in vision, perform an over refraction, and rely on the lens powers that give the best visual acuity.*

Clinical Pearl: *When a confident and accurate retinoscopy finding is available, all the steps of trial frame subjective refraction may not be necessary to follow, particularly for a young child with short attention span and limited ability to provide reliable subjective responses.*

Clinical Pearl: *Subjective refraction in a trial frame is less intimidating than a phoropter for a child and allows the clinician greater ability to observe the child's eyes during testing and to monitor head tilt.*

Clinical Pearl: *Use a single letter/symbol presentation with surround crowding bars rather than a whole chart presentation for a young child when measuring visual acuities with subjective refraction.*

Subjective Refraction with Phoropter

Equipment:

1. Phoropter (Figure 20 shows phoropter and JCC power and axis labels)
2. Distance Acuity Chart

Figure 20. Picture shows phoropter JCC knob with power and axis labels (P = power and thumb wheel knob = axis)

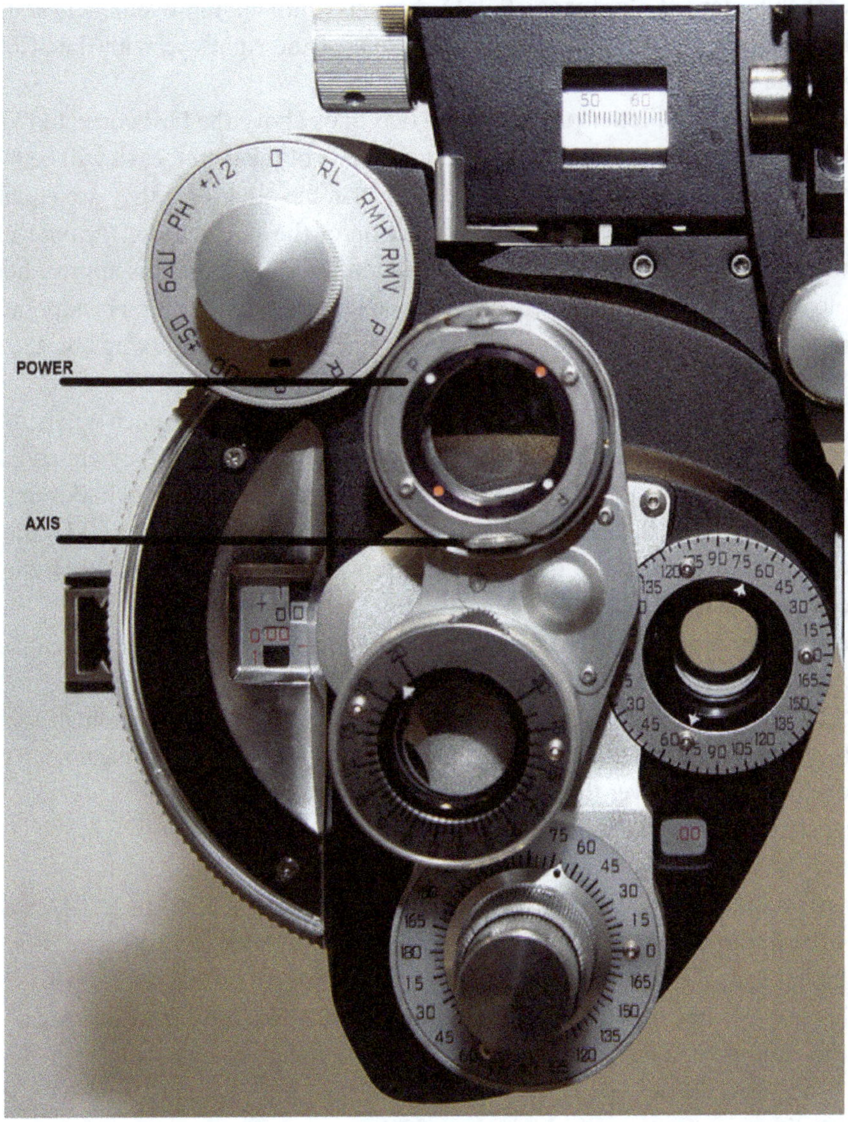

Procedure

Step 1: After retinoscopy, remove half the working distance power in both eyes (e.g., +0.75 D for a 67 cm working distance or a +1.00 D for a 50 cm working distance). This leaves the eyes partially fogged to begin the procedure

Step 2: Occlude the left eye

Step 3: Take distance visual acuity for right eye. The right eye should be fogged at this point and the vision should be 20/40 or slightly worse. If the vision is 20/30 or better, add +0.25 D increments until the acuity is 20/40 or slightly worse

Step 4: Remove 0.25 D steps of plus (or add 0.25D of minus) until no improvement in acuity is obtained.

Step 5: If cylinder is present, introduce the JCC in front of the right eye with the JCC thumb wheel aligned with the phoropter cylinder axis

Step 6: Display a single line of letters that is one to two lines above the best corrected visual acuity

Step 7: Provide these instructions "I will show you two views of the target, each will be slightly blurred, but tell me if one view appears clearer and darker than the other or if they are equal"

Step 8: Move the phoropter cylinder axis in the direction of the JCC red dot. Axis refinement should begin with larger step sizes and the step sizes reduced as the endpoint is approached.

Step 9: When no difference is reported between the two presentations, the axis endpoint is reached

Step 10: To continue with cylinder power refinement, line up the "P" markings on the JCC dial with the phoropter cylinder axis

Step 11: Provide these instructions "I will show you two views of the target, each will be slightly blurred, but tell me if one view appears clearer and darker than the other or if they are equal"

Step 12: If the line is clearer with the red dots aligned with the phoropter cylinder axis, increase the minus cylinder power by 0.25 D. If the cylinder power is increased by 0.50 D, the sphere power should be increased by +0.25 D. If the cylinder power is decreased by 0.50 D, the sphere power should be decreased by +0.25 D

Step 13: When no difference is reported between the two presentations, the power endpoint is reached

Step 14: To refine the final sphere in the right eye, add +1.00 D to fog the eye

Step 15: Remove 0.25 D steps of plus (or add 0.25D of minus) until no improvement in acuity is obtained. The final sphere is the most plus or least minus spherical lens for best visual acuity

Step 16: Remove the occluder over the left eye and occlude the right eye

Step 17: Repeat steps 3-15 for the left eye

Step 18: Remove the occluder over the right eye

Step 19. Perform binocular balance using the Prism Dissociation method. Add +1.00 D lenses to both eyes

Step 20: Add 4 prism diopters base down in front of the right eye, and add 4 prism diopters base up in front of the left eye

Step 21: Display a single line of letters that is one to two lines above the best corrected visual acuity

Step 22: Ask the child if there are two images. If only one image is seen, stop the test. If two images are seen, proceed to the next step

Step 23: Provide these instructions "Which line of letters is clearer, the top, the bottom, or are they equally blurry?"

Step 24: If the top line is clearer, add +0.25 D sphere to the right eye. If the bottom line is clearer, add +0.25 D sphere to the left eye. If the lines are equally blurry, skip step 25 and proceed to step 26

Step 25: Repeat step 24 until no difference is reported

Step 26: Remove the prisms in front of both eyes

Step 27: Reduce the sphere in both eyes at the same time in 0.25 D steps until the best VA is obtained. The least plus to obtain the best VA is the end point

Clinical Pearl: *When performing JCC cylinder axis refinement, use the bracketing technique to minimize the number of presentations and maintain patient attention. When bracketing, the author recommends initially moving the axis by 10-15 degrees in the direction of the preferred axis. In the next presentation, move the axis 5-7 degrees in the direction of the preferred axis. Repeat these steps bracketing the axis by halving the degrees that are moved until both presentations are reported as equal or until the patient's choice is between a narrow range, and the axis in the middle of the range is chosen.*

Clinical Pearl: *The Prism Dissociation method is performed under binocular conditions and is preferred over the Successive Alternate Occlusion method.*

Clinical Pearl: *Subjective refraction performed in a phoropter has advantages over a trial frame because the phoropter provides the changing comparison of different lens quickly and easily to provide a prescription that offers optimal distance vision.*

Clinical Pearl: *Binocular balance is reserved for older children. For younger children, it can be difficult to obtain reliable responses on binocular balance. In these situations, use a more objective method to check if accommodation is the same in the two eyes, such as MEM retinoscopy or Nott's retinoscopy (See chapter on Accommodation).*

Clinical Pearl: *During subjective refraction, when the eye is over minused, the child will report the letter appearing darker and/or smaller but there is no improvement in measured distance visual acuity.*

Clinical Pearl: *While performing JCC cylinder axis refinement, a child's responses may go back and forth within a narrow range of axis locations. In this situation, select the axis in the middle of this range.*

Clinical Pearl: *When performing JCC power refinement, a child's responses may go back and forth within a narrow range of powers. In this situation, select the cylinder power in the middle of this range. Alternatively, remove the JCC and increase/decrease the cylinder power while asking the child to read the line of letters. The final astigmatic correction is the lowest cylinder lens that provides the best acuity.*

CONCLUSION

It is important to accurately determine the refractive error of a child during an eye exam. Depending on the age and maturity of the patient, the clinician can perform retinoscopy and subjective refraction to achieve quick and accurate refractive findings. Cycloplegic retinoscopy using a cycloplegic agent is especially useful to allow for a more accurate retinoscopy measurement in children with poor cooperation, poor fixation, strabismus, amblyopia, latent hyperopia and anisometropia. Early detection and diagnosis of visually significant refractive error can provide for prompt treatment and better prognosis.

REFERENCES

American Optometric Association. (2017). *Evidence-Based Clinical Practice Guideline Comprehensive Pediatric Eye and Vision Examination*. Author.

Bartolone, A., & Rutner, D. (2020). Quantification of Refractive Error. In P. Schnell, M. Taub, & R. H. Duckman (Eds.), *Visual Development, Diagnosis, and Treatment of the Pediatric Patient* (pp. 300–316). Wolters Kluwer.

Bausch & Lomb. (2019). *Tropicamide ophthalmic solution*. Retrieved on September 28, 2021, from https://www.bausch.com/Portals/77/-/m/BL/United%20States/Files/Package%20Inserts/Pharma/Rx-Generics/Tropicamide-package-insert.pdf?ver=2016-08-26-133847-873

Bausch & Lomb. (2021). *Cyclopentolate hydrochloride*. Retrieved on September 28, 2021, from https://www.bausch.com/Portals/77/-/m/BL/United%20States/Files/Package%20Inserts/Pharma/Rx-Generics/Cyclopentolate-Hydrochloride-Solution.pdf?ver=2016-09-13-101701-047

Borchert, M., Wang, Y., Tarczyy-Hornoch, K., Cotter, S., Deneen, J., Azen, S., & Varma, R.The Multi-Ethnic Pediatric Eye Disease Study Group. (2008). Testability of the Retinomax Autorefractor and IOL Master in preschool children. *Ophthalmology*, *115*(8), 1422–1425. doi:10.1016/j.ophtha.2007.10.036 PMID:18164067

Frazier, M., & Jaanus, S. D. (2008). Cycloplegic Refraction. In Clinical Ocular Pharmacology 5th Edition (pp.133). Butterworth Heinmann Elsevier.

Good-lite. (2021). *Retinoscopy paddles with axis compass*. Retrieved on September 28, 2021, from https://www.good-lite.com/products/506600

Iuorno, J., Grant, W., & Noel, L. P. (2004). Clinical Comparison of the Welch Allyn SureSight Handheld Autorefractor Versus Cycloplegic Autorefraction and Retinoscopic Refraction. *Journal of AAPOS*, *8*(2), 123–127. doi:10.1016/j.jaapos.2003.10.006 PMID:15088044

Kauser, F., Gupta, Y., Amitava, A., Saxena, J., Raza, S., & Masood, A. (2020). Do all children need a cycloplegic refraction? A comparison of Mohindra's versus cycloplegic refraction. *Indian Journal of Ophthalmology*, *68*(11), 2458. doi:10.4103/ijo.IJO_229_20 PMID:33120640

Leat, S. J. (2009). Paediatric Assessment. In Optometry: Science, Techniques and Clinical Management (pp. 451-453). Butterworth Heinemann.

McCullough, S. J., Doyle, L., & Saunders, K. J. (2017). Intra- and inter- examiner repeatability of cycloplegic retinoscopy among young children. *Ophthalmic & Physiological Optics*, *37*(1), 16–23. doi:10.1111/opo.12341 PMID:28030881

National Eye Institute. (2020). *Refractive Error*. Retrieved on September 28, 2021 from https://www.nei.nih.gov/learn-about-eye-health/eye-conditions-and-diseases/refractive-errors

Retinomax Autorefractor. (n.d.). http://www.righton-oph.com/en/product/objective/

Saunders, K. J., & Westall, C. A. (1992). Comparison between near retinoscopy and cycloplegic retinoscopy in the refraction of infants and children. *Optometry and Vision Science, 69*(8), 615–622. doi:10.1097/00006324-199208000-00004 PMID:1513557

System Vision. (n.d.). *PlusoptiX A12R & A12C.* Retrieved on September 28, 2021, from http://www.systemvision.eu/plusoptix-a12c-a12r.html

Welch Allyn. (2018). *Spot® Vision Screener-Autorefractor*. Retrieved on September 28, 2021, from https://www.hillrom.com/en/products/spot-vision-screener-autorefractor/

Wickum, S. M., & Amos, J. F. (2008). Cycloplegic Refraction. In Clinical Ocular Pharmacology 5th Edition (pp.344-346). Butterworth Heinmann Elsevier. doi:10.1016/B978-0-7506-7576-5.50026-4

ADDITIONAL READING

Ciuffreda, K. J., & Rosenfield, M. (2015). Evaluation of the SVOne: A Handheld, Smartphone-Based Autorefractor. *Optometry and Vision Science, 92*(12), 1133–1139. doi:10.1097/OPX.0000000000000726 PMID:26540478

Harvey, E. M., Dobson, V., Miller, J. M., Clifford-Donaldson, C. E., Green, T. K., Messer, D. H., & Garvey, K. A. (2009). Accuracy of the Welch Allyn Suresight for measurement of magnitude of astigmatism in 3- to 7-year-old children. *AAPOS, 13*(5), 466–471. doi:10.1016/j.jaapos.2009.08.013 PMID:19840726

Peterseim, M. M. W., Papa, C. E., Wilson, M. E., Davidson, J. D., Shtessel, M., Hasair, M., Cheesemar, E. W., Wolf, B. J., & Trivedi, R. (2014). The effectiveness of the Spot Vision Screener in detecting amblyopia risk factors. *Journal of AAPOS, 18*(6), 539–542. doi:10.1016/j.jaapos.2014.07.176 PMID:25498463

Rosenfield, M., & Cuiffreda, K. (2017). Evaluation of the SVOne Handheld Autorefractor in a Pediatric Population. *Optometry and Vision Science, 94*(2), 159–165. doi:10.1097/OPX.0000000000000999 PMID:27668640

Rosenfield, M., & Logan, N. (Eds.). (2009). *Optometry: Science, Techniques and Clinical Management* (2nd ed.). Heinemann.

Vricella, M., FitzGerald, D. E., & Krumholtz, I. (2002). Effectiveness of the Welch Allyn SureSight Autorefractor as a Screening Tool in a sample of children aged 3-69 months. *Journal of Behavioral Optometry, 13*, 123–125.

KEY TERMS AND DEFINITIONS

Astigmatism: A refractive error where the eye is not spherical due to an irregular cornea of curvature of the lens.

Binocular Balance: Is a subjective technique used to ensure the two eyes are accommodating equally when determining the final refraction.

Cycloplegic Retinoscopy: A technique to measure the refractive state of an eye while controlling accommodation with a cycloplegic eye drop.

Hyperopia: A refractive error where the eye is shorter and light rays focus behind the retina.

Jackson Cross Cylinder (JCC): Is a tool that is used to refine the axis and power of astigmatism.

Mohindra Retinoscopy: A near retinoscopy technique that provides a distance value.

Myopia: A refractive error where the eye is elongated, and light rays focus in front of the retina.

Objective Retinoscopy: A technique to measure the refractive state of an eye without the need for responses from the patient.

Phoropter: An instrument that a patient sits behind which allows the examiner quick access to changing of lenses all incorporated in the instrument.

Subjective Refraction: A technique to measure the refractive state of an eye with responses from the patient.

Chapter 9
Binocular Examination in Children

Surbhi Bansal
Stanford University, USA

Ruth Y. Shoge
University of California, Berkeley, USA

Siva Meiyeppen
Pennsylvania College of Optometry, Salus University, USA

ABSTRACT

This chapter introduces the reader to tests commonly performed in a binocular vision examination to determine a child's binocular status. The testings introduced in this chapter are all chairside techniques that do not involve a significant amount of extra equipment or time. The binocular examination consists of determining the ocular position and then accommodation, vergence, and ocular motor statuses. The ocular position consists of determining where the eyes point in space and if they are correctly aligned. Evaluation of ocular alignment and the ability to move the eyes with coordination can be determined with various techniques, including Hirschberg, Krimsky, cover test, as well as Modified Thorington, motor testing, and vergence ranges. This chapter will familiarize the clinician with the basics of binocular vision testing and improve the reader's comfort with the various elements of the binocular vision examination.

INTRODUCTION

This chapter introduces the reader to tests commonly performed in a binocular vision examination, including various techniques the clinician can use to determine a child's binocular status. The testing introduced in this chapter are all chairside techniques that do not involve a significant amount of extra equipment or time intensive elements. Therefore, they can be easily included into the clinician's eye examination. The objectives of this chapter are to familiarize the clinician with the basics of binocular vision testing and to improve the reader's comfort with this testing.

DOI: 10.4018/978-1-7998-8044-8.ch009

BACKGROUND

Most patients will benefit from a thorough binocular vision evaluation, which should be performed after the correct determination of the child's refractive error. The binocular examination consists of determining the ocular position, and then accommodation, vergence, and ocular motor statuses. The ocular position consists of determining where the eyes point in space, and if they are correctly aligned. Ocular alignment can be determined with various techniques, including Hirschberg, Krimsky, cover test, as well as Modified Thorington. Motor testing, or the evaluation of the ability to move the eyes with coordination, can be determined with vergence assessment. Vergences can be performed in phoropter with Risley prisms or out of phoropter in free space with prism bars. This chapter will familiarize the reader with the various elements of the binocular vision examination.

HIRSCHBERG TEST

Indication

The Hirschberg test allows for an estimated objective assessment of ocular alignment. It is very useful in infants, toddlers, and children with developmental delays. It determines the presence of strabismus, as well as the direction, laterality, frequency, and magnitude of the deviation.

Background

The Hirschberg test estimates the amount of strabismus present based on the first Purkinje image. That is, the decentration of the corneal light reflex produced by a light source (e.g., a transilluminator) in the deviating eye compared to the corneal light reflex of the fixating eye. An equal or symmetrical corneal light reflex indicates alignment. An asymmetric Hirschberg reflex is confirmed by occluding each eye separately to determine the fixating eye and assessing angle kappa. Angle kappa (angle lambda) is the angle between the visual line and the pupillary axis. A positive angle kappa (displacement toward the nose indicated by a "+" sign) of up to 5 degrees can be physiologic. This slightly decentered reflex nasally is often noted as +0.5 mm. A negative angle kappa is when the reflex is displaced temporally and is recorded with a "-" sign. A positive angle kappa may mask a small angle esotropia or cause pseudoexotropia, whereas a negative angle kappa may simulate esotropia or mask exotropia. A 1 mm displacement is approximately 22 prism diopters (Δ) in misalignment (Caloroso, EE and Rouse MW, 1993). The position of the corneal light reflex indicates the type of deviation (Table 1).

Table 1a. Position of corneal light reflex and type of deviation

Position of Corneal Light Reflex	Type of Deviation
Nasal	Exo
Temporal	Eso
Above	Hypo
Below	Hyper

Table 1b.

	OD	OS
Hirschberg test (binocular)	+0.5 mm	–2.5 mm
Kappa test (monocular)	+0.5 mm	+0.5 mm
Total deviation		–3.00 mm = 66 Δ

Table 1c.

	OD	OS
Hirschberg test (binocular)	+2.5 mm	+0.5 mm
Kappa test (monocular)	+0.5 mm	+0.5 mm
Total deviation	+2.00 mm = 44 Δ	

Advantages

The advantages of Hirschberg are that it is a quick screening tool, provides an objective measure of binocular alignment, requires minimal attention and cooperation, and is especially useful for the infant, toddler, and special needs population.

Disadvantages

A disadvantage of Hirschberg is that it can only detect deviations 22 Δ or greater. Small angle deviations may be easily missed.

Equipment

1. Transilluminator
2. Occluder

Procedure

Step 1: The Hirschberg test can be performed with or without correction

Step 2: Room illumination is dim, however moderate room illumination may also be used for better reflex position observation

Step 3: The examiner holds a transilluminator approximately 50 cm away from the child, aimed directly at the bridge of the nose. Ask the child to fixate on the light

Step 4: A symmetric displacement of the reflexes indicates binocular alignment, and the test is complete. The patient does not have strabismus

Step 5: The examiner observes the location of the corneal light reflex in relation to the center of the pupils:

(+) = Nasal displacement

(–) = Temporal displacement

1 mm displacement ≈ 22 Δ

Step 6: If a deviation is observed with the patient viewing the fixation light binocularly, then the test can be repeated monocularly to establish angle kappa and to identify the deviated eye

Step 7: The fixating eye is the eye in which the corneal reflex location is the same on the Hirschberg and Kappa tests. The strabismic eye is the eye in which there is a difference (Figure 1, Figure 2, and Figure 3)

Figure 1. Left esotropia: A total of 3 mm displacement temporally indicates 66 prism diopters of esotropia in the left eye

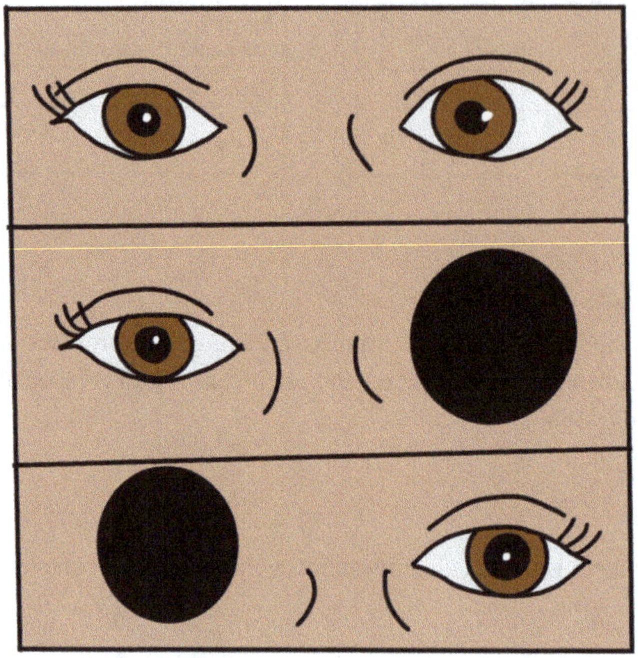

Figure 2. Right exotropia: A total of 2 mm displacement nasally indicates 44 prism diopters of exotropia in the right eye

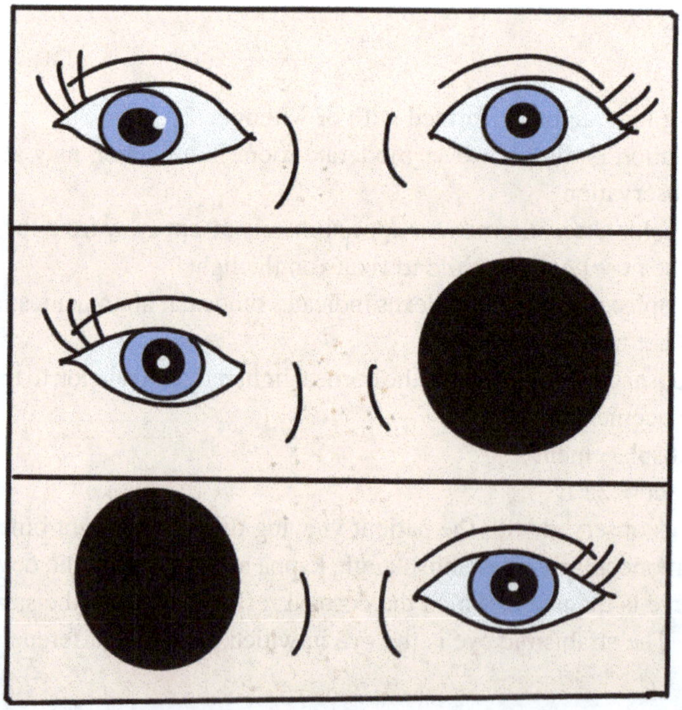

Figure 3. Hirschberg reflex seen nasally in the right eye (compared to left eye); this can indicate a right exo deviation

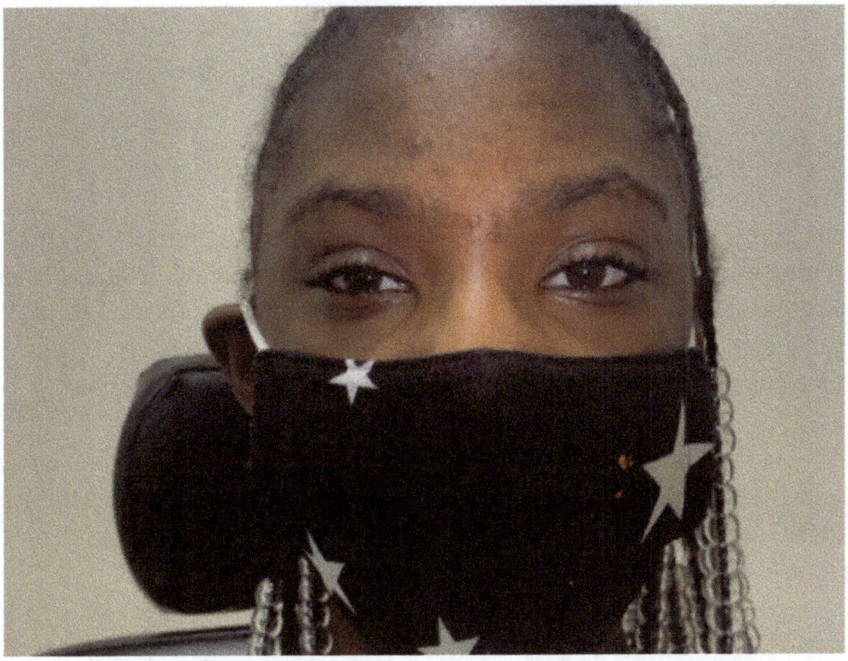

KRIMSKY TEST

Indication

The Krimsky test can be used to evaluate the ocular deviation when cover test cannot be accurately performed.

Background

The Krimsky test is based on the principle of Hering's law of equal innervation. It can improve the quantification of the Hirschberg test.

Advantages

Krimsky is a quick screening assessment of strabismic deviation on a young child, or a child where sustained attention and fixation are difficult.

Disadvantages

Varying results based on primary or secondary deviation if child has a non-comitant strabismus.

Equipment

1. Transilluminator
2. Prism Bar or Loose Prism

Procedure

Step 1: Perform the Hirschberg test

Step 2: Place increasing prism over the fixating eye until the corneal light reflex is centered on the pupil of the deviating eye (Figure 4) (von Noorden, GK and Campos, EC, 2002). Placing the neutralizing prism over the non-strabismic eye while the strabismic eye is fixating on the target gives the secondary angle of deviation

Step 3: Record the amount of prism from step 2. Note the eye and prism direction

Note: In another version of this test, placing the neutralizing prism over the strabismic eye while the non-strabismic eye is fixating on the target gives the primary angle of deviation. However, observation of the corneal reflection through prisms is difficult, which is why the preferred clinical procedure is outlined above (von Noorden, GK and Campos, EC, 2002).

Figure 4. The Krimsky test: increasing amounts of base-in prism is placed over the fixating right eye until the corneal light reflex is centered in the pupil of the deviating eye (left eye)

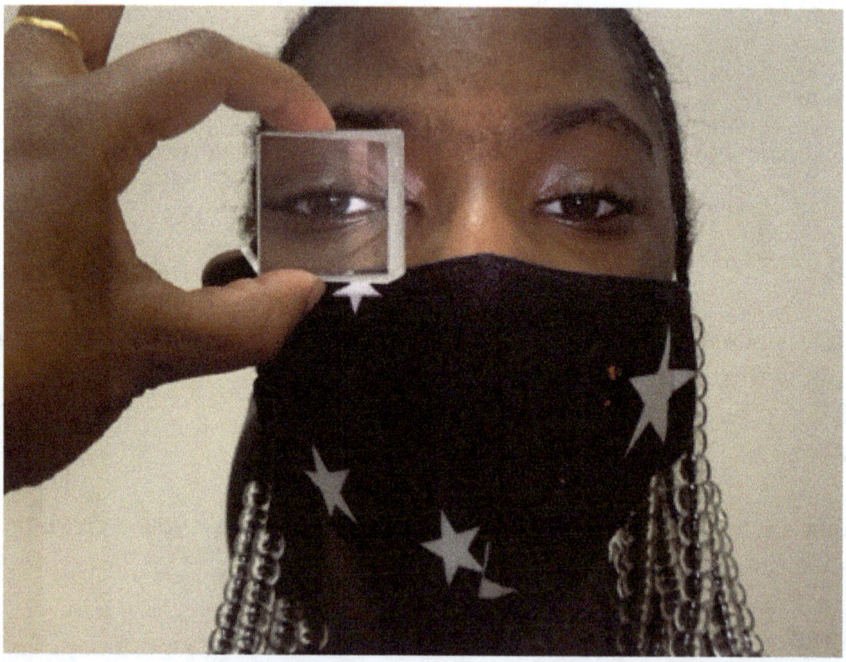

Clinical Pearl: *In non-comitant deviations where there is a paretic muscle, if the neutralizing prism is placed before the non-strabismic eye, with the strabismic eye fixating, the measured deviation (known as the secondary angle of deviation) is much larger than the primary angle of deviation. The explanation for this is due to Hering's law of equal innervation to yoked muscles. With the strabismic eye fixating and using the affected muscle, Hering's law of equal innervation will make the non-strabismic eye move in the same direction with increased force, resulting in a larger angle of deviation.*

BRUCKNER TEST

Indication

The Bruckner test can be used to evaluate binocular alignment in the infant/toddler population and rule out vision—and potentially life threatening—abnormalities (American Academy of Pediatrics, 2008). By comparing the relative brightness and color of the red reflex between the two eyes, the examiner can detect the presence of strabismus, anisometropia, anisocoria, media opacities, or posterior pole abnormalities (Subhi et al., 2021).

Background

The light from the direct ophthalmoscope is transmitted through all the transparent structures of the patient's eyes: tear film, cornea, aqueous humor, lens, and vitreous humor (Alhammouri et al., 2011). The light is reflected from the posterior segment of the eye and is transmitted back through the ocular media and the aperture of the direct ophthalmoscope to the examiner's eye (Alhammouri et al., 2011). If the two reflexes are equally bright, the child is fixating binocularly. An equally bright reflex of both eyes is an expected finding. In strabismus, the deviating eye will appear brighter, and the fixating eye will have a dimmer red reflex due to increased light absorption from stronger pigmentation in the foveal area (Alhammouri et al., 2011). It is important to note that an obstruction in the ocular media, or anisometropia can result in an abnormal red reflex. A cataract and vitreous hemorrhage may have a dark or dull reflex. Retinoblastoma will appear as a white or yellow reflex. Anisometropia will result in an asymmetrical red reflex. A white reflex (leukocoria) warrants an immediate referral.

Advantages

Bruckner is a quick screening tool and provides an objective assessment of a patient's binocular alignment, refractive error, and clarity of ocular media. The Bruckner reflex is easily observed in infants and toddlers and requires minimal patient attention and cooperation.

Disadvantages

The Bruckner test is an estimation test and does not replace a dilated fundus evaluation. The Bruckner reflex is less observable in older children and adults.

Equipment

1. Direct ophthalmoscope

Procedure

Step 1: The Bruckner test is performed on undilated or dilated pupils
Step 2: Dim the room illumination and stand approximately 100 cm (~3 feet) from the child
Step 3: Select the large spot beam of the direct ophthalmoscope. Aim the light at the bridge of the child's nose to illuminate both pupils simultaneously. Instruct the child to look at the light while the examiner looks through the direct ophthalmoscope
Step 4: Dial in the lens power in the direct ophthalmoscope that provides a clear view of the child's eyes and face (approximately +1.00 D to partially compensate for the working distance)
Step 5: Compare the relative brightness of the red reflexes to determine if there is strabismus, anisometropia, refractive errors, or ocular pathology
Step 6: The eye with the brighter reflex is presumed strabismic. The strabismic eye will appear brighter because of the fundus reflection emanating from outside of the pigmented macula region (Figure 5)
Step 7: The location of the crescents and the placement of the red- reflex can indicate the type of refractive error

1. Inferior crescents indicate myopia
2. Superior crescents indicate hyperopia
3. Decentered crescents indicate astigmatism

Figure 5. Left exotropia

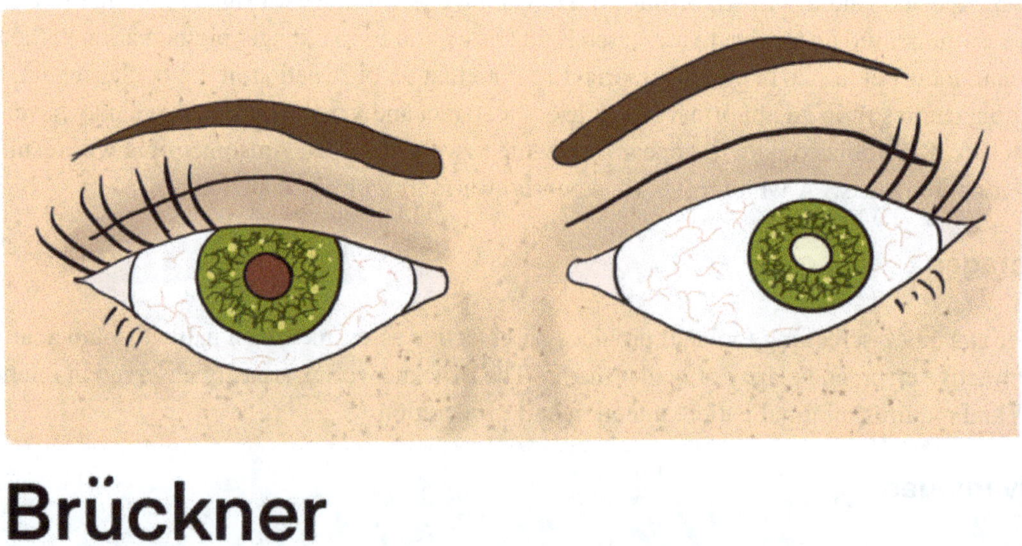

Expected Findings

Equally bright reflex in both eyes.

Clinical Pearl: *A false positive response may occur if there is anisocoria or media opacity. For example, with anisocoria, the eye with the larger pupil will appear brighter, and with media opacity, the affected eye will appear darker.*

Clinical Pearl: *Most young children have some degree of hyperopia, as their eyes are small and still growing. This makes the Bruckner test more useful for picking up myopic errors, but overall, the test is not very accurate for detection of refractive errors in undilated pupils since they can accommodate.*

COVER TEST

Indication

Cover test is used to evaluate the presence and magnitude of a heterophoria or a heterotropia (strabismus). The unilateral cover test (UCT) delineates a heterotropia from a heterophoria. In a heterotropia, the UCT determines the direction, frequency, laterality, and estimated magnitude of the deviation. The alternate cover test (ACT) measures the magnitude of the deviation and any latent component.

Background

The cover test is performed both at distance (6 meters) and at near (40 cm). The unilateral cover test is followed by the alternate cover test. The unilateral cover test determines the presence of a heterotropia. That is, under associated or binocular viewing conditions, the foveal line of sight of one eye fails to fixate on the object of interest. Following the unilateral cover test, the alternate cover test is performed to determine the magnitude of the heterophoria or heterotropia. The heterophoria represents the relative position of the eyes under dissociated viewing conditions. The alternating cover test will not differentiate a heterophoria from a heterotropia.

Advantages

This is the only test that differentiates between a heterotropia and heterophoria and objectively determines the magnitude, laterality, frequency, and direction of the heterotropia and heterophoria.

Disadvantages

This test requires the child to fixate on a target. It can be difficult to use in infants and toddlers who have short attention spans.

Equipment

1. Occluder
2. Distance fixation target(s)
3. Near fixation target(s)
4. Horizontal and vertical prism bars

Procedure

Unilateral Cover Test: Testing for Distance Heterotropia

Step 1: Child is wearing the appropriate habitual correction for the distance being tested
Step 2: Isolate a letter or target that is one line larger than the visual acuity in the poorer seeing eye
Step 3: Ensure adequate room illumination
Step 4: Instruct the child to look at the target and keep it clear
Step 5: Cover the right eye and observe the left eye for movement. If there is no movement, this indicates that the left eye is accurately fixating the target prior to occlusion
Step 6: Remove the occluder and allow a sufficient time for the eye to re-establish fixation
Step 7: Cover the left eye while observing the right eye
Step 8: Any movement of the unoccluded eye will indicate the presence of strabismus (Figure 6)
Step 9: Repeat a few times to confirm your observation (Table 2)
Step 10: If there is movement in both eyes, the patient has alternating tropia
Step 11: Repeat the same steps for testing of near heterotropia with a near target (one line larger than the visual acuity of the poorer eye) or a modified fixation target using colorful, detailed stickers for younger children

It is also important to note upon removal of the cover, the eye that was behind the occluder may take up fixation again. As illustrated in Figure 7, when the cover is removed from the right eye, the right eye resumes fixation while the left eye returns to its strabismic position, this is a unilateral strabismus. If the left eye continues to fixate on the target and the right eye remains in a strabismic position upon removal of the paddle, then this is an alternating strabismus. In an alternating strabismus, either eye may individually fixate the target, as illustrated in Figure 8.

In both figures 7 and 8, the child presented with the left eye turned inward. Figure 7 demonstrates a unilateral esotropia and Figure 8 demonstrates an alternating esotropia. By repeating the test several times, the clinician can determine the frequency of the deviation (intermittent or constant).

Clinical Pearl: *For a child with very reduced acuities, such as an uncorrected high myope, cover testing should be performed with the refractive correction in place.*

Clinical Pearl: *When performing cover testing on a child with strabismus and eccentric fixation, be aware a non-foveal point is used to fixate on the target, which can affect the interpretation of the cover test.*

Clinical Pearl: *The Intermittent Exotropia Control Scale, from 0 to 5, can be used to evaluate and monitor the level of control in children with intermittent exotropia (Mohney and Holmes, 2006).*

Figure 6. Classification of Strabismus

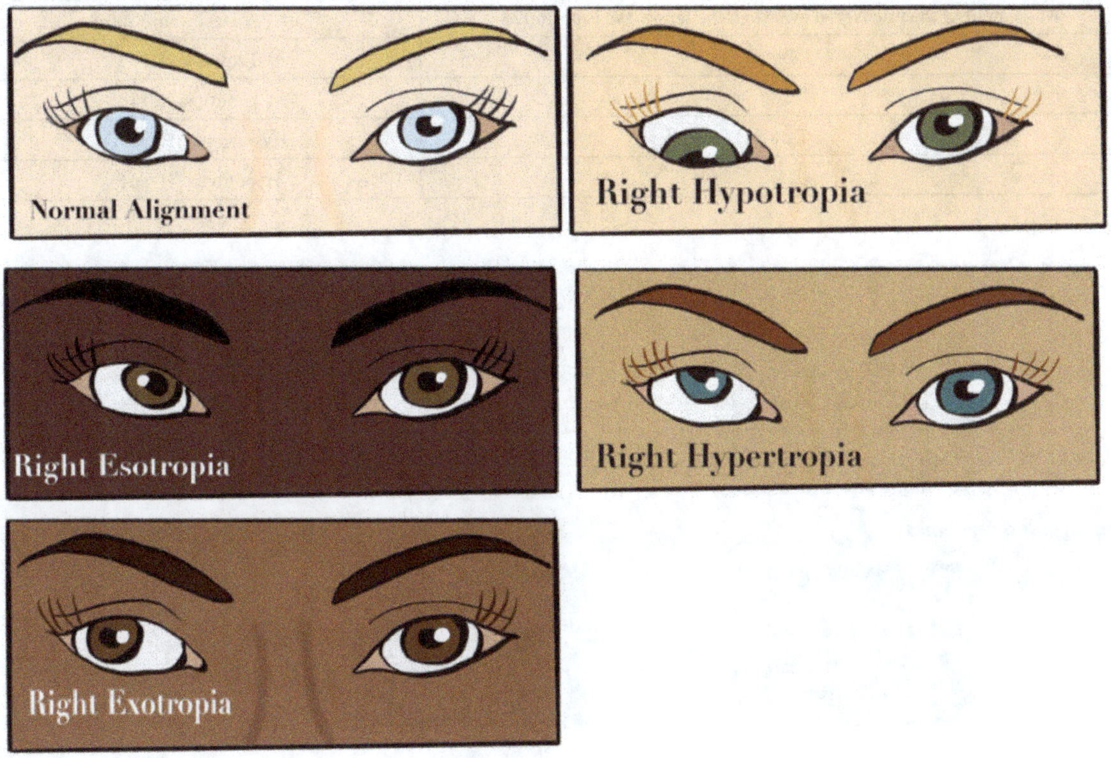

Figure 7. Constant left esotropia

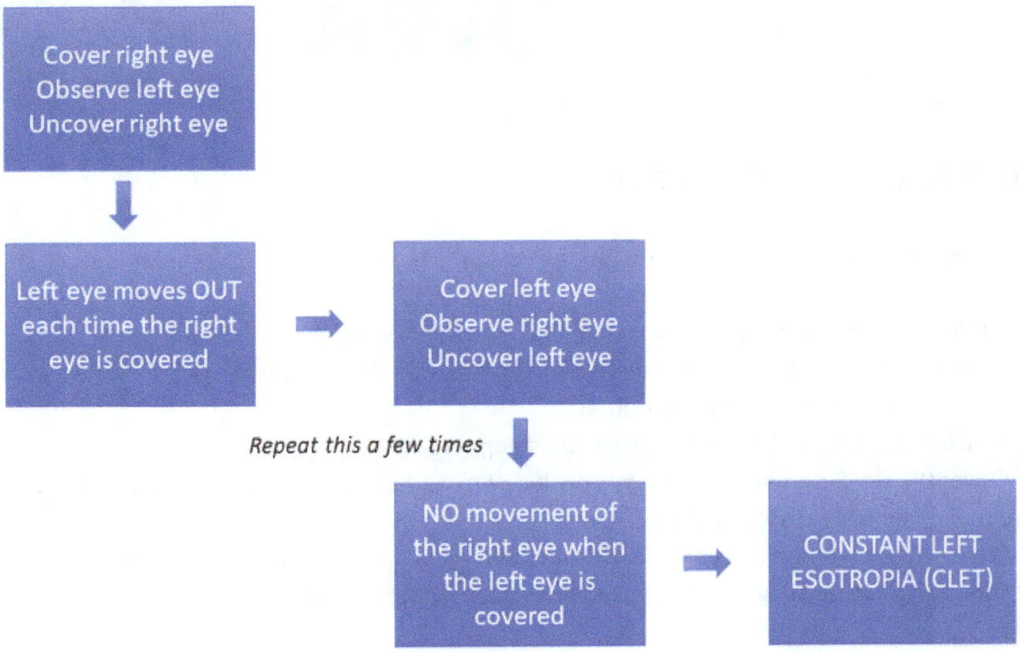

Table 2. Classification of heterotropia

Movement of the uncovered eye when the fellow eye is occluded	Deviation
Out	Esotropia (ET)
In	Exotropia (XT)
Down	Hypertropia (HyperT)
Up	Hypotropia (HypoT)

Figure 8. Constant alternating esotropia

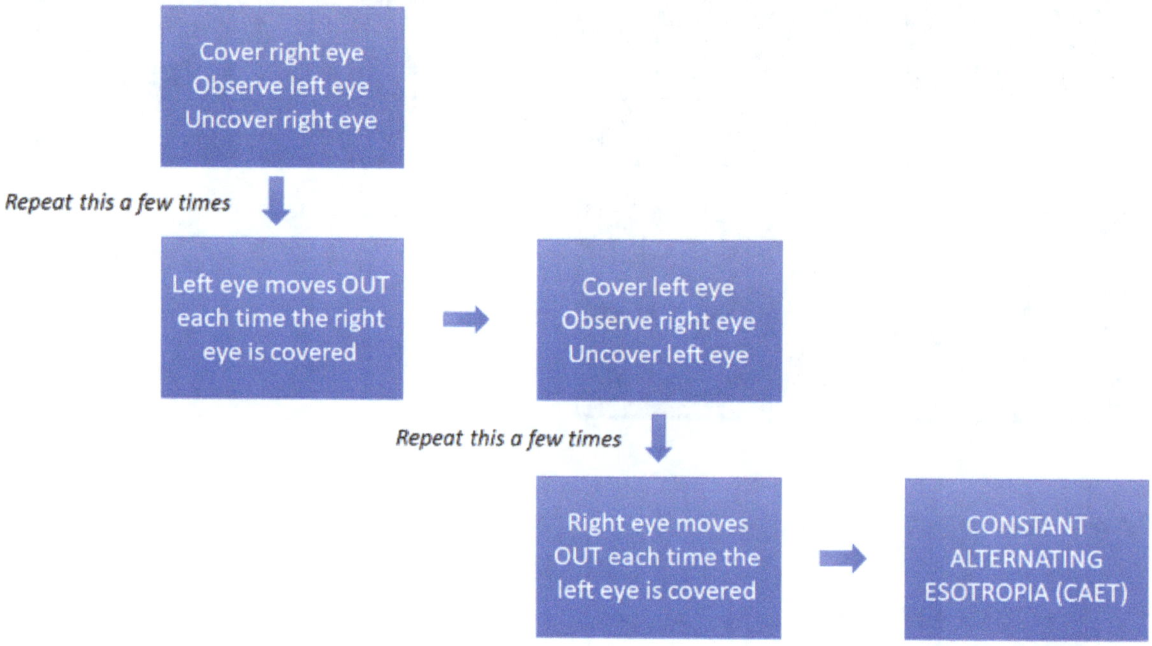

ALTERNATE COVER TEST (ACT)

Perform after the unilateral cover test: Testing for distance heterophoria

Step 1: Child is wearing the appropriate habitual correction for the distance being tested
Step 2: Isolate a letter or target that is one line larger than the visual acuity in the poorer seeing eye
Step 3: Ensure adequate room illumination
Step 4: Instruct the child to look at the target and keep it clear
Step 5: Cover the right eye and leave the eye occluded for at least 3-5 seconds. This will allow the right eye to deviate to its dissociated position
Step 6: Observe the ***right eye on removal of the occluder*** as it is placed over the left eye. Any movement of this eye to regain fixation indicates the presence of heterophoria

Step 7: Occlude the left eye for at least 3-5 seconds. This will allow the left eye to deviate to its deviated position

Step 8: Observe the ***left eye on removal of the occluder*** as it is placed over the right eye

Step 9: Repeat steps 5 through 9 several times or until you have confirmed the direction of movement (Table 3)

Step 10: A prism bar or loose prism can be used to neutralize the magnitude of the movement observed using alternate cover test (Figure 9 and Figure 10)

Step 11: The amount of prism recorded with the alternate cover test (Table 4) is the amount of both the manifest and latent deviation. To neutralize the magnitude of a heterotropia with the alternate cover test, assess both the primary deviation (non-strabismic eye fixating) and secondary deviation (strabismic eye fixating)

Step 12: Repeat the same steps for testing of near heterophoria with a near target (one line larger than the visual acuity of the poorer eye). For infants and toddlers, targets such as stickers and colorful objects can be used as fixation targets (Figure 11)

Table 3. Classification of heterophoria

Movement of the eye following removal of the occluder	Deviation
Out	Esophoria (EP)
In	Exophoria (XP)
Down	Hyperphoria (HyperP)
Up	Hypophoria (HypoP)

Figure 9. Alternate cover test (ACT) and prism neutralization for exophoria

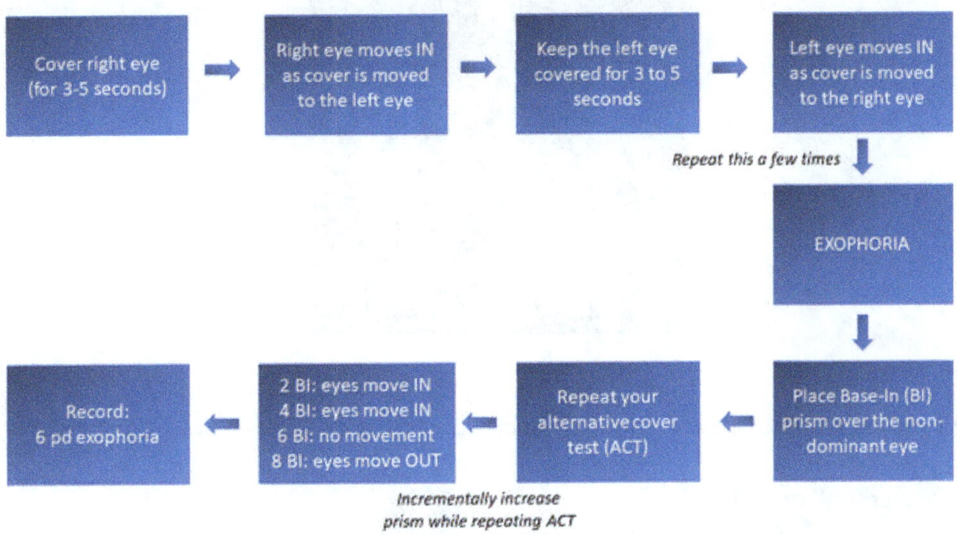

Figure 10. Alternate cover test (ACT) and prism neutralization for esophoria

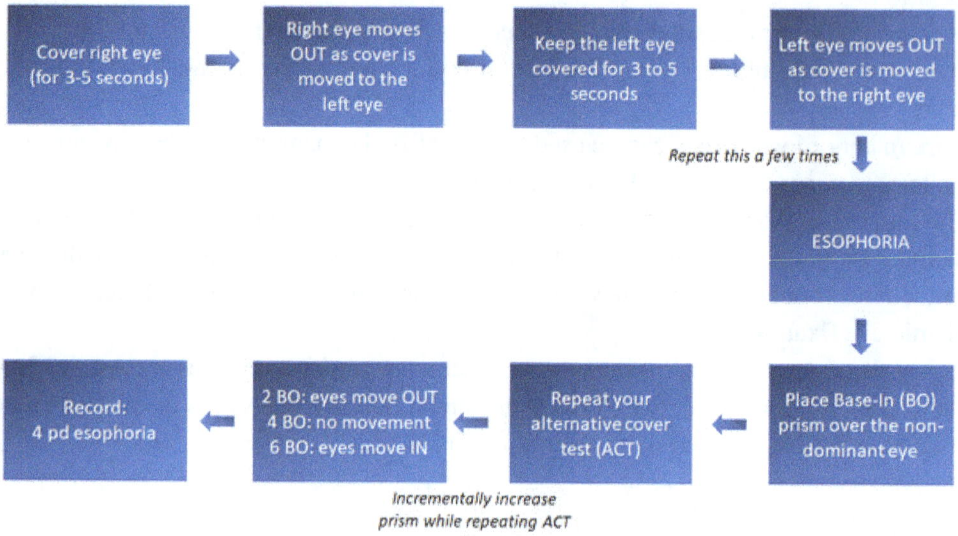

Figure 11. Fixation targets for cover test

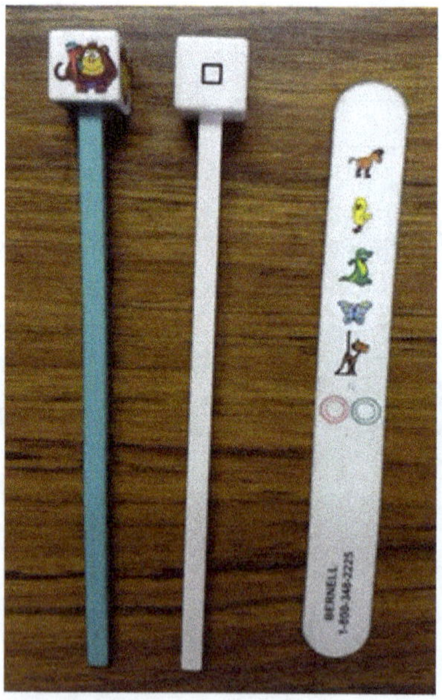

Recording Findings (abbreviations may vary among clinicians)

1. Write "cover test" or "CT"
2. Record CT findings for distance (DCT) and near (NCT)

3. If a heterotropia is present, record the type of deviation (e.g., esotropia), magnitude (amount), the laterality (left, right, or alternating) and the frequency (constant or intermittent). For example, 20^ CLET (20 prism diopters constant left esotropia).
4. If a heterophoria is present, just record esophoria (EP) or exophoria (XP); record orthophoria if there is no presence of a heterophoria.
5. For vertical deviation, indicate right or left vertical phoria (right hyper, right hypo, left hyper or left hypo). The term hypertropia is reserved for unilateral upward deviating tropias.

Expected Findings

At distance: 1 exophoria ± 2 pd
At near: 3 exophoria ± 3 pd

SUBJECTIVE COVER TEST

While performing the ACT, and heterophoria is present, the child may report an apparent *jump* in the fixation object when the cover is removed. In the case of exophoria, the child will report the target moving in the same direction as the movement of the occluder. Conversely in the case of esophoria, the child will report the target moving in the opposite direction as the movement of the occluder. Similarly, for a right hyper, the child will report a downward movement of the target and for a left hyper, the child will report an upward movement of the target as the occluder is moved from the child's right eye to the left eye. The subjective movement of the fixation target can occur when cover test is performed at distance and at near.

NEAR POINT OF CONVERGENCE

Indication

The near point of convergence (NPC) is used to determine the magnitude of convergence amplitude.

Background

The near point of convergence (NPC) is used to diagnose a vergence dysfunction. It is one of the hallmark findings in diagnosing Convergence Insufficiency. This test uses both an accommodative target and a non-accommodative target (transilluminator with red/green glasses). The benefit of an accommodative target is that it combines fusional and accommodative convergence, whereas a transilluminator does not include accommodative convergence. This test can be repeated to assess for stamina of convergence amplitude.

Advantages

NPC is an easy, quick and low-cost test. Normative data is available.

Disadvantages

Poor attention to the target can underestimate the patient's true convergence amplitude.

Equipment

1. Near accommodative target (e.g., isolated 20/50 target on Gulden fixation stick)
2. Penlight or transilluminator
3. Red/green glasses
4. Measuring tape/ruler

Procedure

Step 1: Patient must wear habitual correction for near work
Step 2: Starting at 40 cm, slowly bring the target toward the patient and remind them to keep the target single for as long as possible (Figure 12)

Clinical Pearl: *To obtain a true measure of NPC, the examiner should use an accommodative target, remind the child to maintain fusion, and encourage the child to regain fusion when diplopia is observed.*

Step 3: Ask the child to report when the target breaks into two (subjective break of NPC) or if you observe one or both eyes drifting out (objective break of NPC), record which eye(s) deviated and in which direction

Clinical Pearl: *Some children will never report diplopia due to suppression of one eye.*

Step 4: Then move the target away from the child's eyes and record the distance at which the two images fuse into one (subjective recovery) or the distance at which the deviated eye(s) regained fixation (objective recovery)
Step 5: NPC should be measured from the outer canthus of the eye which approximates the plane of the center of rotation of the eye
Step 6: Repeat testing three times or more if you want to test for fatigue factors and the ability to sustain convergence.
Step 7: Record break and recovery with the appropriate measurement scale (e.g., cm, mm, inches). If the patient can converge up to the nose, record "TTN" (to the nose). Indicate whether it's a subjective or objective result
Step 8: If the near point of convergence is normal with an accommodative target but convergence insufficiency is suspected, repeat testing under dissociated conditions (using red/green glasses and transilluminator) to eliminate the accommodative component
Step 9: If the NPC is receded, and you suspect an accommodative problem (rather than a convergence problem), place +1.00 lenses over each eye and repeat testing with an accommodative target

1. If the NPC findings improve, your patient has a pseudo-convergence insufficiency (that is, they have an underlying accommodative dysfunction)

2. If the findings remain the same or worsen, your patient may have a true convergence insufficiency

Expected Findings

With an Accommodative target: 2.5 cm break (+/- 2.5 cm) /4.5 cm recovery (+/-3.0 cm)
With Penlight and Red/Green Glasses: 2.5 cm break (+/- 4.0 cm)/4.5 cm recovery (+/-5.0 cm)

Table 4. Prism base direction used to neutralize various heterophorias on alternating cover test

Deviation	Base Direction
Eso	Base Out
Exo	Base In
Hyper	Base Down
Hypo	Base Up

Figure 12. Measuring near point of convergence

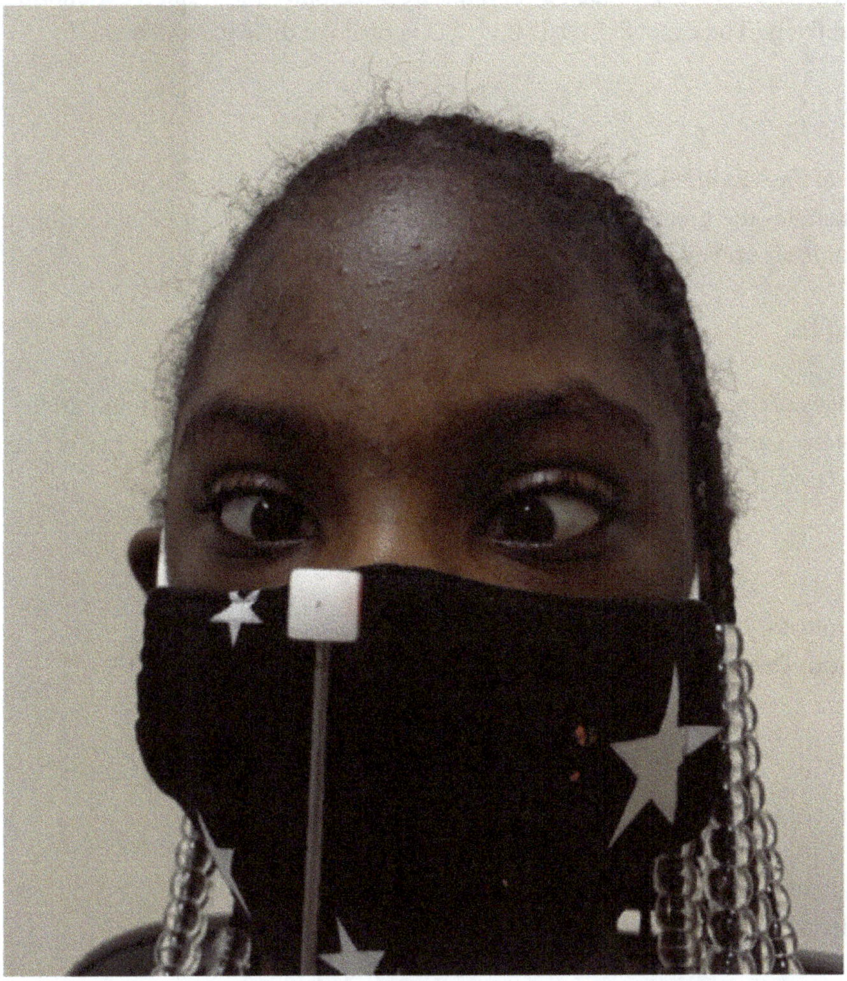

MODIFIED THORINGTON (MT)

Indication

Modified Thorington (MT) is used as an alternative subjective method to determine the presence, direction, and magnitude of a horizontal and vertical phoria.

Background

The Modified Thorington test is used to measure a subjective phoria at distance and near. The test uses the Maddox rod which is a series of high-powered cylinders aligned in parallel. When placed over one eye and fixating on a light source, the Maddox rod forms a streak perpendicular to the cylinders. This results in the patient seeing two dissimilar objects: 1) a spot of light and 2) a streak perpendicular to the lines on the Maddox Rod.

MT is performed through the child's habitual correction. The near lateral phoria can be re-measured through a +1.00 lens to determine the accommodative-convergence/accommodation (AC/A) ratio. In addition, the phoria can be re-measured through lenses (e.g., prism lenses, near addition lenses) to determine the final prescription. The expected findings are 1 exophoria ± 1 and 3 exophoria ± 3 at distance and near, respectively. The expected vertical phoria is ortho at distance and near.

Advantages

The advantage of the Modified Thorington test is that it does not require the phoropter. It is a free space test that demonstrates the greatest repeatability of subjective tests to assess motor alignment. It is easy and fast to administer on young children.

Disadvantages

The disadvantages of the Modified Thorington test are that the clinician must remind the patient to keep the numbers on the Thorington card clear during the entire procedure. Also, some MT cards go up to 12 prism diopters only, limiting their use for higher deviations.

Equipment

1. Transilluminator or penlight
2. Maddox rod: Distance (3m) and near (40 cm) Thorington card (Figure 13)

Procedure

Distance Phoria (3m)

Step 1: The patient must wear their habitual correction at distance
Step 2: The Maddox rod is held over the patient's right eye

Step 3: When the grooves or lines on the Maddox Rod are oriented horizontally, the patient sees a vertical streak (Figure 14). This measures the lateral phoria. The horizontal numbers on the Thorington card are used to measure the lateral phoria

Step 4: When the grooves or lines on the Maddox rod are oriented vertically, the patient sees a horizontal streak (Figure 15). This measures the vertical phoria. The vertical numbers on the Thorington card are used to measure the vertical phoria

Step 5: Place the transilluminator behind the hole in the center of the card

Step 6: Instruct the patient to tell you where the streak is in relation to the light (Maddox rod over right eye) (Figure 16):

1. Streak is through the light source = orthophoria
2. Streak is to the right of the light source = eso
3. Streak is to the left of the light source = exo
4. Streak is above the light source = left hyper or right hypo
5. Streak is below the light source = right hyper or left hypo

* The patient will report opposite findings if the Maddox rod is over the left eye

Step 7: Instruct the patient to tell you which number the streak is going through

Step 8: Record the magnitude (number on Thorington card) and direction of phoria

Near Phoria (40 cm)

Step 1: Child wears habitual correction at near

Step 2: The Maddox rod is held over the child's right eye

Step 3: When the grooves or lines on the Maddox Rod are oriented horizontally, the child sees a vertical streak. This measures the lateral phoria. The horizontal numbers on the Thorington card are used to measure the lateral phoria

Step 4: When the grooves or lines on the Maddox rod are oriented vertically, the child sees a horizontal streak. This measures the vertical phoria. The vertical numbers on the Thorington card are used to measure the vertical phoria

Step 5: Place the transilluminator behind the hole in the center of the card

Step 6: Instruct the child to tell you where the streak is in relation to the light

1. Streak is through the light source = orthophoria
2. Streak is to the right of the light source = eso
3. Streak is to the left of the light source = exo
4. Streak is above the light source = left hyper or right hypo
5. Streak is below the light source = right hyper or left hypo

*The child will report opposite findings if the Maddox rod is over the left eye

Step 7: Instruct the child to tell you which number the streak is going through

Step 8: Record the magnitude (number on Thorington card) and direction of phoria

Step 9: To measure the accommodative-convergence/accommodation (AC/A) ratio, add +1.00 lenses to the near prescription and re- measure the horizontal phoria

Note: The difference in phoria with and without the +1.00 lenses at near is the AC/A ratio

Figure 13. There are two modified types of Modified Thorington card, one for distance and one for near

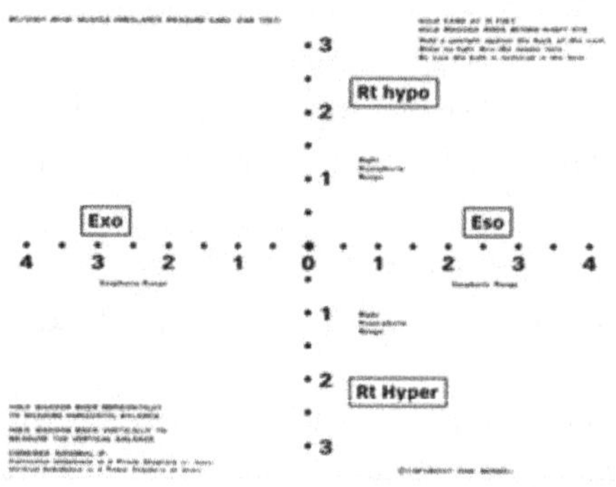

Distance card is held at 10 feet

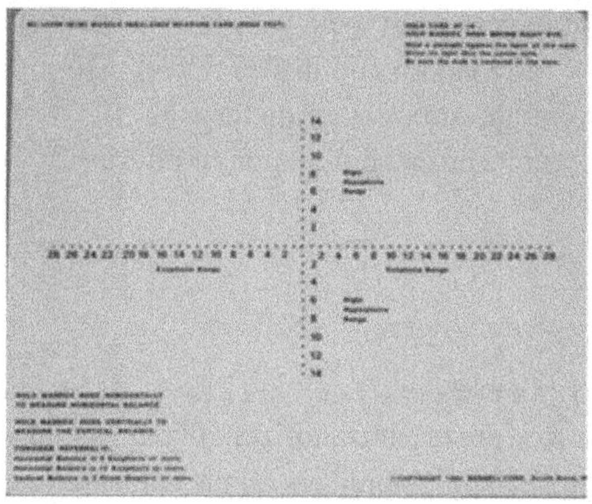

Near card is held at 16 inches

VON GRAEFE PHORIA

Indication

The Von Graefe phoria test is a subjective method to determine the presence, direction, and magnitude of a horizontal and vertical phoria.

Background

The Von Graefe phoria test is used to measure a subjective phoria at distance and near. It is performed in the phoropter through the patient's best corrected manifest refraction. The near lateral phoria can be re-measured through a +1.00 ADD to determine the accommodative-convergence/accommodation (AC/A) ratio. In addition, the phoria can be re-measured through lenses (e.g., prism, near addition lenses) to determine the final glasses prescription.

Figure 14. Horizontal Maddox Rod (patient sees vertical line)

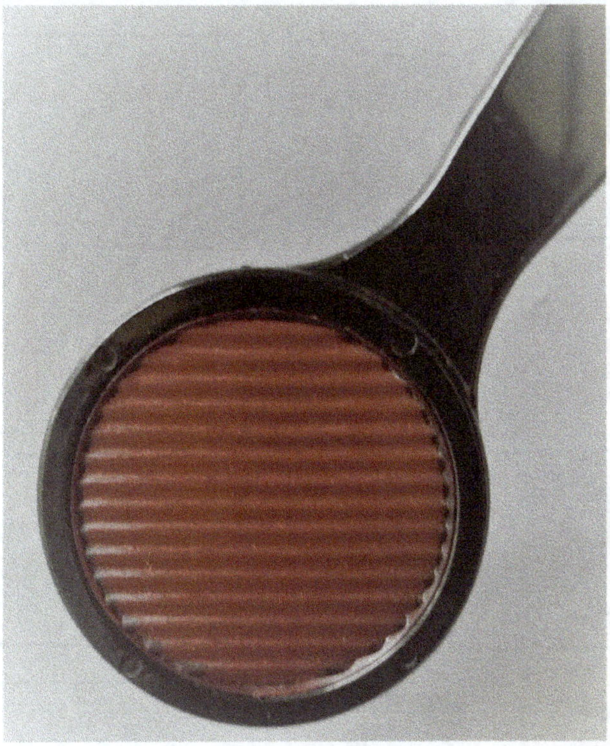

Figure 15. Vertical Maddox Rod (patient sees horizontal line)

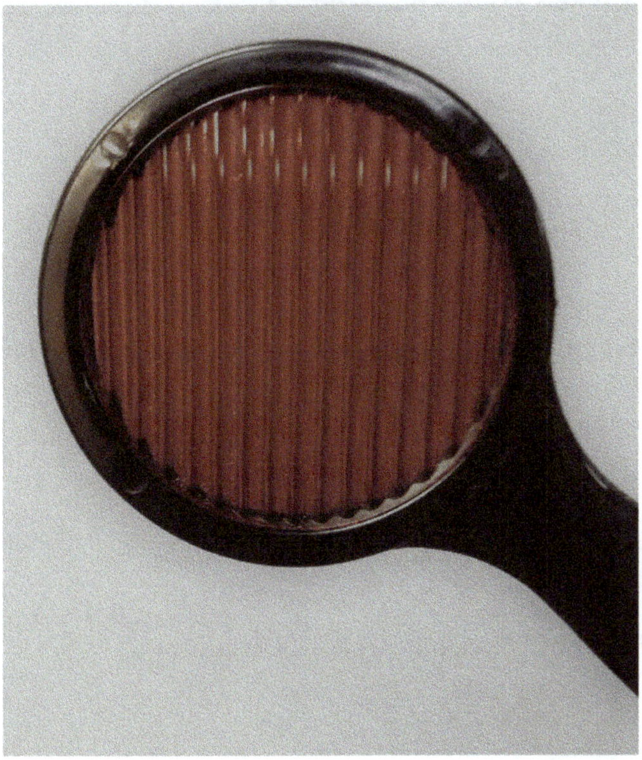

Figure 16. Image viewed by the patient with the Maddox rod test (Maddox rod over the right eye)

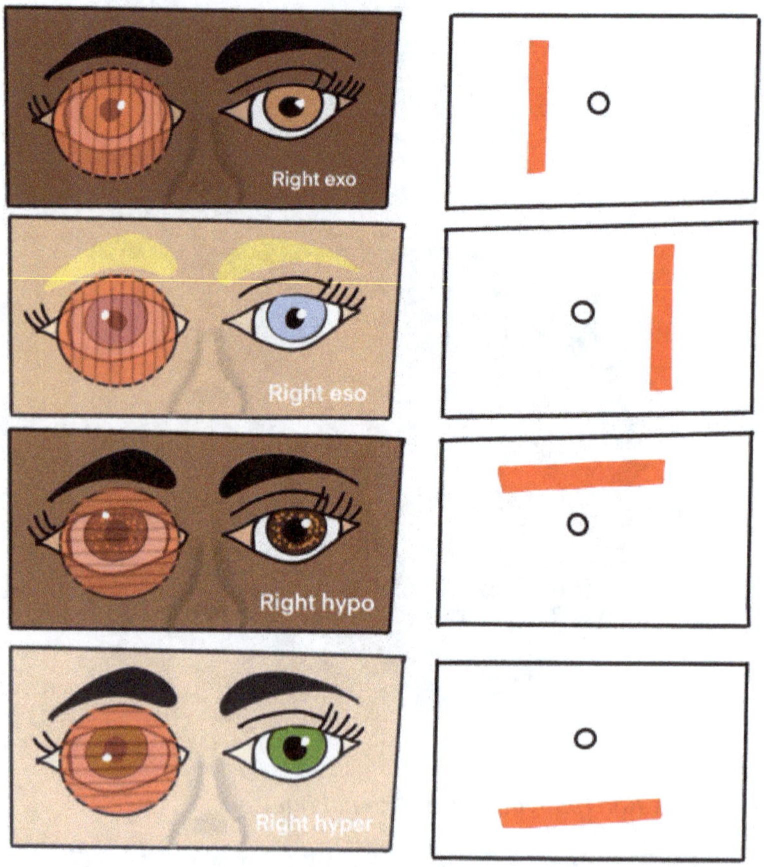

Advantages

There are standardized norms available for Von Graefe testing.

Disadvantages

The test is difficult to perform in younger children (<7 years). This test has low repeatability for measuring heterophoria.

Equipment

1. Phoropter (Risley prisms)
2. A distance acuity chart
3. Near point rod
4. Near point card with a small block of letters (~20/30 in size)

Procedure (Carlson NB and Kurtz D, 2004)

Distance Lateral Phoria

Step 1: Place child's distance correction in the phoropter
Step 2: Isolate a single letter one line larger than the best corrected visual acuity of the poorer eye
Step 3: Instruct child to close eyes
Step 4: Place the rotary Risley prisms in the phoropter before both eyes. Set the prism at 12 Δ base-in (BI) over the right eye and 6 Δ base-up (BU) over the left eye (Figure 17)

Clinical Pearl: *When measuring the lateral phoria, the 12 Δ BI is the measuring prism and the 6 Δ BU is the dissociating prism*

Figure 17: Phoropter set-up for von Graefe phoria (12 Δ BI and 6 Δ BU)

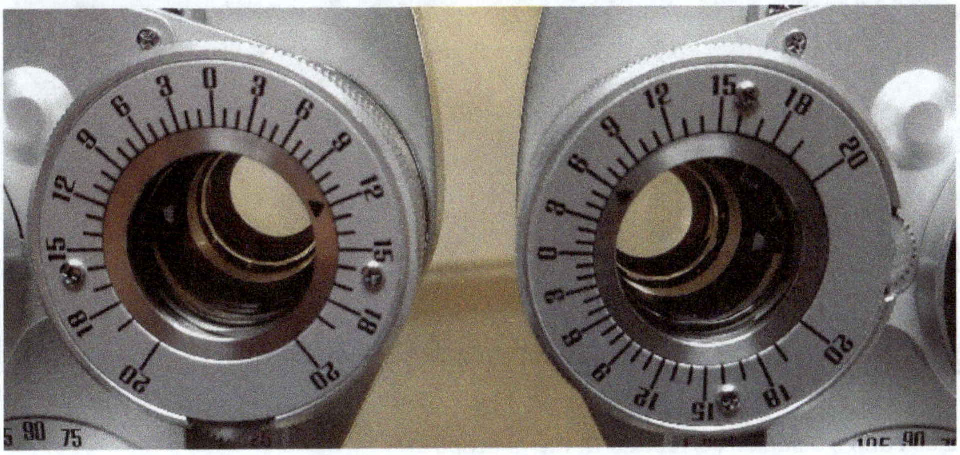

Step 5: Instruct the child to open eyes and ask them how many targets she/he sees and where they are in relation to one another

1. The response should be: "I see two targets, one up and to the right, one down and to the left"
2. If child does not see two targets, alternately occlude each eye to bring awareness to each target. If the patient continues to see one target, increase the amount of either prism
3. At this point child should see one image down and to the left and the other up and to the right

Step 6: Instruct child to look at the lower target and keep it clear while being aware of the upper target
Step 7: Inform child that the upper target will be moving. Ask child to tell you when the two targets are "lined up on top of each other, like buttons on a shirt"

Clinical Pearl: *Remind child to fixate on the stationary target while being aware of the moving target*

Step 8: Slowly reduce the base-in prism until child reports that the targets are vertically aligned, e.g., stopping at 3 Δ BI OD indicates 3 Δ exo deviation (Figure 18)

Expected Finding

The expected finding is 1 exophoria ± 2 at distance.

Clinical Pearl: *You can also overcorrect the phoria by advancing the measuring prism beyond the point of image alignment and re- measuring the phoria by rotating the prism in the opposite direction (the result will be the mean of the two values).*

Figure 18. Example of von Graefe lateral phoria testing endpoint of 3 Δ base-in = 3 Δ exo

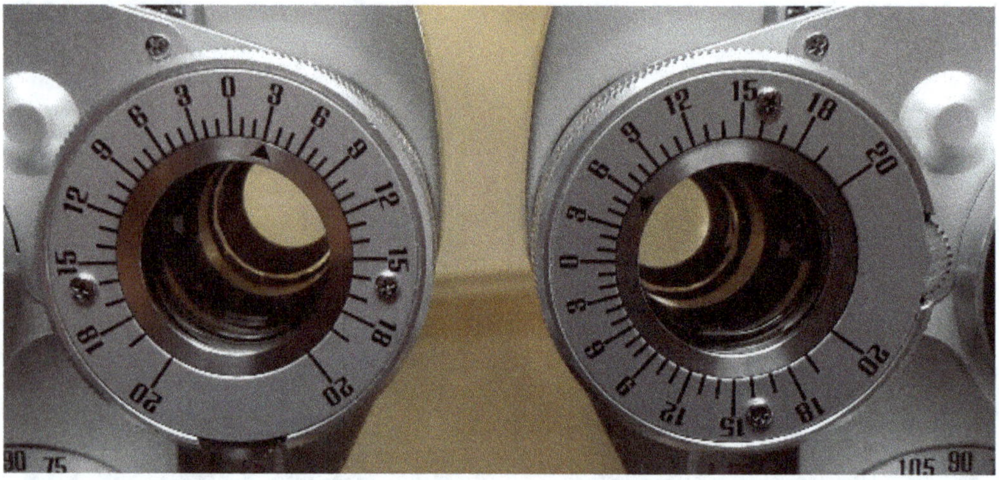

Distance Vertical Phoria

Step 1: Place child's distance correction in the phoropter
Step 2: Isolate a single letter one line larger than the best corrected visual acuity of the poorer eye
Step 3: Instruct child to close eyes
Step 4: Place the Risley prisms before both eyes. Introduce 12 Δ base-in (BI) over the right eye and 6 Δ base-up (BU) over the left eye
Step 5: When measuring the vertical phoria, the 12 Δ BI is the dissociating prism and the 6 Δ BU is the measuring prism
Step 6: Instruct child to open eyes and ask how many targets does she/he see and where they are in relation to one another

1. The response should be: "I see two targets, one up and to the right, one down and to the left"
2. If child does not see two targets, alternately occlude each eye to bring awareness to each target. If child continues to see one target, increase the amount of either prism by using the phoropter auxiliary lens knob

Step 7: Instruct child to look at the upper target and keep it clear while being aware of the lower target
Step 8: Inform child that the lower target will be moving. Ask child to tell you when the two targets are "lined up side by side, like headlights on a car"

Clinical Pearl: *Remind child to fixate on the stationary target while being aware of the moving target*

Step 9: Slowly reduce the base-up prism OS until child reports that the targets are horizontally aligned. This will be the amount needed to correct the hyper deviation, e.g., 2 Δ BU OS = 2 left hypo deviation or 2 right hyper deviation (Figure 19)

Figure 19. Example of von Graefe vertical phoria testing endpoint of 2 Δ base-up over the left eye = 2 Δ Right Hyper

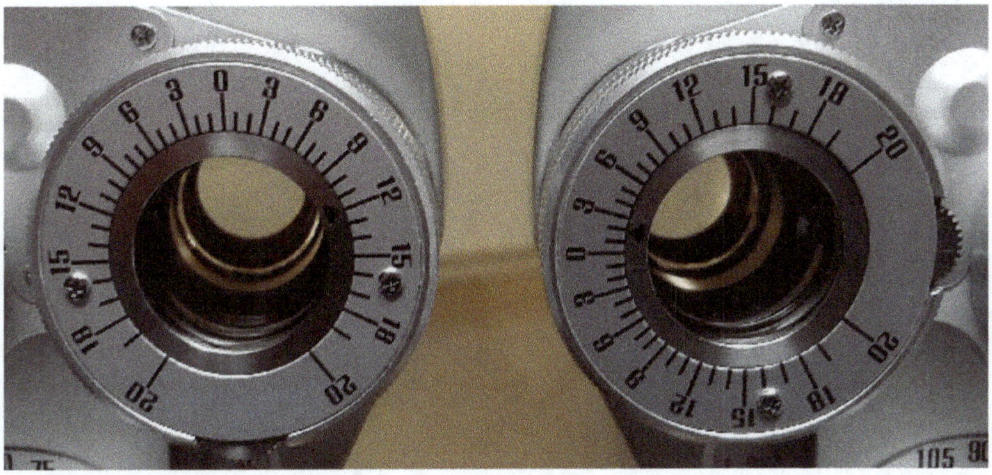

Expected Finding

The expected finding is ortho at distance.

Clinical Pearl: *You can also overcorrect the phoria by advancing the measuring prism beyond the point of image alignment and re- measuring the phoria by rotating the prism in the opposite direction (the result will be the mean of the two values).*

Near Lateral Phoria

Measuring the near deviations is similar to the distance deviations except for the change in fixation target. The near target should be a good stimulus of accommodation such as the 7x7 square of letters found on the phoropter near point card (Figure 20). A single letter or line target can also be used, as it is easier for patients to note separation. Place the best corrected visual acuity refraction for near in the phoropter and near pupillary distance (PD). The gradient AC/A ratio can be calculated by adding +1.00 over the patients near correction. The difference between the lateral phoria without +1.00 and with +1.00 is the AC/A ratio.

Expected Finding

The expected finding is 3 exophoria ± 3 pd at near.

Example

Lateral phoria: 4 exo
Lateral phoria with +1.00: 10 exo
AC/A: 6/1
Normal value: 4/1 ± 2

Figure 20. Fixation target for near lateral phoria and near vertical phoria

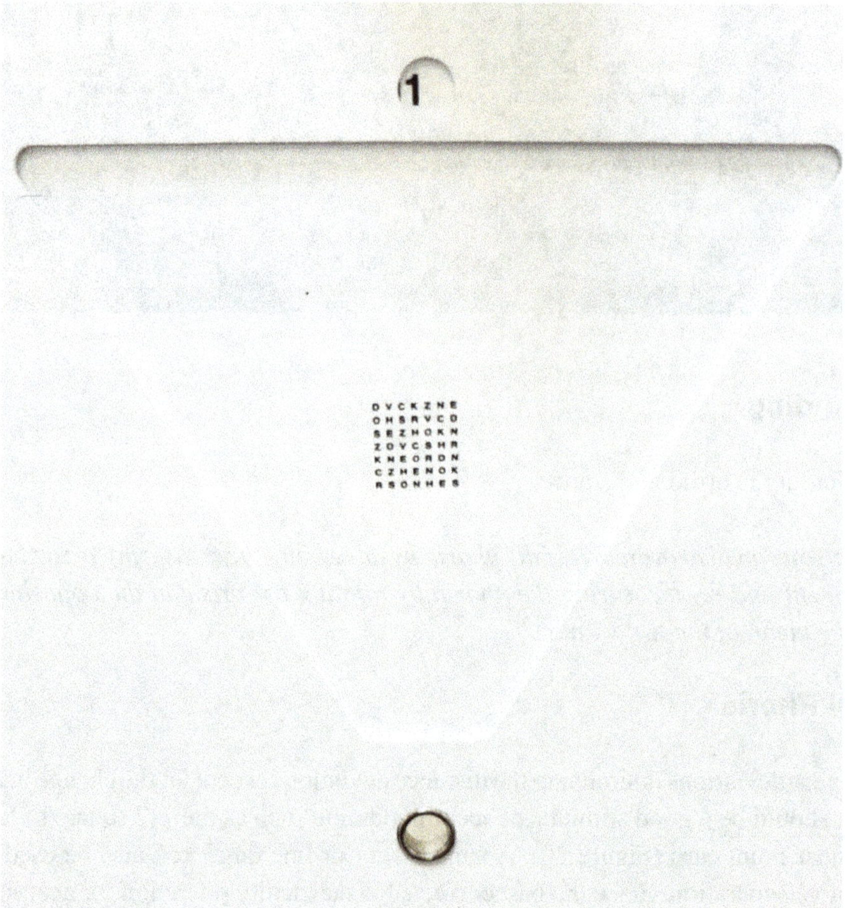

Near Vertical Phoria

Measuring the near deviations is similar to the distance deviations except for the change in fixation target. The near target should be a good stimulus of accommodation such as the 7x7 square of letters found on the phoropter near point card. A single letter or line target can also be used, as it is easier for patients to note separation. Place the best corrected visual acuity refraction for near in the phoropter and near pupillary distance (PD).

Expected Finding

The expected vertical phoria is ortho at near.

Clinical Pearl: *Measurement of near deviation should be done with the habitual working distance rather than the standard 40 cm and with the habitual near correction especially with symptomatic patients where their symptoms relate to their visual demand, e.g., tablet and phone use.*

FUSED CROSS CYLINDER (FCC)

Indication

This is a subjective method to evaluate the accuracy of the accommodative response.

Background

The Fused Cross Cylinder (FCC) test is used to determine the amount of accommodation in play at near when blur no longer provides a stimulus for accommodation but disparity vergence is fully functional. The stimulus configuration (cross grid) is intended to break the feedback loop by reducing the contrast and causing astigmatic blur on the cross-hatched target. FCC is an accommodative test that also indirectly measures positive and negative fusional vergence abilities because it is performed under binocular conditions. The result of this test, therefore, can be used to confirm or deny a particular clinical hypothesis of a binocular vision disorder. It is also a way of determining plus acceptance for a tentative add power in a near-point prescription.

Advantages

The findings from this test can be used as a tentative add prescription under binocular/fused conditions.

Disadvantages

FCC is difficult to perform on young patients. It produces variable accommodative results in non-presbyopes due to their active accommodation systems.

Equipment

1. Phoropter with 0.50 Jackson Cross Cylinders (Figure 21)
2. Cross grid on near-point card (Figure 22)
3. Near-point rod

Procedure

Step 1: Place child's optimum, balanced distance prescription in the phoropter, and set the interpupillary distance (IPD) for near viewing

Step 2: Choose dim illumination, both for the room and for the overhead lamp. Direct the overhead lamp from the side and provide sufficient illumination for child to see the target clearly. Dim illumination is used to minimize the depth of focus by achieving the largest pupillary diameter

Step 3: Insert the 0.50 cross cylinder mounted on the auxiliary wheel of the phoropter in front of both eyes

Step 4: Direct child to view the cross-grid pattern on the near-point card (see picture of target below) at 40 cm from the eyes

Step 5: Ask child, "Are the lines running up and down (the vertical lines) or the lines running side to side (horizontal lines) sharper and clearer?" If child is accommodating exactly in the plan of the target, then following the introduction of the cross-cylinder, the circle of least confusion will lie on the retina and child will report that both sets of lines are equally clear or equally blurred

1. If child was under accommodating for the target (lag of accommodation), then child will report the horizontal lines are clear since the horizontal focal line is closer to the retina
2. If child was over accommodating for the target (lead of accommodation), then child will report that the vertical lines are clearer

Step 6: If child reports that the vertical lines are sharper, add minus lens in 0.25 D steps until both sets of lines appear equally distinct

Step 7: If child reports that the horizontal lines are clearer, add plus lens in 0.25 D steps until both sets of lines appear equally distinct. This is the endpoint.

1. On occasion, no equal point is reached, for example the horizontal lines appear clearer through +0.50 D but with the addition of +0.25 D makes the vertical lines clearer, record this as +0.50 H or +0.75 V indicating that the horizontal lines were clearer through t+0.50 lens but an additional +0.25 D makes the vertical lines clearer
2. In young children, it is common for their accommodative response to fluctuate where it is impossible to obtain a clear end point. Record this as "fluctuation of accommodation."

Clinical Pearl: *If there is less plus than expected, it suggests over accommodation and can be indicative of accommodative spasm or excess.*

Clinical Pearl: *If there is more plus than expected, it indicates under-accommodation and can be indicative of accommodative insufficiency.*

Expected Findings

The expected range is +0.50 D ± 0.50 D.

Figure 21. Phoropter with 0.50 Jackson Cross Cylinders

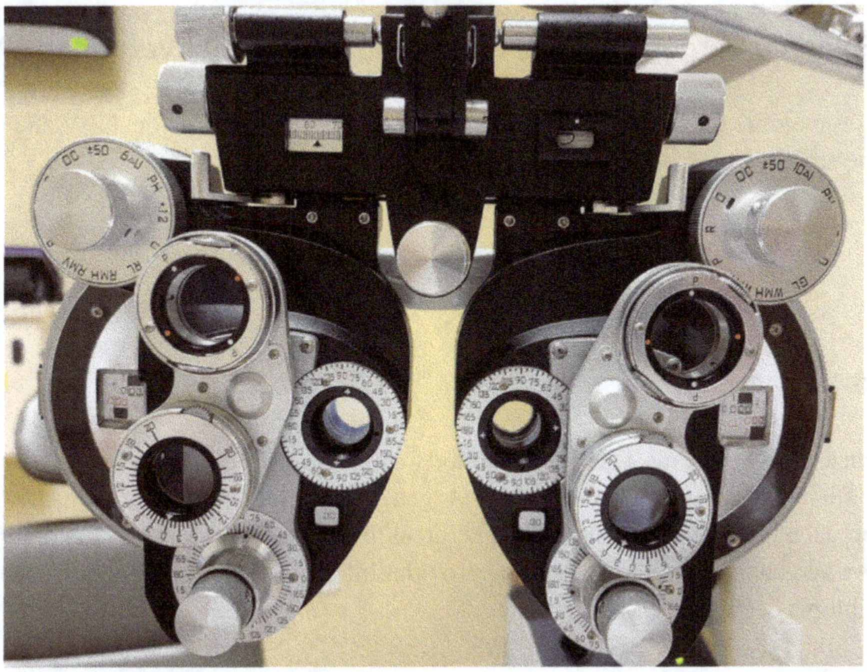

Figure 22. FCC target: Optical condition of the cross cylinder. The vertical myopic meridian corresponds to the horizontal focal line and the horizontal hyperopic meridian corresponds to the vertical focal line

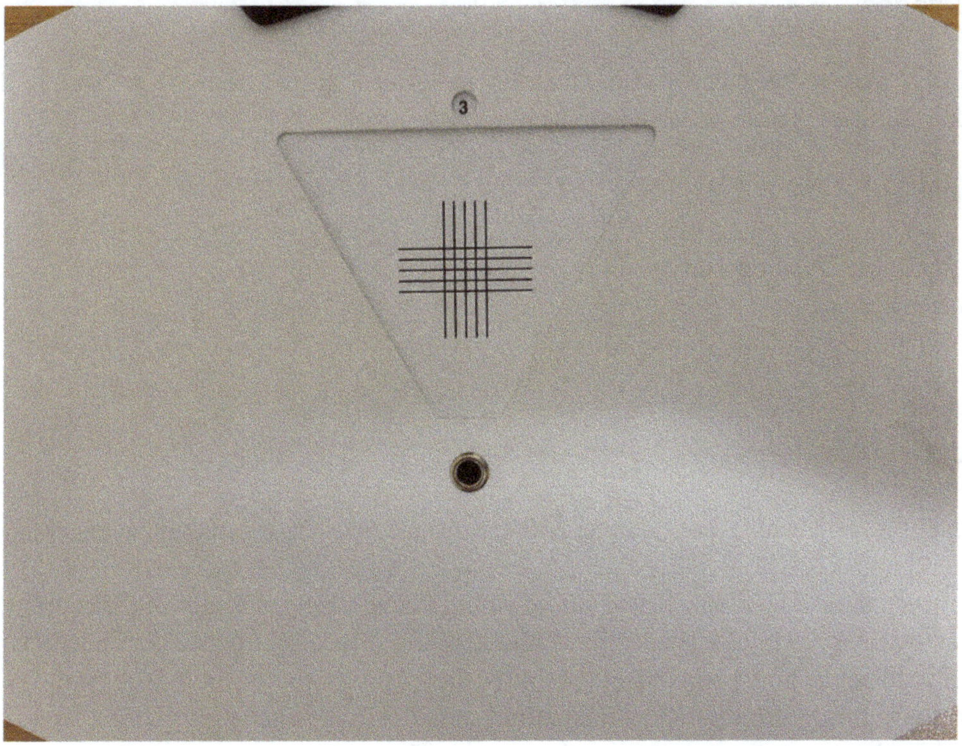

SMOOTH VERGENCE RANGES

Negative Fusional Vergence (NFV) and Positive Fusional Vergence (PFV)

Vergence ranges measure the child's ability to maintain binocular single vision. NFV and PFV are measured while the stimulus to accommodation is held constant.

Indication

Designed to assess the fusional vergence amplitude and recovery at distance and near with rotary prisms.

Background

Smooth vergence testing is the most common method for assessing the amplitude of the fusional vergence response for both positive and negative fusional vergence. The blur finding is a measure of the amount of fusional vergence free of accommodation. The break indicates the amount of fusional vergence and accommodative vergence. The recovery finding provides information about the patient's ability to regain fusion after diplopia occurs.

Advantages

NFV and PFV are relatively fast and easy to administer in the phoropter.

Disadvantages

NFV and PFV may be difficult for young children to perform. It may be more difficult to detect if a patient has a deviated eye during testing in the phoropter.

Equipment

1. Phoropter with Risley prisms
2. Distance acuity chart
3. Near-point card
4. Near point rod

Procedure

Step 1: Place the child behind the phoropter with the distance spectacle refraction in place and the room moderately illuminated

Step 2: Instruct child to view an isolated letter two lines larger than the acuity of the poorer eye

Step 3: Set the right and left Risley prisms at zero marking vertical so that the horizontal prism can be introduced before both eyes

Step 4: Instruct child to keep both eyes open. Child should see only one target. If child reports diplopia, add either base-in or base-out until fusion occurs. This will be your starting point for the test

Step 5: Instruct child to report immediately if the target becomes blurred or breaks into two

Step 6: Positive fusional vergence (PFV) should be performed after negative fusional vergence (NFV) assessment in routine testing; otherwise, the patient's compensating range should be measured first, for example BI for eso and BO for exo. Almost all vergence range testing will stimulate vergence adaptation, whichever range is measured second may be biased by this adaptation

Step 7: Measure the BI or divergence ranges

1. Slowly and smoothly introduce BI prism before both eyes, try to keep the amount of prism equal before each eye. Rotate both prisms in a BI direction at a rate of about 2 Δ per second, and ask child to tell you when the letters blur, split into two columns, or begin to move
2. If child reports a blur, stop rotating the prism, and ask whether she/he can clear the target. The criterion is first sustained blur; note this prism amount as the *blur* point. (Most do not report a blur on the distant BI vergence test). If child does report a blur, suspect an under correction for hyperopia or an overcorrection for myopia. A blur at distance during divergence (BI) fusional measurements means that accommodation was not entirely relaxed. The refraction should be rechecked to confirm accurate refractive findings
3. Continue adding BI prism until child reports that the target becomes and remains double (diplopia) or that the column has begun to move left or right. Record this prism amount as the break point

Note: if the target is moving to the right then the left eye is suppressing and if the target is moving to the left then the right eye is suppressing

4. Continue 2 to 4 Δ past the break point, then reduce the BI prism, and instruct child to report when the two images just fuse and binocular single vision is recovered (single target). Record this as the *recovery* point
5. Record the total prism in place when child reported first slight sustained blur, diplopia, and recovery of fusion (blur/break/recovery). If any of the prism values are BO, use negative numbers
6. For example: if the target breaks with 4 Δ BI OD and 4 Δ BI OS, the total amount of the horizontal prism is 8 Δ BI

Step 8: Measure the BO or convergence ranges

1. Slowly and smoothly introduce BO prism before both eyes, try to keep the amount of prism equal before each eye. Rotate both prisms in a BO direction at a rate of about 2 Δ per second
2. When child reports a blur, stop adding prism, and ask whether the target can be cleared. The criterion is first sustained blur; this is the blur point
3. Continue adding BO prism until child reports that the target becomes and remains double (diplopia) or that the column is moving left or right (suppression). This prismatic amount defines the break point
4. Continue 2 to 4 Δ past the break point, and then reverse the direction of the prism rotation, thereby reducing the amount of BO prism in effect, and instruct child to report when the images just fuse and binocular single vision is recovered (single target). Note the prism amount as the recovery point
5. Record the distant BO vergence finding in the form of blur/ break/recovery. In the event child reported no blur but only a break and recovery, record the blur finding as an X. If the recovery is obtained with the prism base in the opposite direction to that originally used, record as a

negative value, for example: when testing BI, the recovery was 2 Δ BO, there was no blur point and the break is 8 Δ BI, record as x/8/–2

Step 9: Repeat these steps at near using the near card with an isolated letter two lines larger than the best corrected visual acuity

Clinical Pearl: *Control accommodation by stressing the importance of keeping the target clear.*

Clinical Pearl: *If child reports movement rather than diplopia as you attempt the break measure, suppression is the most likely reason whereby the target seen by the non-suppressed eye appears to move.*

Clinical Pearl: *If suppression is present, try to complete the measurement by using an anti-suppression technique, such as reducing input to the non-suppressed eye by putting the polarized filter from the phoropter in front of the eye to act as a neutral density filter. If this technique doesn't work, simply note the suppression and discontinue the test.*

Table 5.

Expected Findings: (Scheiman and Wick, 2019)	**Smooth Vergence**	
	Average Value	Standard Deviation
Base out (distance):	9/19/10	± 4/8/4
Base in (distance):	x/7/4	± x/3/2
Base out (near):	17/21/11	± 5/6/7
Base in (near):	13/21/13	± 4/4/5

SMOOTH VERGENCE RANGES

Supra- and Infra Vergence Ranges

Vergence ranges measure the patient's ability to maintain binocular single vision.

Indication

Designed to assess the vertical fusional vergence amplitude and recovery at distance and near with rotary prisms.

Background

Smooth vergence testing is the most common method for assessing the amplitude of both supra-vergence and infra-vergence. The break indicates the point where the patient can no longer maintain single vision. The recovery finding provides information about the patient's ability to regain fusion after diplopia occurs. There is no blur finding for vertical vergence testing.

Advantages

Vertical vergences ranges are relatively fast and easy to administer in the phoropter.

Disadvantages

It may be more difficult to detect if a patient has a deviated eye during testing; this test may be difficult for young children to perform.

Equipment

1. Phoropter with Risley prisms
2. Distance acuity chart
3. Near-point card
4. Near point rod

Procedure

Step 1: Place child behind the phoropter with the distance spectacle refraction in place and the room moderately illuminated
Step 2: Instruct child to view an isolated letter two lines larger than the acuity of the poorer eye
Step 3: Set the right and left Risley prisms at zero marking horizontal so that the vertical prism can be introduced before one eye (Figure 23)
Step 4: Instruct child to keep both eyes open. Child should see only one target. If child reports diplopia, add either base-up or base-down until fusion occurs. This will be your starting point for the test
Step 5: Slowly introduce base-up (BU) prism over the right eye (rate = 1 prism diopter per second). BU prism over the right eye is measuring right infra-vergence
Step 6: Instruct the patient to report immediately when the target breaks into two. This will be the *break* point
Step 7: Continue 2 to 4 Δ past the break point, then reduce the BU prism over the right eye, and instruct child to report when the two images just fuse and binocular single vision is recovered (single target). Record this as the *recovery* point
Step 8: Repeat the steps above by introducing base-down (BD) over the right eye. This is measuring right supra-vergence.
Step 9: Repeat these steps at near using the near card with an isolated letter two lines larger than the acuity of the poorer eye

Expected Findings

Break: 3-4 prism diopters
Recovery: 1-2 prism diopters

Figure 23. Risley prism set-up to measure vertical vergence ranges

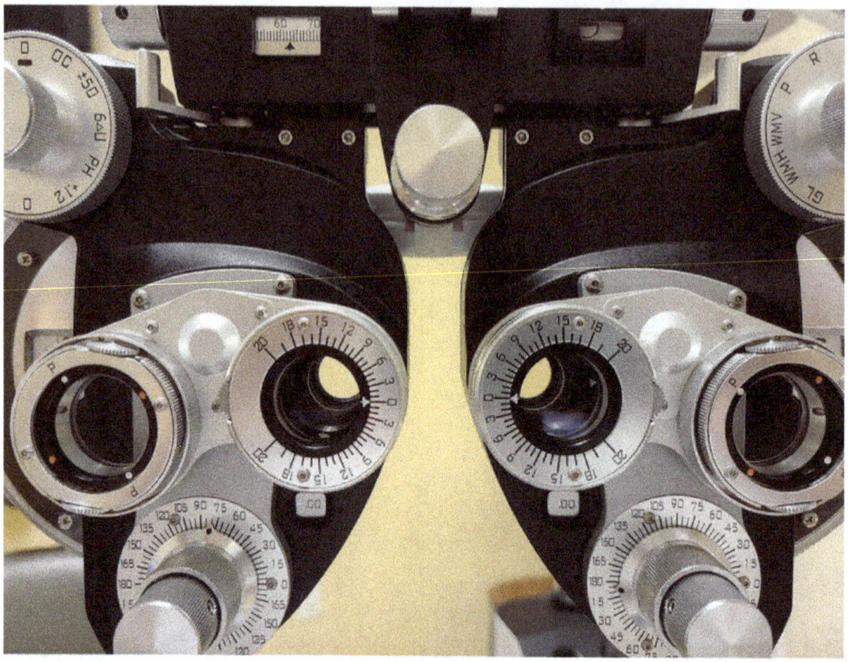

RELATIVE ACCOMMODATION

Negative Relative Accommodation (NRA) and Positive Relative Accommodation (PRA)

Indication

The purpose of this test is to measure the patient's ability to increase (PRA) and decrease (NRA) accommodation under binocular conditions when the convergence demand is held constant at 40 cm. It can be used to check if the near add for is balanced and to determine a tentative add.

Background

Testing of relative accommodation assesses the flexibility in the inextricable link between accommodation and vergence. This test is done under fused or binocular conditions. Under these conditions, changes in accommodative convergence are compensated for by changes in fusional vergence. When the clinician binocularly introduces either plus (NRA) or minus (PRA) lenses, the accommodative response alters, while vergence is maintained within Panum's fusional area. It is important to remember that as the lenses are introduced, there is a transient change in eye posture to maintain single vision. For example, when minus lenses are added, the eyes are transiently driven to converge by the increased accommodation and corresponding accommodative vergence. Maintaining fusion requires an immediate compensatory stimulus of negative fusional vergence (NFV) to place the target back to the center of Panum's area.

The endpoint of a relative accommodation procedure signals one of three possible events: 1) the ability of the fusional vergence system to provide countering innervation to accommodative convergence has been exceeded; 2) the ability of the accommodative system to react to the stimulus has been exceeded; 3) the accommodative system does not respond to blur. All three possible events signaled by the blur point revealed by the relative accommodation measurements can be more directly determined by other tests (such as accommodative amplitude, fusional vergence testing, and monocular accommodative facility) that offer better diagnostic information and arrive at a more precise differential diagnosis. Thus, the magnitude of the relative accommodation finding is determined by the vergence range and AC/A ratio.

Advantages

NRA and PRA are good tools to help determine the tentative add. Also helps determine if the distance prescription has been over-minused or over-plused.

Disadvantages

NRA and PRA findings provide inconclusive diagnostic information if used alone. Balancing the NRA and PRA findings to determine an optimal add prescription works best in patients with presbyopia and does not work as well for non-presbyopes.

Equipment

1. Phoropter
2. Near-point card
3. Near point rod

Procedure

Negative Relative Accommodation

Step 1: Adjust the phoropter for near-point (40 cm) viewing by adjusting the PD and place the near-point card on the near-point rod. Choose a reduced Snellen chart, a box of 20/30 letters, or a similar arrangement of small letters

Step 2: Direct the overhead lamp onto the near-point card, and set the lamp on high illumination

Step 3: Put the child's near-point prescription (usually the distance spectacle refraction) into the phoropter

Step 4: Ask child to tell you when the letters begin to blur as you add plus power in 0.25 D steps at the rate of one step every 1-2 seconds binocularly. When blur is reported, ask child to clear the target, if possible. Note the number of 0.25 DS steps until the point of first sustained blur. Some clinicians reverse the process and reduce the relative plus power to determine the negative relative accommodation (NRA) recovery finding. They ask the patient to report when the letters are once again clear

Step 5: Record the amount of relative plus power added until first sustained blur. For example, child might report that the target has just blurred and cannot be cleared with +2.25 D over the distance spectacle refraction. The NRA would be recorded +2.25 D. If an NRA recovery finding was determined, perhaps at +1.75 D, the complete NRA measurement result would be recorded as +2.25/+1.75

Positive Relative Accommodation

Step 1: The procedure for testing PRA is the same as that for testing NRA (described above) except that minus power is used in place of plus power

Step 2: Record the amount of minus power added until the first sustained blur occurs. Then, if you wish, reduce the minus until clear vision is recovered. For example, child might report that the target has just blurred and cannot be cleared with – 2.50 D over the distance spectacle refraction. You would then reduce the relative minus power until the patient reports clarity at, for example, –2.00 DS over the distance refraction. The PRA measurement would be recorded as –2.50/–2.00

Clinical Pearl: *As a practical point, there is rarely a reason to measure PRA past the –3.00 D level.*

Clinical Pearl: *An NRA higher than +2.75 D suggests that the prescription may be under corrected for hyperopia or over minused for myopia.*

Expected Findings

NRA: +2.00 D ± 0.50
PRA: –2.37 D ± 1.00

STEP VERGENCES

Positive Fusional Vergence (PFV) and Negative Fusional Vergence (NFV) Testing

Indication

To measure the horizontal vergence ranges at distance and near in free space with a prism bar.

Background

The purpose of vergence eye movements is to provide appropriate convergence and divergence of the eyes at a given distance. Specifically, fusional vergence is a flexible and powerful component that alters the vergence level of the eyes to achieve fusion, or binocular vision. It adds convergence or acts to diverge the eyes when tonic, proximal, and accommodative vergence either does not provide sufficient convergence or provides excessive convergence of the eyes for a given stimulus.

Advantages

This technique is particularly useful when the use of a phoropter is not practical such as in young patients. It is also great for objective measurements of vergence ranges by observing the fixation patterns of the eyes through the prism bar lenses.

Disadvantages

The only disadvantage is that the clinician must hold the prism bar lenses to measure the range and hold the target at the same time when measuring near vergence ranges, there will be no free hand available for other tasks.

Equipment

1. Horizontal prism bar
2. Near fixation target
3. Distance fixation target

Procedure

Distance Step Vergences

Step 1: Ensure child is adequately corrected for refractive error
Step 2: Using moderate room lighting, project an isolated letter 2 line above BCVA onto the wall screen or monitor
Step 3: Position the prism bar in front of one of the child's eyes, beginning with the lowest power placed BI or BO. Increase the BI or BO power of the prism bar, at the rate of 2 Δ per 1-2 seconds (this allows for the opportunity to fuse if possible)
Step 4: The vergence ranges can be determined objectively or subjectively

Objective Measurement (BI)

1. Instruct child to keep the target clear and single as long as possible
2. Watch the eyes behind the prism as you increase the prism amount. The eye will make a series of small abduction movements (BI prism will make the eyes diverge) until it makes a large adduction movement, when diplopia occurs. This indicates fusion is broken. Note the amount of prism to cause the break point
3. Now, decrease the BI power at the same rate that you increased it, and wait for a fusion movement to occur. The movement may be in the eye with the prism, or it may consist of a version-vergence movement of both eyes. The version-vergence movement is observed as an initial version of both eyes (conjugate eye movement), closely followed by a vergence movement (disconjugate eye movement of one or both eyes). Some movements are small and subtle so watch closely
4. Record the break and recovery findings. (A blur point cannot be objectively determined)

Subjective Measurement (BI)

1. Instruct child to keep the chart as clear as possible.
2. Instruct child to tell you when the target becomes blurred, double, or starts to move.
3. Begin to increase the power of the prism bar before one eye. When child reports a blur, give them a few seconds to clear it before moving on to the next incremental increase in prism. The recorded

blur is the first sustained blur. Remember, a blur at distance during negative fusional vergence measurement means the accommodation was not entirely relaxed. Note: while we may record a blur finding for step vergences, there are no expected norms for blur

4. Continue to increase the prism power until child reports double vision, or the target starts to move to the left or right
   Note: if the prism bar is placed over the right eye and the target is moving to the right then the left eye is suppressing. If the target is moving to the left (and the prism bar is placed over the right eye) then the right eye is suppressing
5. Record the magnitude of the prism as the break point
6. Begin to decrease the power of the prism until child reports that the two images have become one (single), and record this as the recovery finding

Objective Measurement (BO) and Subjective Measurement (BO)

1. Position the prism bar BO in front of one of the child's eyes
2. Increase the BO prism at the same rate that you increased BI prism
3. Once again, you may make either objective or subjective measurements
4. Increase the BO prism power until one of the eyes (usually the eye under the prism) makes an abduction movement. Record that point as the break point
5. Reduce the prism power until the eyes are seen to recover fusion. Again, this may be a simple vergence movement, or it may be a version followed by a vergence of one or both eyes
6. Note the break and recovery points
7. Some movements are small and subtle so watch closely

Procedure

Near Step Vergences

Step 1: Place target (Gulden Fixation Stick with single column of 20/30 letters) in primary gaze 40 cm from child's eyes (Figure 24)
Step 2: Make sure ambient and overhead lighting provide good illumination
Step 3: Follow the procedure as listed above in the procedures for distance step vergence testing
Step 4: Figure 25 illustrates negative fusional vergence testing (base-in prism over the right eye)
Step 5: Figure 26 illustrates positive fusional vergence testing (base-out over the left eye)

Clinical Pearl: *Positive fusional vergence (PFV) should be performed after the negative fusional vergence (NFV) assessment in routine testing; otherwise, the child's compensating range for phoria should be tested first. The examiner should wait 30 seconds after the NFV measure before performing the PFV measures.*

Clinical Pearl: *The blur finding indicates the limits of fusional vergence, the break finding indicates the limits of accommodative and fusional vergence, and the recovery finding indicates the magnitude in which child is able to regain fusion.*

Clinical Pearl: *If child is able to fuse the largest (45 Δ) prism, record >45 for the break value and have child close or cover one eye to break fusion so that recovery can be measured. Record the amount of prism through which child was able to regain fusion.*

Clinical Pearl: *You may have to use minus numbers if child does not fuse entirely in the divergence or convergence range. That is, if the recovery is obtained with the prism base in the opposite direction to that originally used, record the finding as a negative value.*

Clinical Pearl: *If diplopia is not reported but examiner notes loss of fusion, the prism through which fusion is lost will be recorded as the break finding. Likewise, an examiner observation or recovery of fusion will be recorded as recovery.*

Figure 24. Fixation targets for near step vergence testing

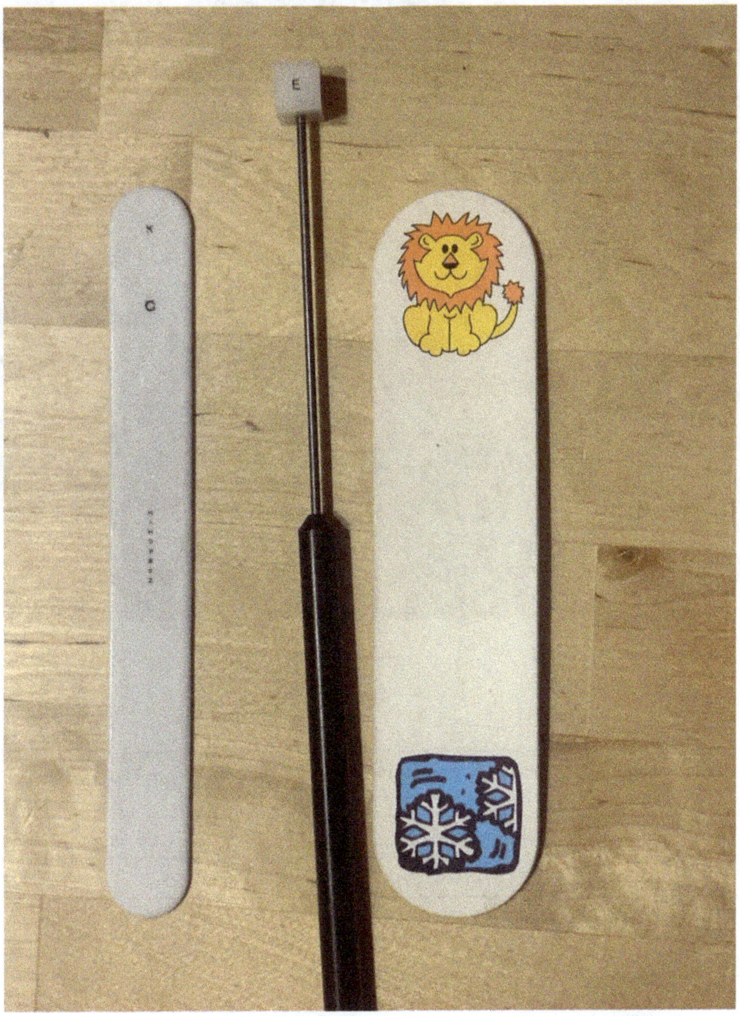

Figure 25. Negative fusional vergence testing at near with prism bar

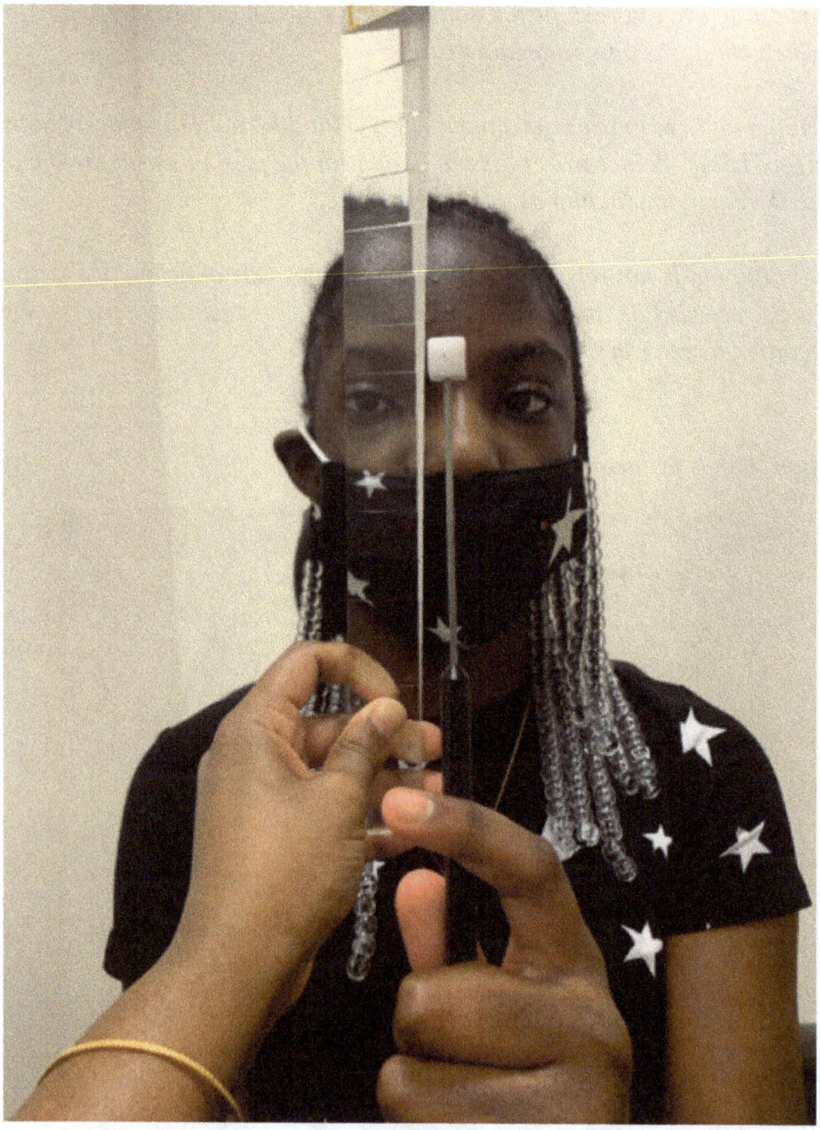

Table 6.

Expected Findings: Vergence Amplitudes for Children 4.5-5.5 Years Old (Lam et al., 1996)		
	Average Value	Standard Deviation
Base out (distance):	x/14.5/10.6	± x/5.5/5.2
Base in (distance):	x/8.9/5.7	± x/2.7/2.9
Base out (near):	x/28.9/23.4	± x/5.6/5.1
Base in (near):	x/15.5/12.3	± x/4.5/4.3

Figure 26. Positive fusional vergence testing at near with prism bar

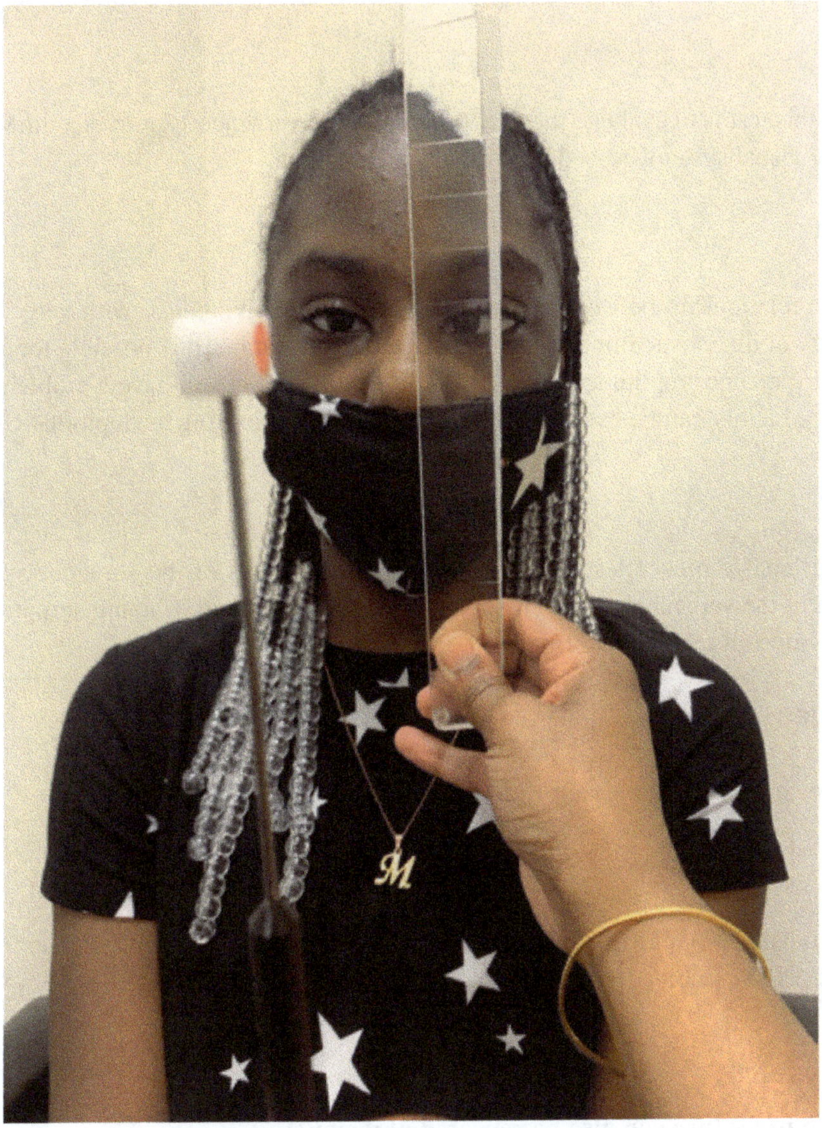

Table 7.

Expected Findings: Step Vergence for Children 7-12 years old (Scheiman and Wick, 2019)		
	Average Value	Standard Deviation
Base out (near):	x/23/16	± x/8/6
Base in (near):	x/12/7	± x/5/4

VERGENCE FACILITY

Indication

The purpose of this test is to evaluate the performance of the vergence system in a time-dependent task to determine the visual system's speed and resistance to fatigue.

Background

There is a close relationship between symptoms and vergence dynamics, with vergence latency and vergence velocity of diagnostic importance in a binocular evaluation. It is possible for a patient to have normal fusional vergence amplitudes (PFV and NFV findings) and still have a problem with vergence facility. Vergence facility can be used to differentiate symptomatic from asymptomatic patients.

Advantages

It is the only fusional vergence test which measures the dynamics of the vergence system. This will test the stamina of the vergence system. It should be tested in patients who are symptomatic and their vergence ranges are still relatively normal.

Disadvantages

This test may be challenging for young children.

Equipment

1. Near fixation target (Gulden fixation stick)
2. 3 Δ BI/12 Δ BO combination prism

Procedure

Near only, same procedure can also be repeated at distance
Step 1: Direct child to observe the fixation target through the habitual correction
Step 2: Make sure ambient and overhead lightings provide good illumination
Step 3: Place target (Gulden Fixation Stick with single vertical column of 20/30 letters) in primary gaze 40 cm from child's eyes.
Step 4: Place 3 Δ BI side of the prism in front of child's eyes. Ask child to try to make the letters single and clear as quickly as possible. Instruct child to say "now" as soon as the letters are single and clear.
Step 5: When letters are reported to be single and clear, quickly move the prism up to the 12 Δ BO side, again instructing child to report when letters are single and clear.
Step 6: Once you have confirmed child understands and is able to perform the task, prepare to begin timing for one minute using a stopwatch
Step 7: Start timing as you place the BI side of the prism in front of child's eyes

Step 8: Continue to alternate sides of the prism for 1 minute, while counting the number of sides of the prism child is able to make single and clear

Step 9: This test can also be performed objectively or subjectively. Watch for the child's eyes to diverge/converge appropriately through the prism when performing objectively. See the instructions for objective measurement in the fusional vergence section for more details.

Step 10: Record number of prism cycles as cycles per minute (cpm)— total number of times child cleared the prism sides divided by 2, or the number of times the patient cleared both BI and BO prisms.

Expected Findings

15 cpm ± 3

Clinical Pearl: *Vergence facility can be tested at far and near, but it is most commonly measured at near. In both cases, the fixation target must be large enough and detailed. For instance, at distance a vertical column of small (20/30) letters is preferred. At near, a vertical column or a block of small letters (also 20/30) makes an ideal target.*

Clinical Pearl: *Even if child has difficulty (i.e., is slow or takes a while to clear) making the target single and clear through the prism, testing should be continued for a full minute. However, if child cannot clear the BI or BO prism in one minute, then 0 cpm will be recorded.*

CONCLUSION

Binocular examination is an important part of the functional vision exam for children. It should be performed after refraction is completed to ensure best acuity is achieved before evaluation of binocular function. This chapter introduced the reader to elements of the binocular vision examination involving assessment of the ocular posture as well as vergence testing.

REFERENCES

Alhammouri, Q., Graf, M., & Lorenz, B. (2011). Bruckner Test Sensitivity to Detect Foveal Dimming. *Journal of Research in Medical Sciences*, *18*, 10–15.

American Academy of Pediatrics. (2008). Red Reflex Examination in Neonates, Infants, and Children. *Pediatrics*, *122*(6), 1401–1404. doi:10.1542/peds.2008-2624 PMID:19047263

Caloroso, E. E., & Rouse, M. W. (1993). *Clinical Management of Strabismus* (1st ed.). Butterworth-Heinemann.

Carlson, N. B., & Kurtz, D. (2004). *Clinical Procedures for Ocular Examination* (3rd ed.). McGraw Hill.

Lam, S. R., LaRoche, G. R., De Becker, I., & Macpherson, H. (1996). The range and variability of ophthalmological parameters in normal children aged 4 1/2 to 5 1/2 years. *Journal of Pediatric Ophthalmology and Strabismus*, *33*(5), 251–256. doi:10.3928/0191-3913-19960901-10 PMID:8880619

Mohney, B. G., & Holmes, J. M. (2006). An Office-Based Scale for Assessment Control in Intermittent Exotropia. *Strabismus, 14*(3), 147–150. doi:10.1080/09273970600894716 PMID:16950743

Scheiman, M., & Wick, B. (2019). *Clinical Management of Binocular Vision Heterophoric, Accommodative, and Eye Movement Disorders* (5th ed.). Lippincott Williams & Wilkins.

Subhi, Y., Schmidt, D. C., Al-Bakri, M., Bach-Holm, D., & Kessel, L. (2021). Diagnostic Test Accuracy of the Red Reflex Test for Ocular Pathology in Infants. *JAMA Ophthalmology, 139*(1), 33–40. doi:10.1001/jamaophthalmol.2020.4854 PMID:33180103

von Noorden, G. K., & Campos, E. C. (2002). *Binocular Vision and Ocular Motility: Theory and Management of Strabismus* (6th ed.). Mosby, Inc.

ADDITIONAL READING

Benjamin, W. J. (2006). *Borish's Clinical Refraction* (2nd ed.). Butterworth-Heinemann.

Braddick, O., Atkinson, J., French, J., & Howland, H. C. (1979). A photorefractive study of infant accommodation. *Vision Research, 19*(12), 1319–1330. doi:10.1016/0042-6989(79)90204-9 PMID:532100

Chung-Lock, I., & Han, S. (2019). Evaluation of Accommodation. In P. Schnell, M. B. Taub, & R. Duckman (Eds.), *Visual Development, Diagnosis, and Treatment of the Pediatric Patient* (2nd ed.). Lippincott Williams & Wilkins.

Hasebe, S., Ohtsuki, H., Tadokoro, Y., Okano, M., & Furuse, T. (1995). The Reliability of a Video-Enhanced Hirschberg Test under Clinical Conditions. *Investigative Ophthalmology & Visual Science, 36*, 2678–2685. PMID:7499090

LaMattina, K. C., Vagge, A., & Nelson, L. B. (2019). Can the Red Reflex Test Detect Unequal Refractive Error? *The Journal of Pediatrics, 214*, 175–177. doi:10.1016/j.jpeds.2019.06.051 PMID:31378518

Rosenbloom, A. A., & Morgan, M. W. (1990). *Principles and Practice of Pediatric Optometry*. J.B. Lippincott Company.

Scheiman, M., & Wick, B. (2008). *Clinical Management of Binocular Vision. In Heterophoric, Accommodative, and Eye Movement Disorders* (3rd ed.). Lippincott Williams & Wilkins.

KEY TERMS AND DEFINITIONS

Accommodation: The process in which the eye changes optical power to maintain focus on an object at varying distances. This is measured in diopters and decreases predictably with age.

Angle Kappa: The angle between the visual line or line of sight (which connects the point of fixation with the nodal points and the fovea) and the pupillary axis (which is a line through the center of the pupil perpendicular to the cornea).

Binocular Vision: The ability to maintain visual focus on an object in one's visual field with both eyes, creating a single visual percept.

Cover Test: Technique performed to evaluate the presence and magnitude of a heterophoria or a heterotopia (also commonly known as strabismus). A unilateral cover test determines the presence of a strabismus, and an alternating cover test determines the presence of a heterophoria.

Fused Cross Cylinder: A subjective in phoropter method to evaluate the accuracy of the accommodative response.

Heterophoria: A latent deviation that occurs when binocular viewing is disrupted, observed during an alternating cover test. Phorias include exophoria (eyes drift outward), esophoria (eyes drift inwards), hypophoria (eyes drift downward), hyperphoria (eyes drift upward).

Modified Thorington: A subjective method of determining the presence, direction, and magnitude of a horizontal and vertical phoria utilizing a Maddox Rod, transilluminator and Modified Thorington Card.

Strabismus (Heterotropia): A manifest deviation of ocular alignment that is present during binocular viewing conditions, observed during unilateral cover test. Tropias include exotropia (eye sits out), esotropia (eye sits in), hypotropia (eye sits down), hypertropia (eye sits up).

Vergence: The simultaneous disconjugate movement of both eyes to maintain bifoveal fixation and fusion on a target. Convergence (eyes moving inward together). Divergence (eyes moving outward together).

Chapter 10
Testing Accommodation in Children

Ida Chung
Western University of Health Sciences, USA

ABSTRACT

Accommodation disorders are associated with a host of etiologies. Children with accommodative disorders can present with various symptoms including blur, fluctuating vision, eye pain, burning sensation, tired eyes, asthenopia, headaches, fatigue with near work, and excessive rubbing, blinking, or tearing. This chapter provides an overview of accommodation testing on pediatric patients in the clinical setting. The author describes the indications for accommodation testing and provides clinical pearls for testing accommodative function in children. The chapter covers the specific tests, equipment required, and step-by-step procedures for testing accommodative amplitude, accommodative response, and accommodative facility.

INTRODUCTION

The purpose of ocular accommodation is to maintain clear vision at variable distances to resolve objects through changes in the refractive power of the crystalline lens.

Patients who have asthenopia such as headaches, eye fatigue and eye pain that are worst at the end of the day and blurred vision at near, especially with prolonged near work, or intermittent distance blur after sustained near work may indicate one or more forms of accommodative dysfunctions (Daum, 1983). It is more important today to test for accommodative dysfunction as the world has shifted its emphasis from distance to near vision tasks such as reading, smart phones, tablets, computer and desk work (Rosenfield, 2016).

Evaluation of accommodation should be a part of a comprehensive eye examination, including a baseline cycloplegic refraction to quantify significant refractive error in children (American Optometric Association, 2017). Symptomatic patients who have accommodative dysfunction may also have binocular dysfunctions and vice versa because the two systems, accommodative and vergence, are controlled by an interactive negative feedback loop (Ciuffreda and Tannen, 1995).

DOI: 10.4018/978-1-7998-8044-8.ch010

Young children with accommodative problems may be asymptomatic (US Preventive Services Task Force, 2011). Reliance on symptoms to drive testing for accommodative dysfunction for younger children may be misleading due to younger patients' inability to relate performance with visual dysfunction. Children may not report blurred vision at near because of their lack of awareness of what clarity is or they avoid the tasks that make them uncomfortable. It is important to include a test of accommodation for all school-aged children even if the patient does not report symptoms.

The varied causes of accommodative dysfunction make it essential for the clinician to evaluate accommodative dysfunction by selecting the appropriate tests and interpreting the test findings in the context of the patient's symptoms, ocular health, and systemic health to reach an appropriate management plan.

This chapter covers the specific tests, equipment required, and provides step-by-step procedures for testing accommodative amplitude, accommodative response, and accommodative facility.

BACKGROUND

Accommodation disorders are associated with a host of etiologies. In healthy children, accommodative disorders are associated with convergence disorders, emotional stress and uncorrected refractive errors, particularly hyperopia (Chrousos et al., 1988). Associated ocular conditions include ocular inflammation and sclerosis of the crystalline lens. Neurologic conditions including head trauma, cranial nerve III palsy, pharmacologic agents, and encephalitis, can negatively affect accommodation. Additionally, systemic conditions that can affect accommodation include myasthenia gravis, diabetes, hypertension, Gillian Barr syndrome, tuberculosis, endocrine disorders, and syphilis (Cooper and Panariello, 1988; DeRespinis et al, 1989; Master et al., 2016; Moss et al., 1987).

The eye structures involved in accommodation are the crystalline lens, ciliary muscle, and zonule fibers which attach the lens to the ciliary muscle. Figure 1 shows the ocular structures involved in accommodation.

Figure 1. Anatomy of the accommodation structures

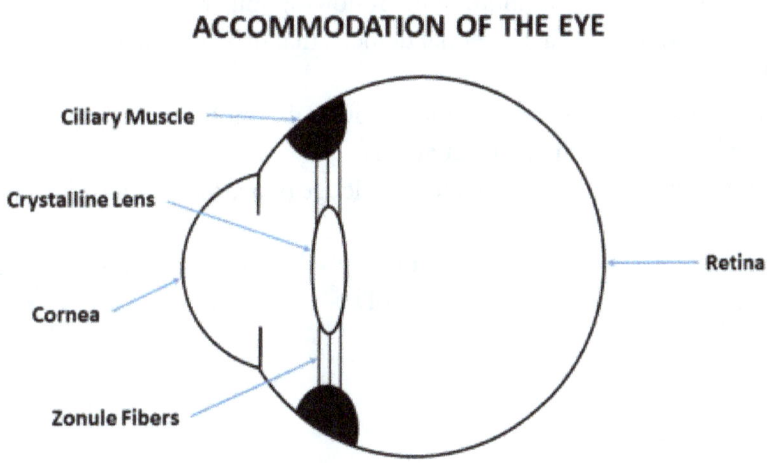

Optical accommodation occurs to keep an object in focus on the retina while the distance from the object to the eye changes. With the eyes viewing a distant object, light rays are nearly parallel and accommodation is not needed to bring objects into focus. When the eye is relaxed, in the unaccommodated state, the ciliary muscles are relaxed, the zonule fibers are taut, and the lens is less convex. Figure 2 shows the eye in an unaccommodated state.

Figure 2. The eye in an unaccommodated state

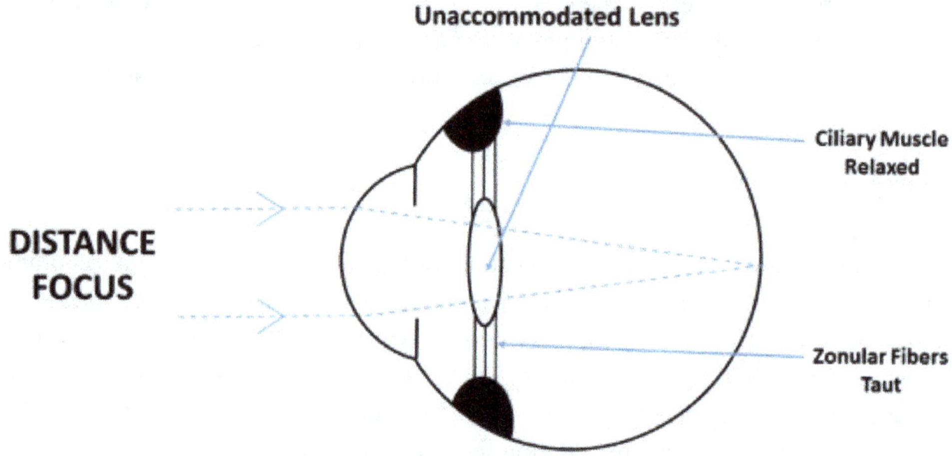

With the eyes viewing a near target, light rays diverge and require accommodation for focusing objects. Ocular accommodation is accomplished by an increase in convexity of the crystalline lens located posterior to the iris. This increase in refractive power is achieved by stimulation and contracture of the ciliary muscle, followed by a relaxation of the zonule fibers attached to the crystalline lens, resulting in a more convex lens. Figure 3 shows the eye in an accommodated state.

Accommodation is activated by one or more of the following four ways:

1. Blur-driven accommodation. This is retinal defocus that drives a change in accommodation effort to clear an object.
2. Convergent accommodation. This is accommodation driven from convergence when maintaining single vision while focusing on an object at near.
3. Proximal accommodation. This is from the knowledge of nearness of an object due to its proximity to the eye.
4. Tonic accommodation. This is the ciliary muscle innervation or tonus in the absence of visual stimulation. The average amount is 0.5D to 1.0D.

Figure 3. The eye in an accommodated state

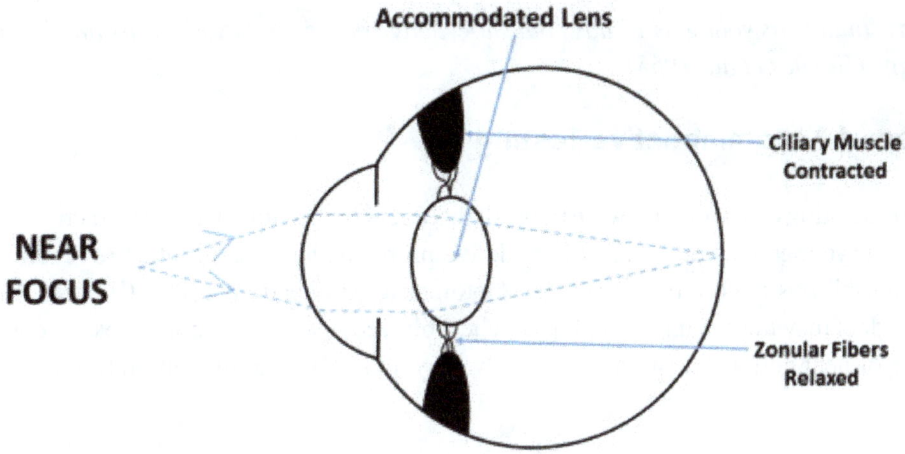

The accommodative response to a blur-driven stimulus is more accurate with both proximity and convergence accommodation together than with blur alone.

Three components of accommodation tested clinically are:

1. Amplitude of accommodation

Amplitude of accommodation is the maximum amount of refractive power the eye can stimulate at a given distance. A problem with amplitude of accommodation is called Accommodative Insufficiency, a condition in which the patient has difficulty with stimulating accommodation. Ill-Sustained Accommodation, a subset of Accommodative Insufficiency, is diagnosed when the symptoms or signs of accommodative insufficiency worsen over time associated with prolonged near work.

2. Accuracy of accommodation

Accuracy of accommodation is the measured lag or lead of the accommodative response to a stimulus at near. The normal lag of accommodation finding in school-age children are +0.25D to +0.75D. When accommodation response exceeds the stimulus demand required to focus, this is called Accommodative Excess or Accommodative Spasm. Accommodative Spasm is often used interchangeably with Accommodative Excess, with the former being a more severe form.

3. Facility of accommodation

Facility of accommodation is the ability of the eye to alternately stimulate and relax focus to changes in stimuli. A problem of facility in accommodation is called Accommodative Infacility. Accommodative facility is important for a child's ability to quickly and accurately shift focus from distance to near, such as copying from the board, and vice-versa.

Clinical Pearl: *One diopter (1D) of accommodation is required to focus an object 1 meter from the eye.*

Clinical Pearl: *Infants as young as 15 days old show active accommodation ability and is adult-like by 4 months of age (Haynes et al., 1965).*

Advantages of Accommodative Testing

Accommodative testing can confirm a wide range of disorders such as uncorrected refractive errors, latent hyperopia, and psychogenic factors. Accommodative problems have been linked to reading problems and learning disabilities in children (American Optometric Association, 2008). Children with accommodative disorders may have symptoms of headaches, blurred vision, asthenopia, loss of concentration, and avoidance of near activity. Testing is relatively easy and cost of equipment to test accommodation is inexpensive.

Disadvantages of Accommodative Testing

Accommodative testing does require additional chair time and responses may be variable due to age limitations. For the younger child, the selection of a more objective test is preferred.

ACCOMMODATIVE AMPLITUDE TESTING

Diagnosis of Accommodative Insufficiency

Accommodative insufficiency is by far the most frequently reported of the accommodative dysfunctions (Daum, 1983). The single clinical finding to diagnose accommodative insufficiency is a finding of an accommodative amplitude of at least 2.00 D below the minimal age-appropriate amplitude (Cacho et al., 2002).

Norms for Accommodative Amplitude

Table 1 provides Hofstetter's formulas for calculating minimal, average, and maximal amplitudes of accommodation based on age in years. Table 2 provides the average amplitudes of accommodation for 5 through 18 years of age.

Table 1. Hofstetter's formulas for calculating amplitudes of accommodation

Minimal amplitudes of accommodation	15 D-1/4(age)
Average amplitudes of accommodation	18.50 D -1/3(age)
Maximal amplitudes of accommodation	25 D-1/4(age)

Table 2. Age-expected amplitude of accommodation for age 5 through 18 years

Table of Age-Expected Amplitude of Accommodation Avg amplitude of accommodation = 18.5 D -1/3(age)			
AGE (yr)	**AMPLITUDE (D)**	**AGE (yr)**	**AMPLITUDE (D)**
5	16.8	12	14.5
6	16.5	13	14.2
7	16.2	14	13.8
8	15.8	15	13.5
9	15.5	16	13.2
10	15.2	17	12.8
11	14.8	18	12.5

Tests for Accommodative Amplitude

There are three clinical tests to measure accommodative amplitude (Taub & Shallo-Hoffmann, 2012). For older children responsive to testing, the minus lens method performed in the phoropter is used. For younger children, and when performing testing without the phoropter in free space, the push-up test is used. For children of any age whose subjective responses are questionable, the pull-away test is preferred over the push-up test and minus lens method.

Minus Lens Test for Accommodative Amplitude

Equipment

(Figure 4 shows the equipment used for minus lens test for accommodative amplitude)

- Phoropter
- Near point rod
- Eye patch (optional)

Figure 4. Equipment for minus lens test for accommodative amplitude

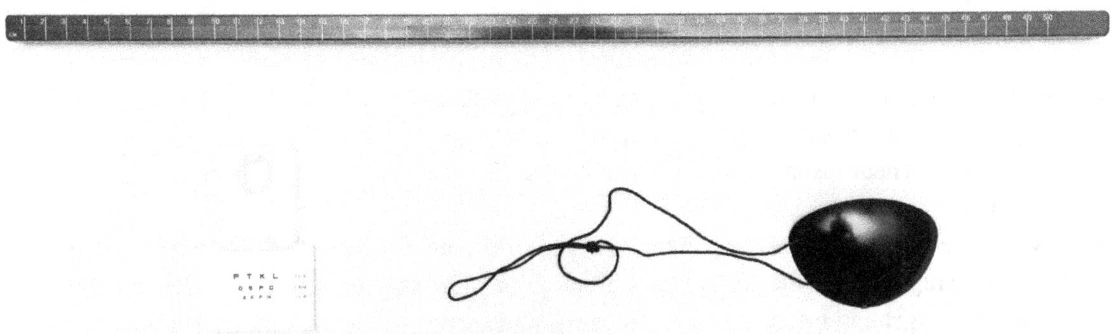

Procedure

Step 1: Begin with the patient's distance manifest refraction in the phoropter
Step 2: Set the near point rod at 40cm
Step 3: Select a single line of 20/30 letters (If the visual acuity is less than 20/20, choose a target that is two lines larger than the best acuity)
Step 4: Occlude the left eye
Step 5: Instruct the patient to keep the letters clear. Add lenses in -0.25D steps until the patient reports first sustained blur
Step 6: The total amplitude for that eye is the power of the minus lens added, plus +2.50 D (to account for the 40 cm test distance)
Step 7: Occlude the right eye. Repeat Steps 5-6

Clinical Pearl: *Change the lenses at a rate of 1 second per 0.25 D lens change. Be sure to allow the child sufficient time to clear the target, or to report blur.*

Clinical Pearl: *When the patient first reports blur, ask the patient if s/he can clear the target. If the patient's answer is yes, continue adding lenses until patient reports the letters stay blurred. The test end point is when the patient reports slight blur even if the letters are still readable.*

Clinical Pearl: *When performing minus lens amplitude of accommodation test, encourage the patient to always keep the target clear. This is particularly important in children whose attention to the target may drift if not reinstructed to attend. Poor attention may result in a reduced measured amplitude of accommodation.*

Push-Up Method for Accommodative Amplitude

Equipment

(Figure 5 shows the equipment used for push-up test for accommodative amplitude)

1. Near target with 20/20 letters or symbols
2. Ruler (cm)
3. Eye patch or occluder

Procedure

Step 1: Perform the test monocularly. Use a patch to cover the patient's left eye. Hold a target with 20/20* letters or symbols at 40 cm directly in front of the patient's unoccluded eye
*If the patient's near visual acuity is worse than 20/20, use a target that is two lines larger than the best acuity.
Step 2: Move the target towards the patient at a rate of 5 cm/s. Instruct the patient to keep the target clear and to report when the target first starts to blur. When the patient reports sustained blur, stop moving the target and measure the distance from the target to the patient's lateral canthus**

**If the patient is wearing spectacles, measure the distance from the target to the patient's spectacle plane.

Step 3: The maximal amplitude of accommodation is the calculated inverse of the measured distance in meters and expressed in diopters

Step 4: Transfer the occluder or patch to the right eye. Repeat Steps 1-3 for the other eye

Figure 5. Equipment for push-up test for accommodative amplitude

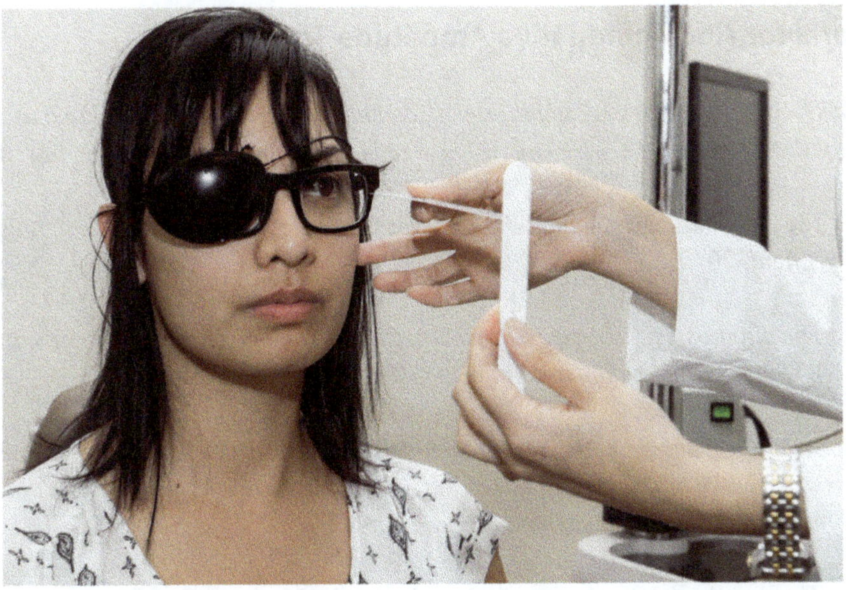

Pull-Away Method for Accommodative Amplitude

The pull-away test is a variation of the push-up test, and is performed under similar conditions except the target is moved away from the patient.

Equipment

1. Near target with 20/20 letters or symbols
2. Ruler (cm)
3. Eye patch

Procedure

Step 1: Perform the test monocularly. Use a patch or occluder to cover the patient's left eye. Hold a target with 20/20* letters or symbols at 40 cm directly in front of the patient's unoccluded eye

*If the patient's near visual acuity is worse than 20/20, use a target that is two lines larger than the best acuity.

Step 2: Move the target away from the patient at a rate of 5cm/s. Instruct the patient to report when s/he can identify the letter or symbol. When the patient is able to identify the target, stop moving the target and measure the distance from the target to the patient's lateral canthus**
**If the patient is wearing spectacles, measure the distance from the target to the patient's spectacle plane.

Step 3: The maximal amplitude of accommodation is the calculated inverse of the measured distance in meters and expressed in diopters

Step 4: Transfer the occluder or patch to the right eye. Repeat Steps 2-3 for the left eye

Clinical Pearls for Accommodative Amplitude Testing

Clinical Pearl: *The average expected amplitude of accommodation can be calculated using Hofstetter's formula: Amplitude (D) = 18.50 D -1/3 (age). The age is expressed in years of the past birthday.*

Clinical Pearl: *The amplitude of accommodation is known to decrease with age, starting at age 5 years (Benzoni & Rosenfield, 2012).*

Clinical Pearl: *The diagnosis of accommodative insufficiency is made if the patient's amplitude of accommodation is at least 2D below the minimum amplitude for patient's age.*

Clinical Pearl: *Always test accommodation monocularly; this separates the accommodative system from the binocular system (when both eyes are tested together) and therefore removes possible influences of an inefficient binocular system on accommodation.*

Clinical Pearl: *The amplitude of accommodation obtained with the pull-away test is comparable with the conventional push-up test. Take accurate measures of the distance from the target to the eye since small mm changes can translate into large dioptric values.*

Clinical Pearl: *The pull-away method is advantageous over the push-up method because the correct identification of the target gives a more reliable finding in patients with questionable subjective responses.*

Clinical Pearl: *For patients with amblyopia, only the minus lens method is valid. Use of the push-up or pull-away tests on patients with amblyopia will result in an erroneously higher amplitude of accommodation finding (Hokoda & Ciuffreda, 1982).*

Clinical Pearl: *Accommodative amplitudes obtained by the push-up method can increase with repeated testing; therefore, if initial findings are below 12D, the clinician should repeat the test (Adler, et al., 2013).*

Clinical Pearl: *A change of at least 1.50 D is considered a significant variation on repeat amplitude of accommodation testing (Rosenfield & Cohen, 1996).*

ACCOMMODATIVE RESPONSE TESTING

Diagnosis of Accommodative Response Inaccuracy

Accommodative response measures the accuracy of a patient's accommodative system when viewing a target at near. The response can be a lag (accommodation is behind the plane of convergence) or a lead (accommodation is in front of the plane of convergence). A lag is measured and neutralized with plus power lenses. A lead is measured and neutralized with minus power lenses.

A lead of accommodation is the hallmark finding in the diagnosis of accommodative excess. Accommodative spasm, a more severe form of accommodative excess, is a condition in which accommodation is maintained in the absence of a stimulus, or the accommodative response to a near stimulus demand is excessive.

Norms for Accommodative Response

The normal expected accommodative response finding is a lag of +0.25 D to +0.75 D. A lag of accommodation of +1.00 or greater is considered higher than normal, indicating a plus prescription acceptance for near work. A finding of plano or a lead of accommodation indicates accommodative excess or accommodative spasm. In this situation, plus lenses are not indicated for near. If symptoms persist, vision therapy is an indicated treatment (Scheiman, et al., 2011).

Tests of Accommodative Response

There are several clinical methods to measure accommodative response. Two methods are performed objectively: Monocular Estimate Method (MEM) retinoscopy and Nott retinoscopy. The third method is fused cross-cylinder (FCC) which is a subjective technique used more often in older children.

MEM Retinoscopy for Accommodative Response Testing

Equipment

(Figure 6 shows the equipment used for MEM retinoscopy)

1. Retinoscope
2. Age-appropriate accommodative target*
3. Plus and minus power lenses

*For preverbal children, a modified target such as pictures or a detailed finger puppet that engages the patient's attention can be utilized for fixation. Figure 7 contains examples of suitable targets for performing modified MEM retinoscopy on younger children.

Figure 6. Equipment for MEM retinoscopy test of accommodative response

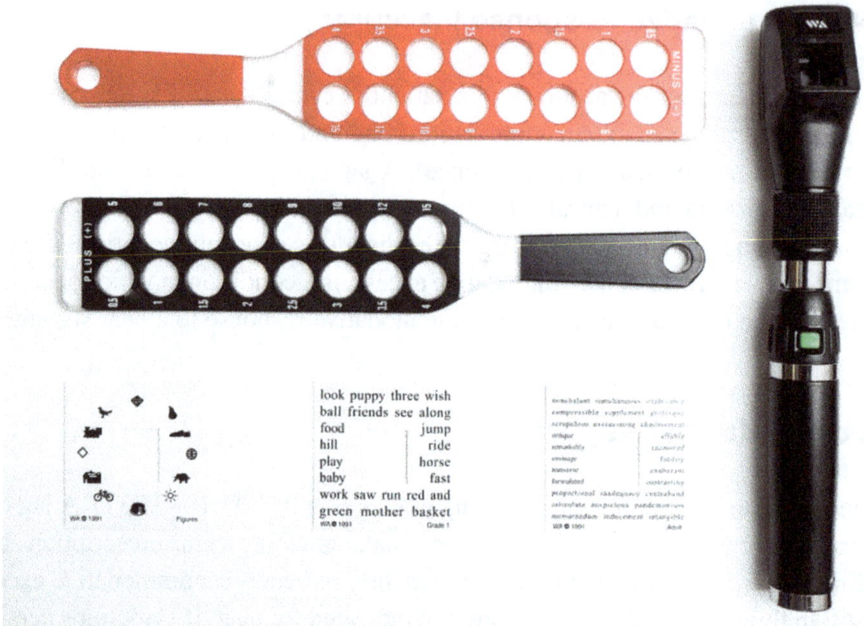

Figure 7. Equipment for modified MEM retinoscopy test for accommodative response

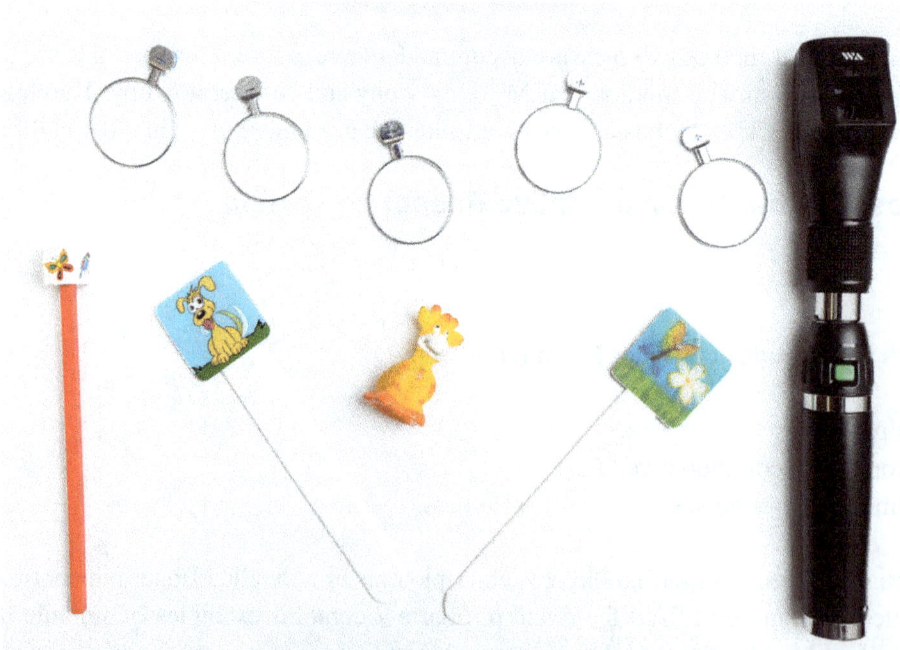

Procedure

Step 1: MEM retinoscopy is performed with an age-appropriate reading material at the plane of the retinoscope light held at the patient's habitual near working distance (as determined by asking the patient to hold reading material and noting the distance), or at the patient's Harmon distance (the distance from the patient's elbow to the third knuckle)

Step 2: Hold the retinoscope and target at the patient's midline and slightly below patient's eye level, similar to a normal reading posture. Set room illumination such that the reading target is adequately illuminated while allowing the clinician to easily view the retinoscopic reflex

Step 3: The patient wears the appropriate lenses for near. This can be the patient's distance correction, a tentative near prescription, or no lenses

Step 4: Instruct the patient to begin reading the words or identifying the pictures out loud

Step 5: With both eyes open, neutralize one eye at a time with lenses. Quickly interpose lenses to neutralize the reflex in the right eye, leaving the lens in place no longer than half a second. The lens power that neutralizes the reflex is the measured accommodative response

Step 6: Repeat Steps 4-5 for the left eye

Clinical Pearls for MEM Retinoscopy

Clinical Pearl: *Placement of the lens in front of the eye has to be quick. Leaving the lens in place for more than a half second will change the accommodative response and lead to an erroneous measurement (Haynes, 1960).*

Clinical Pearl: *Prior to interposing lenses, note the reflex first. If "with" motion is seen, select a plus lens. If "against" motion is seen, select a minus lens to achieve neutralization of the reflex.*

Clinical Pearl: *If using single loose lenses, hold in the hand two lenses at a time to quickly estimate the reflex. For example if "with" motion is seen, selection of a +0.50 D and a +1.00 D lens allows the clinician to bracket the lens power that neutralizes the reflex.*

Clinical Pearl: *If astigmatism is present, the two major meridians can be neutralized separately. The preference is to correct the astigmatism by having the patient wear a trial frame and then perform MEM retinoscopy over the lenses.*

Clinical Pearl: *The Harmon working distance is estimated to be 20 to 25cm for a young child. The Harmon working distance is considered the optimal visual distance for reading and close work (Bieber, 1974). It is measured by placing a closed fist under the chin and then holding a book or reading material at the tip of the elbow.*

Clinical Pearl: *Some retinoscopes have MEM fixation cards with pre-manufactured square cut-outs that attaches to the scope and facilitates MEM retinoscopy. The Welch Allyn Retinoscope has magnetic fixation cards, and the Heine Retinoscope has a card clip.*

Clinical Pearl: *The choice of fixation target for performing MEM retinoscopy can affect the measurements. A more challenging target (such as smaller and/or higher grade level words) may result in a lower lag of accommodation, while the use of larger or easier to read targets may result in a higher lag of accommodation finding.*

Clinical Pearl: *Inaccuracy in accommodative response can be due to poor localization of the target actual distance from the eye, i.e. a target proximity error. Having the patient touch the target can correct for this error and result in an increase in accommodative response (i.e., less lag of accommodation).*

Nott Retinoscopy for Accommodative Response Testing

Equipment

1. Retinoscope
2. Age-appropriate accommodative target
3. Ruler (cm)

Procedure

Step 1: Performed with patient wearing the appropriate lenses for near. This can be the patient's distance correction, a tentative near prescription, or no lenses
Step 2: The clinician holds an age-appropriate reading material or accommodative target at the patient's midline and slightly below patient's eye level. Instruct the patient to fixate on the target held at 40 cm from the patient
Step 3: With the other hand, the clinician holds the retinoscope 10 cm directly behind the target and observes the reflex of the right eye. Set room illumination such that the target is adequately illuminated while allowing easy view of the retinoscopic reflex
Step 4: Instruct the patient to begin reading the words or identifying the pictures out loud
Step 5: Move the retinoscope away from the patient if with motion is seen, or closer to the patient if against motion is seen, until the reflex is neutral
Step 6: Measure the distance in cm between the target and the retinoscope position at the point of neutrality. The inverse of the distance in meters is the accommodative lag (if retinoscope is behind the target), or accommodative lead (if retinoscope is in front of the target) in diopters.
Step 7: Repeat Steps 3-6 for the left eye

Clinical Pearls for Nott Retinoscopy

Clinical Pearl: *When performing Nott retinoscopy, align the retinoscope beam within 10 degrees of the target to avoid inducing erroneous findings (Haynes, 1985).*

Clinical Pearl: *Nott retinoscopy does not present possible contamination of results from a neutralizing lens, an advantage over MEM retinoscopy.*

Fused Cross-Cylinder (FCC) for Accommodative Response Testing

Equipment

1. Phoropter with +/-0.37 D cylinder lenses
2. Cross-cylinder grid target composed of vertical and horizontal sets of lines
3. Nearpoint rod with clip

Procedure

Step 1: Start with patient's distance prescription in the phoropter
Step 2: Affix the cross-cylinder grid target at 40 cm on a nearpoint rod
Step 3: Dim room illumination to ensure light is not shining directly on the cross-cylinder target
Step 4: Binocularly add +0.25 D lenses at a time until the patient reports the lines are equally dark and sharp, or if the vertical lines are darker and sharper
Step 5: The added lens that gives this endpoint is the measured accommodative lag

Clinical Pearls for Fused Cross-Cylinder (FCC) Testing

Clinical Pearl: *A response of vertical lines being darker and sharper before any lenses are added indicates a lead of accommodation. Do not proceed with the test.*

Clinical Pearl: *The FCC test can also be performed monocularly to determine the accommodative lag in each eye.*

Clinical Pearl: *The FCC test relies on subjective responses and the ability of the patient to sit behind a phoropter. If the patient's responses are not reliable, perform MEM retinoscopy or Nott retinoscopy instead.*

ACCOMMODATIVE FACILITY TESTING

Diagnosis of Accommodative Infacility

Accommodative facility is the ability to stimulate and inhibit accommodation. It is a measure of accommodative facility and stamina either monocularly or binocularly.

If the patient has difficulty clearing plus and minus lenses, this is an indication of accommodative infacility. If a patient passes the monocular accommodative facility test it is unlikely an accommodative facility problem exists.

Ease in clearing the plus lens, and failure with the minus lens, is indicative of difficulty with stimulation of accommodation and points to an accommodation insufficiency.

Ease in clearing minus lens, and failure with plus lens, is indicative of difficulty with relaxation of accommodation and points to an accommodative excess/spasm.

Norms for Accommodative Facility

Accommodative facility is usually tested over a 1-minute period. The normal findings are 11 cycles per minute monocularly and 8 cycles per minute binocularly (Zellers et al., 1984).

Children do not perform as many cycles on facility testing as do adults, which is attributed to slower verbal responses. Therefore, using a different failure criterion for children 12 years and under is suggested.

For children 8-12 years of age, the failure criterion is less than 4.5 cycles per minute monocularly. For children 6-7 years of age the failure criterion is below 3 cycles per minute monocularly (Scheiman et al., 1988).

For binocular accommodative facility testing, using a failure criterion of 3 cycles per minute or less differentiates symptomatic from asymptomatic children (Hennessey et al., 1984).

Table 3 summarizes the accommodative facility norms for age 6 to18 years.

Table 3. Norms for accommodative facility

Norms for Accommodative Facility		
AGE (yr)	MONOCULAR (cpm)	BINOCULAR (cpm)
6	5.5	3
7	6.5	3.5
8-12	7	5
13-18	11	8

Tests for Accommodative Facility

The +/- 2.00 D lens flipper test is used to measure accommodative facility. Accommodative facility tested under monocular conditions is the primary method of diagnosing accommodative infacility. Performing the test monocularly removes the influence of the binocular system on accommodation. Patient wears the distance correction when performing accommodative facility.

Lens Flipper Test for Accommodative Facility

Equipment

(Figure 8 shows the equipment used for lens flipper test of accommodative facility)

1. Plus and minus 2.00 D lens flipper
2. Near target with 20/30 letters or symbols
3. Timer or stopwatch
4. Eye patch or handheld occluder (for monocular testing)
5. Pen or pencil (for binocular testing)
6. SOV9 acuity suppression vectogram and polaroid glasses (for binocular testing)

Figure 8. Equipment for lens flipper test of accommodative facility

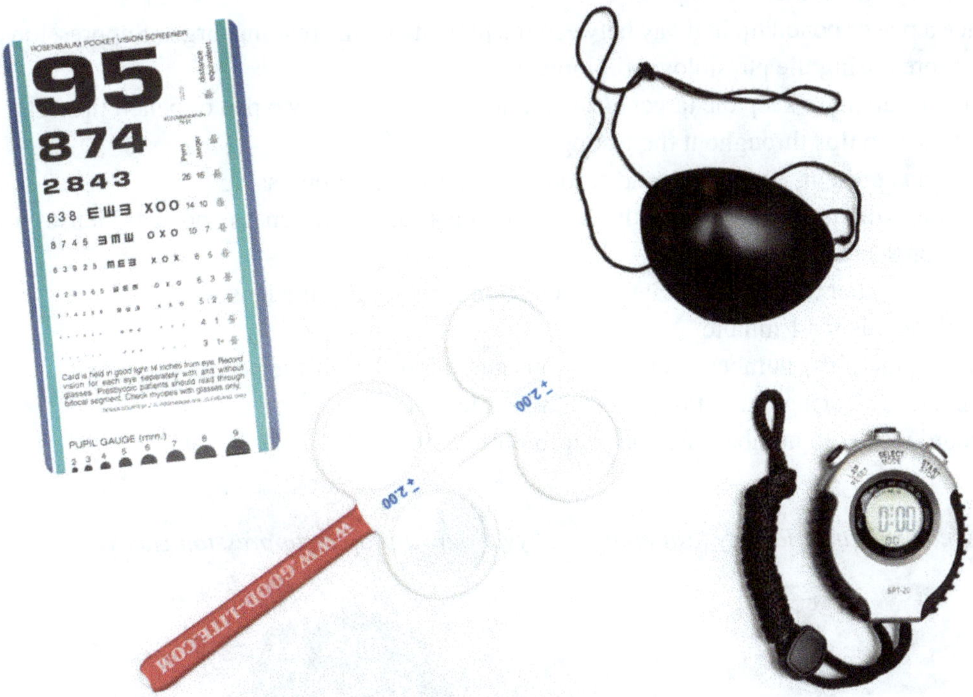

Procedure for Accommodative Facility (Monocular)

Step 1: Start with patient wearing distance prescription
Step 2: Place the 20/30 letter target at 40cm from the patient
Step 3: Occlude the left eye
Step 4: Place the plus 2.00 D lenses binocularly in front of the patient's eyes
Step 5: Ask the patient to report when the letters are clear and single
Step 6: Once the patient reports the letters are clear and single, flip the lenses to the minus 2.00 D side.
Step 7: Ask the patient to report when the letters are clear.
Step 8: Continue this for 1 minute, alternately flipping the +2.00 and -2.00 lenses
Step 9: Keep count of the number of cycles of plus and minus lenses the patient can clear within 1 minute (One cycle is clearing one set of plus and minus lenses)
Step 10: Record results in number of cycles per minute (cpm)
Step 11: Transfer the occluder or patch to the right eye. Repeat Steps 4-10 for the left eye

Procedure for Accommodative Facility (Binocular)

Option A: Use pen or pencil for suppression control.(Figure 9 shows the set up for binocular accommodative facility testing using physiologic diplopia as suppression check)

Step 1: For binocular testing present the lenses binocularly without occlusion and a suppression check is necessary for accurate testing

Step 2: Place a pen or pencil tip halfway between the patient and the reading target. Suppression control is monitored using the physiologic diplopia technique

Step 3: Ask the patient to keep the target clear and notice if there are two pen or pencil tips. The patient should see two tips throughout the testing*

*If suppression is present, end testing and record which eye was suppressing

Step 4: Ask the patient to report when the letters are clear as +2.00 lenses and -2.00 lenses are alternatively presented

Step 5: Once the patient reports the letters are clear and single, flip the lenses

Step 6: Continue this for 1 minute

Step 7: Keep count of the number of cycles of plus and minus lenses the patient clears within 1 minute (One cycle is clearing one set of plus and minus lenses)

Step 8: Record results in number of cycles per minute (cpm)

Figure 9. Accommodative facility testing using physiologic diplopia suppression check

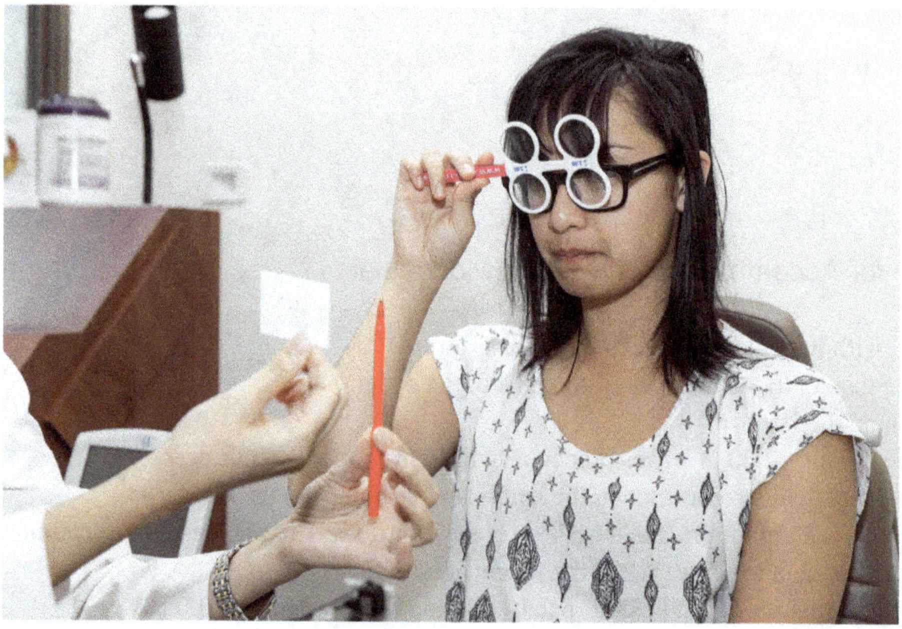

Option B: Use SOV9 acuity suppression vectogram and polaroid glasses (Figure 10 shows the SOV9 vectogram and polaroid glasses for suppression check during binocular accommodative facility testing)

Step 1: For binocular testing present the lenses binocularly without occlusion and a suppression check is necessary for accurate testing

Step 2: The patient wears the polaroid glasses

Step 3: Place the SOV9 acuity suppression vectogram over the 20/30 letter target at 40cm from the patient. The target consists of seven lines, with line number 4 seen by the left eye only and line number 6 seen by the right eye only. All other lines are seen by both eyes

Step 4: Ask the patient to report when the letters are clear as +2.00 lenses and -2.00 lenses are alternatively presented. Additionally, ask the patient to report if the letters disappear, indicating suppression*

*If suppression is present, end testing and record which eye was suppressing

Step 5: Once the patient reports the letters are clear and single, flip the lenses

Step 6: Continue this for 1 minute

Step 7: Keep count of the number of cycles of plus and minus lenses the patient can clear within 1 minute (One cycle is clearing one set of plus and minus lenses)

Step 8: Record results in number of cycles per minute (cpm)

Figure 10. SOV9 acuity suppression vectogram and polaroid glasses equipment for binocular accommodative facility testing

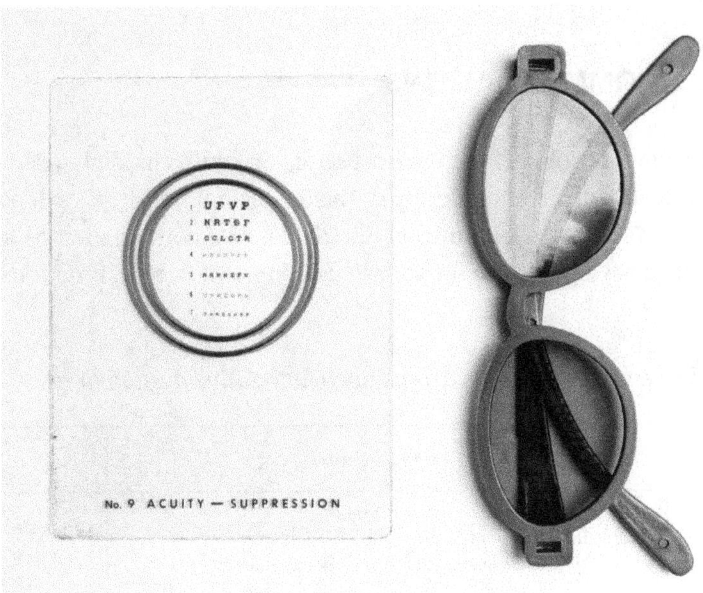

Clinical Pearls for Accommodative Facility Testing

Clinical Pearl: *If the patient's near acuity is worse than 20/20, use a letter target 2 lines above best acuity.*

Clinical Pearl: *To solely test accommodation function, the test must be performed monocularly.*

Clinical Pearl: *Use of an elastic eye patch rather than a handheld occluder to occlude one eye helps to prevent child from peeking.*

Clinical Pearl: *Binocular accommodative lens flipper tests both accommodation and vergence abilities. If patient does well with monocular lens flipper but poorly with binocular lens flipper, the etiology of the problem may be a vergence dysfunction rather than an accommodative dysfunction.*

Clinical Pearl: *For younger children whose responses are questionable, accommodative facility testing can be modified by asking the child to say aloud the letters or symbols on the target rather than simply reporting whether they are clear.*

Clinical Pearl: *Performing the test for 30 seconds compared with 1 minute is acceptable to provide information on accommodative facility, but not for accommodative stamina.*

Clinical Pearl: *Variability on repeat testing of facility is more likely in symptomatic patients.*

Clinical Pearl: *Accommodative infacility problems can be treated with optometric vision therapy when lenses alone are not effective or sufficient.*

SOLUTIONS AND RECOMMENDATIONS

If an accommodative dysfunction of sufficiency, response, or facility is diagnosed utilizing the tests described in this chapter, treatment can include any of the following: prescription lenses with an add for near work; optometric vision therapy (Scheiman et al., 2011); or a combination of lenses and therapy. Table 4 summarizes the primary treatments for various accommodative dysfunctions.

Table 4. Treatment and key test findings for various accommodative dysfunctions

Accommodative Dysfunction	Key Test Finding	Treatment
Accommodative insufficiency	• Reduced amplitude of accommodation • Large lag of accommodation • Inability to clear minus lenses on monocular facility test	• Plus lenses for near • Optometric vision therapy
Accommodative infacility	• Inability to clear minus and plus lenses on monocular facility test	• Optometric vision therapy
Accommodative excess	• Inability to clear plus lenses on monocular facility test • Lead of accommodation	• Optometric vision therapy
Ill-sustained accommodation	• Ability to clear minus and plus lenses on binocular facility test diminishes over time	• Plus lenses for near • Optometric vision therapy

CONCLUSION

Pediatric patients with possible accommodative dysfunction will most often present with symptoms of blurred vision, frontal headaches, eye pain, and tired eyes associated with visually demanding near activities. When accommodative dysfunction is suspected, a comprehensive assessment of a child's accommodative system should include a cycloplegic refraction, and tests of amplitude, response, and facility. Presence of underlying systemic disease and adverse side effects of medications can negatively impact the accommodation system and should be ruled out before initiating treatment of accommodative disorders with lenses or therapy. With well-established and validated tests of accommodation in children, a correct diagnosis of accommodative dysfunction is the first step in providing relief of symptoms and successful treatment of accommodative disorders.

REFERENCES

Adler, P., Scally, A. J., & Barrett, B. T. (2013). Test-retest reproducibility of accommodation measurements gathered in an unselected sample of UK primary school children. *The British Journal of Ophthalmology, 97*(5), 592–597. doi:10.1136/bjophthalmol-2012-302348 PMID:23426733

American Optometric Association. (2008). *Optometric Clinical Practice Guideline: Care of the Patient with Learning Related Vision Problems.* https://www.aoa.org/practice/clinical-guidelines/clinical-practice-guidelines?sso=y

American Optometric Association. (2017). *Evidence-Based Clinical Practice Guideline: Comprehensive Pediatric Eye and Vision Exam.* https://aoa.uberflip.com/i/807465-cpg-pediatric-eye-and-vision-examination/0?m4=

Benzoni, J. A., & Rosenfield, M. (2012). Clinical amplitude of accommodation in children between 5 and 10 years of age. *Optometry and Vision Development, 43*(3), 109–114.

Bieber, J. (1974). Why nearpoint retinoscopy with children. *The Optometric Weekly, 65*(3), 54–57.

Cacho, P., Garcia, A., Lara, F., & Seguí, M. M. (2002). Diagnostic signs of accommodative insufficiency. *Optometry and Vision Science, 79*(9), 614–620. doi:10.1097/00006324-200209000-00013 PMID:12322932

Chrousos, G. A., O'Neill, J. F., Lueth, B. D., & Parks, M. M. (1988). Accommodative deficiency in healthy young individuals. *Journal of Pediatric Ophthalmology and Strabismus, 25*(4), 176–179. doi:10.3928/0191-3913-19880701-07 PMID:3411421

Cooper, J., & Panariello, G. F. (1988). The pathognomonic pattern of accommodative fatigue in myasthenia gravis. *Binocular Vision & Strabismus Quarterly, 3*(3), 141–148.

Ciuffreda, K. J., & Tannen, B. (1995). *Eye movement basics for the clinician.* Mosby.

Daum, K. M. (1983). Accommodative dysfunction. *Documenta Ophthalmologica, 55*(3), 177–198. doi:10.1007/BF00140808 PMID:6884172

DeRespinis, P. A., Shen, J. J., & Wagner, R. S. (1989). Guillain-Barre syndrome presenting as a paralysis of accommodation. Case report. *Archives of Ophthalmology, 105*(4), 508–512. doi:10.1001/archopht.1989.01070020352010 PMID:2783058

Haynes, H. M. (1960). Clinical observations with dynamic retinoscopy. *The Optometric Weekly, 51*, 2243–2246, 2306–2309.

Haynes, H. M., White, B. L., & Held, R. (1965). Visual accommodation in human infants. *Science, 148*(3669), 528–530. doi:10.1126cience.148.3669.528 PMID:14263778

Haynes, H. M. (1985). Clinical approaches to nearpoint lens power determination. *American Journal of Optometry and Physiological Optics, 62*(6), 375–385. doi:10.1097/00006324-198506000-00004 PMID:4014425

Hennessey, D., Iosue, R. A., & Rouse, M. W. (1984). Relation of symptoms to accommodative infacility in school-aged children. *American Journal of Optometry and Physiological Optics, 61*(3), 177–183. doi:10.1097/00006324-198403000-00005 PMID:6720863

Hokoda, S. C., & Ciuffreda, K. J. (1982). Measurement of accommodative amplitude in amblyopia. *Ophthalmic & Physiological Optics, 2*(3), 205–212. doi:10.1111/j.1475-1313.1982.tb00178.x PMID:7177646

Master, C. L., Scheiman, M., Gallaway, M., Goodman, A., Robinson, R. L., Master, S. R., & Gray, M. F. (2016). Vision diagnoses area common after concussion in adolescents. *Clinical Pediatrics, 55*(3), 260–267. doi:10.1177/0009922815594367 PMID:26156977

Moss, S. E., Klein, K., & Klein, B. E. K. (1987). Accommodative ability in younger-onset diabetics. *Archives of Ophthalmology, 105*(4), 508–512. doi:10.1001/archopht.1987.01060040078037 PMID:3566603

Rosenfield, M. (2016). Computer vision syndrome (a.k.a. digital eye strain). *Optometry in Practice, 17*(1), 1–10.

Rosenfield, M., & Cohen, A. S. (1996). Repeatability of clinical measurements of the amplitude of accommodation. *Ophthalmic & Physiological Optics, 16*(3), 247–249. doi:10.1046/j.1475-1313.1996.95000933.x PMID:8977892

Scheiman, M., Cotter, S., Kulp, M.T., Mitchell, G.L., Cooper, J., Gallaway, M., Hopkins, K.B., Bartuccio, M., & Chung, I., the Convergence Insufficiency Treatment Trial Study Group. (2011). Treatment of accommodative dysfunction in children: Results from a random clinical trial. *Optometry and Vision Science: Official Publication of the American Academy of Optometry, 88*(11), 1343-1352. . doi:10.1097/OPX.0b013e31822f4d7c

Scheiman, M., Herzberg, H., Frantz, K., & Margolies, M. (1988). Normative study of accommodative facility in elementary school children. *American Journal of Optometry and Physiological Optics, 65*(2), 127–134. doi:10.1097/00006324-198802000-00009 PMID:3364515

Taub, M. B., & Shallo-Hoffmann, J. (2012). A comparison of three clinical tests of accommodation to Hofstetter's norms to guide diagnosis and treatment. *Optometry and Vision Development.*

US Preventive Services Task Force. (2011). Vision screening for children 1 to 5 years of age: US Preventive Services Task Force Recommendation Statement. American Academy of Pediatrics, 127(2), 340–346. doi:10.1542/peds.2010-3177

Zellers, J. A., Alpert, T. L., & Rouse, M. W. (1984). A review of the literature and a normative study of accommodative facility. *Journal of the American Optometric Association, 55*(1), 31–37. PMID:6699343

ADDITIONAL READING

Chung-Lock, I., & Han, S. (2020). Evaluation of Accommodation. In Visual Development, Diagnosis, and Treatment of the Pediatric Patient (pp. 379-396). Wolkers Kluwer.

Nott, I. S. (1925). Dynamic skiametry, accommodation and convergence. *American Journal of Optometry and Physiological Optics*, *6*(4), 490–503.

Sheard, C. (1929). Dynamic skiametry. *American Journal of Optometry*, *6*(11), 609–623. doi:10.1097/00006324-192911000-00001

Tassinari, J. T. (2002). Monocular estimate method retinoscopy: Central tendency measures and relationship to refractive status and heterophoria. *Optometry and Vision Science*, *79*(11), 708–714. doi:10.1097/00006324-200211000-00008 PMID:12462539

KEY TERMS AND DEFINITIONS

Accommodative Excess: When the accommodation response exceeds the stimulus demand required to focus.

Accommodative Infacility: The inability of the eye to alternately stimulate and relax focus to changes in stimuli.

Accommodative Insufficiency: A visual dysfunction with stimulating accommodation.

Amplitude of Accommodation: The maximum amount of refractive power the eye can stimulate at a given distance.

Fused Cross-Cylinder Test: A method of evaluating accommodative response using ±0.37 D cylinder lenses and a grid target of horizontal and vertical sets of lines.

Lens Flipper Test: An evaluation of accommodative facility utilizing +2.00 D and -2.00 D lenses that are alternately cleared while viewing an accommodative target at near.

MEM Retinoscopy: The Monocular Estimate Method measures the accuracy of a patient's accommodative system when viewing a target at near utilizing lenses to neutralize the retinoscopy reflex.

Minus-Lens Test: A method of measuring accommodative amplitude using concave lenses in increasing power while patient views an accommodative target at near.

Nott Retinoscopy: A method of measuring the accuracy of a patient's accommodative system with a retinoscope held at near and changing the distance of an accommodative target until a neutral reflex is observed.

Push-Up/Pull-Away Method: A test to measure accommodative amplitude utilizing an accommodative target presented at near that is either moved closer, or away from the patient's eye with an endpoint of first sustained blur.

Chapter 11
Diagnostic Agents in the Pediatric Eye Examination

Lily Zhu-Tam
Citywide Eye Care Optometry, USA

ABSTRACT

In this chapter, the author reviews the most common topical ophthalmic drops for diagnostic use in a pediatric eye exam. Topical diagnostic agents have become an integral part of an ocular health examination even in infants and young children. Topical local anesthetics are commonly used for eye procedures such as tonometry, gonioscopy, and minor office procedures. The proper use of mydriatic drugs allows clinicians to identify and diagnose various ocular abnormalities that might otherwise go undetected. Cycloplegic refraction is a reliable procedure to determine the true refractive status of patients with accommodative esotropia, pseudomyopia, and latent hyperopia. Cycloplegic refraction is also useful in non-communicative or uncooperative patients and when a functional vision problem is suspected such as when visual acuities do not correlate with symptoms or clinical expecteds. Many times, diagnostic drops can help a clinician be more confident of the patient's clinical findings.

INTRODUCTION

Topical diagnostic agents have become the mainstream of an ocular health examination. At times, installation of drops in infants, toddlers and preschool children can be quite a challenge. It is useful to utilize the parents as your helper. Parents can cradle the patients like holding a baby and the practitioner can insert the drop on the nasal aspect of the eye. This chapter will present the most commonly used diagnostic drops in clinic and its use for the pediatric population.

DOI: 10.4018/978-1-7998-8044-8.ch011

BACKGROUND

This chapter will discuss topical anesthesia, dilation and diagnostic cycloplegic drops. Different concentrations of diagnostic agents and its usage based on the different age groups and the instillation methods will also be covered.

Prior to instilling diagnostic eye drops in children, we need to obtain parental consent from all children younger than 18 years old. Once verbal consent is obtained, briefly explain to the guardian the side effects of the diagnostic agents. Educate the patient and the parents to avoid near task for the next few hours. They can also stay indoor to avoid light sensitivity if necessary.

ANESTHESIA

Topical anesthesia aids in intraocular pressure (IOP) measurements especially with the Goldmann applanation and the Tonopen technique (see section on IOP measurements). There are two basic ophthalmic anesthesia commonly used in clinic. They are Proparacaine Hydrochloride ophthalmic solutions and Fluress ophthalmic solutions.

Proparacaine Hydrochloride Ophthalmic Solutions

Proparacaine Hydrochloride ophthalmic solutions are topical anesthesia used to anesthetize the eye and increase corneal penetration. For older children one drop of Proparacaine can be used to increase corneal penetration followed by Tropicamide 1% and Phenylephrine 2.5% for dilation. In some children where we have limited opportunity to instill drops, we may skip Proparacaine and go straight to the dilating agents. A fluorescent strip can be added to Proparacaine Hydrochloride to measure intraocular pressure. This is a two-step procedure involving the instillation of topical anesthetic followed by separate application of sodium fluorescein strip to anesthetize the cornea prior to applanation.

Fluress Ophthalmic Solutions

Fluress is an ophthalmic combination drop that consists of fluorescein sodium and benoxinate hydrochloride. It can also be used as an ophthalmic anesthesia prior to tonometry measurements instead of the two-step procedure with Proparacaine Hydrochloride and a fluorescent strip.

Figure 1 shows a picture of Proparacaine HCL ophthalmic solution, Figure 2 shows a picture of Fluress strip and Figure 3 shows a picture of Fluress which is the combination fluorescein and anesthesia.

In clinic we usually use Fluress to measure IOP with Goldmann applanation tonometry followed by dilation drops and cycloplegic drops if needed. In younger children where we are not measuring Goldmann applanation tonometry, we tend to use Proparacaine followed by dilation drops and/or cycloplegic drops such as Tropicamide, Phenylephrine and Cyclopentolate to increase corneal penetration.

Figure 1. Proparacaine

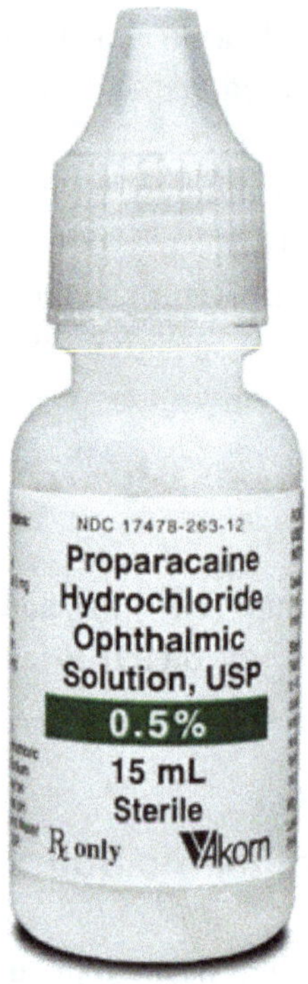

Figure 2. Fluress strip

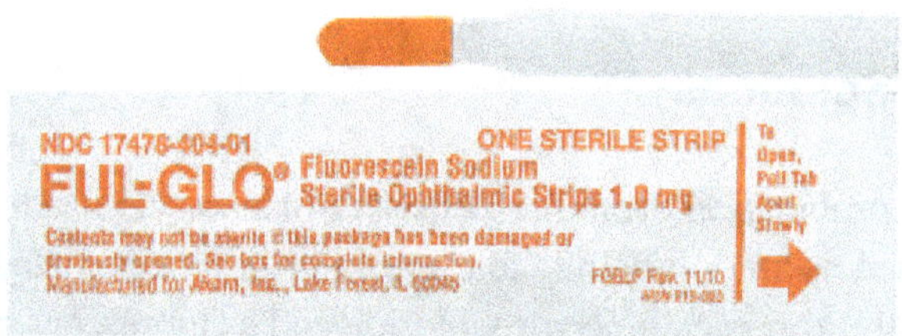

DILATION AND CYCLOPLEGIA

Dilating agents are needed to examine the health of the eye in all children. Dilation is especially crucial in examining premature infants to rule out retinopathy of prematurity.

Cycloplegia plays an important role in the refractive examination of the pediatric population. Children with amblyopia, strabismus, suspected latent hyperopia, pseudomyopia and any unexplained decrease of vision should be cyclopleged.

Figure 3. Fluress
Courtesy of Manufacturer Akorn

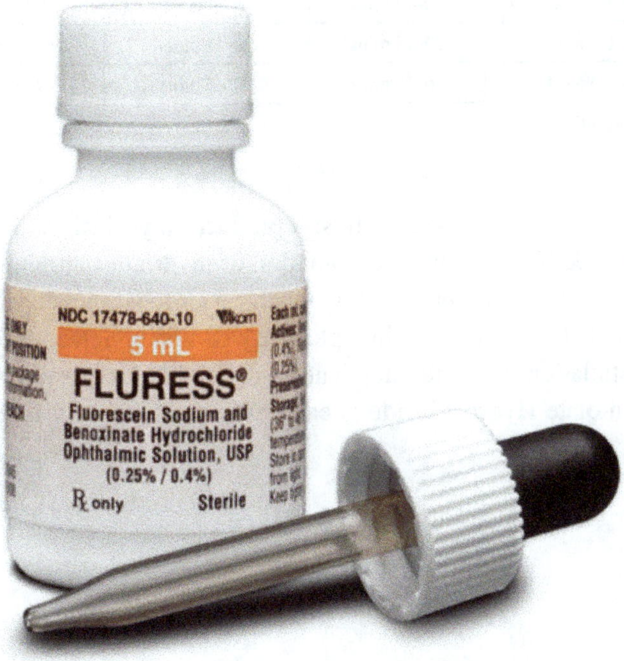

Both Tropicamide and Cyclopentolate are anticholinergic drugs that inhibit the actions of acetylcholine. In clinic they are commonly referred to as mydriatic and cycloplegic agents since they are used for pupillary dilation and cycloplegic refractions. The addition of Phenylephrine to tropicamide should produce a good dilation for the examination. Atropine is the most potent cycloplegic agent currently available but due to its prolonged paralysis of accommodation that causes patients to be visually handicapped at near, Atropine is not typically used for routine cycloplegic refractions in school-age children or adults. The potency of Atropine can last for about 7-12 days compared to Cyclopentolate and Tropicamide which last for about 6 to 24 hours (Blancett, 2001). This makes Cyclopentolate the drug of choice for cycloplegic refraction due to its rapid onset of action, minimal side effects, and minimal residual accommodation. Cyclopentolate is available in 0.5%, 1% and 2% concentration; however, the 2% is rarely used because of its increased risk for significant side effects. Table 1 provides a summary of the effects of cycloplegic drugs based on strength, onset, duration and residual accommodation (Blancett, 2001).

This chapter will only discuss Cyclopentolate and Tropicamide for cycloplegia due to its practicality in clinical settings.

During dilation, use topical anticholinergic drops such as Tropicamide 0.5% or 1% and topical mydriatic drops such as Phenylephrine 2.5%. If a cycloplegic refraction is needed add two drops of 0.5% or 1% Cyclopentolate, 5 minutes apart following the dilating drops.

These drops can be administered individually from each bottle or together as a combination. A spray top cap can be added to the top of the bottle for ease of use as well.

Table 1. The effect of cycloplegic drugs based on strength, its onset, duration and residual accommodation

Drug	Strength	Onset of max mydriasis	Onset of max cycloplegic effect	Duration of cycloplegic effect	Residual accommodation
Atropine	0.5-1.0% ung.	30-40 mins	3-6 hours	7-12 days	Negligible
Cyclopentolate	0.5-1.0% soln.	20-45 mins	20-45 mins	6-24 hours	Minimal
Tropicamide	0.5-1.0% soln.	20-35 mins	20-45 mins	6 hours	moderate

Note: ung = ointment soln = solution

This spray can be applied to the closed eyelids; it produces mydriasis and cycloplegia. This spray is comparable to those provided by the same combination of mydriatics administered as eye drops to the open eye. Many clinicians prefer the spray as it is much easier to administer for young children.

According to a clinical study published in Optometry & Vision Science (Ismail et al., 1994) on the comparison of drop installation and spray application of 1% Cyclopentolate Hydrochloride, the spray application of Cyclopentolate Hydrochloride is easier to administer and is an effective alternative to drop installation.

SPRAY CAPS

Indication

Spray caps are used to replace caps from standard ophthalmic drop bottles. This conversion of ophthalmic drop bottles to spray bottles can easily facilitate dispensing eye drops in uncooperative patients.

Advantages

Instead of trying to instill multiple eye drops, the clinician can spray the solution into the eye or on the eyelid and it will diffuse into the eye creating a clinically equivalent result (Amos, 2001).

Disadvantages

Need to purchase spray caps.

Figure 4 illustrates how a regular capped ophthalmic drop bottle is replaced by a spray cap

Dilation and Cycloplegia for Older Children

In children older than 1 year old, we usually use 1% Tropicamide and 2.5% Phenylephrine to dilate the pupils. 1% Cyclopentolate can be used to create cycloplegia in children older than 3 months. This can be instilled from a bottle as a drop or as a spray.

Figure 4. Procedure for installation of spray cap onto ophthalmic drop bottle
Photo courtesy of Gulden Ophthalmics

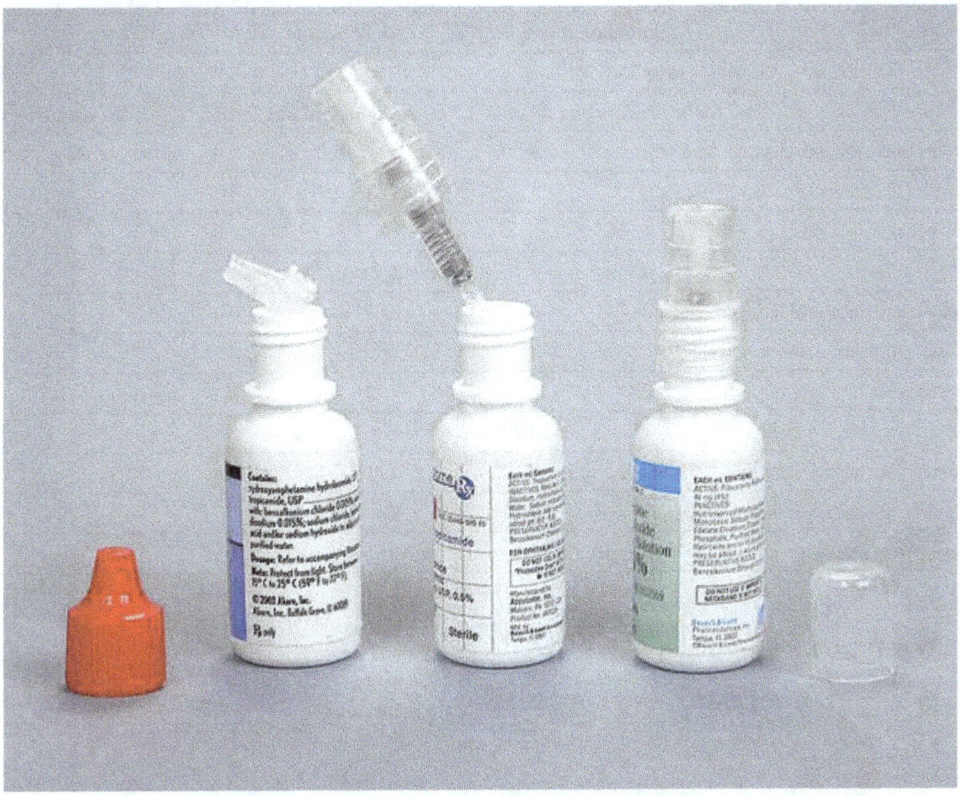

Dilation and Cycloplegia for Neonates and Infants

In neonates and infants, we tend to use a lower concentration. The author recommends the combination drop Cyclomydril for neonates and infants. Cyclomydril solution consists of Cyclopentolate 0.2% and Phenylephrine 1%. This drop is used for dilated exams on premature infants to maximize dilation with minimal risk of systemic side effects. The most effective method for dilation is to use three drops of Cyclomydril, five minutes apart to dilate infants.

In preterm infants, the clinician must observe for adverse cardiovascular effects, elevated blood pressure and heart rate. Due to gastrointestinal effects such as gastric secretory inhibition and the risk of necrotizing enterocolitis in preterm infants, the concentration of cyclopentolate should be limited to 0.25%. Cyclomydril has proven to be effective and has minimal risk of cardiovascular or gastrointestinal effects.

The author also suggests to use 0.5% Tropicamide for infants younger than 1 year old.

Table 2 illustrates recommended types of cycloplegic and dilation drops used in clinic by age category (Bartolone and Rutner, 2006).

Figure 5 shows a picture of Cyclomydril. Figure 6 shows a picture of Cyclopentolate 0.5%. Figure 7 shows a picture of Cyclopentolate 1%.

Figure 8 shows Tropicamide 0.5%. Figure 9 shows Tropicamide 1%. Figure 10 shows Phenylephrine 2.5%.

Table 2. Recommended types of cycloplegic and dilation drops used by age category (Bartolone and Rutner, 2006)

Combination drops for neonates and infants
• Cyclomydril (cyclopentolate 0.2% and phenylephrine 1%)
Cycloplegia and dilation for neonates and infants
• 0.5% Cyclopentolate (infants less than 3 months)
• 0.5% Tropicamide (infants less than 1 year old)
• 2.5% Phenylephrine
Cycloplegia and dilation for older children
• 1% Cycloplentolate (infants older than 3 months)
• 1% Tropicamide (infants older than 1 year)
• 2.5% Phenylephrine
Cycloplegia and dilation for older children
• 1% Cycloplentolate (infants older than 3 months)
• 1% Tropicamide (infants older than 1 year)
• 2.5% Phenylephrine

Figure 5. Cyclomydril

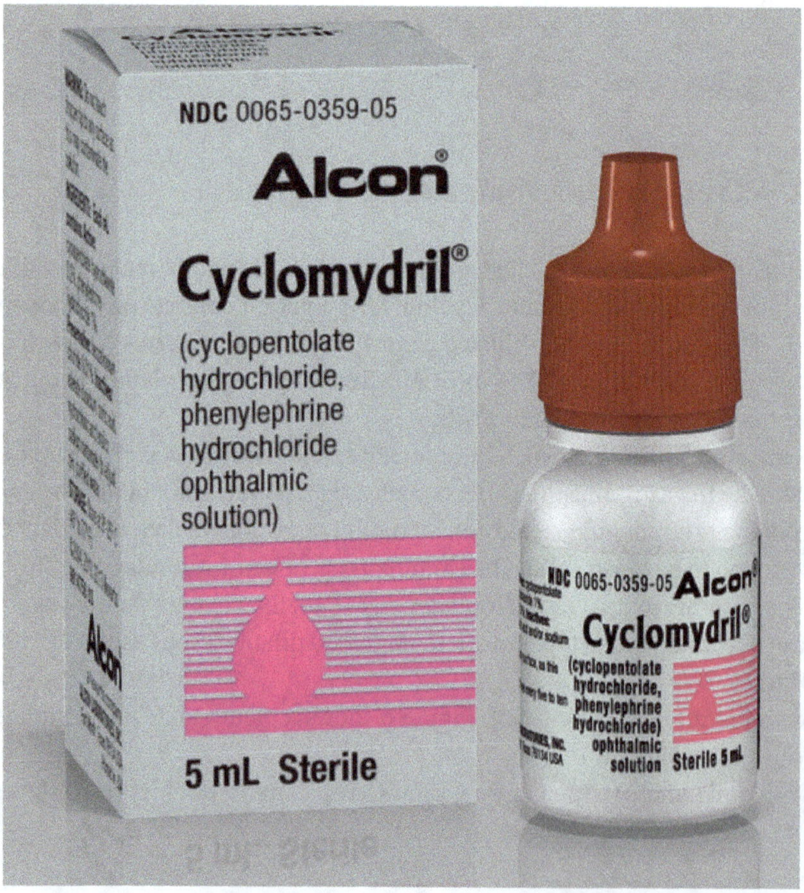

Figure 6. Cyclopentolate 0.5%

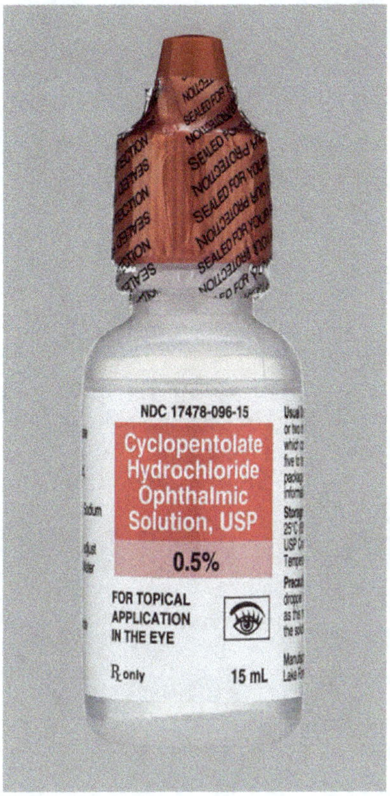

Figure 7. Cyclopentolate 1%
Courtesy of Manufacturer Alcon (Figure 5), Akorn (Figure 6) and Bausch & Lomb (Figure 7)

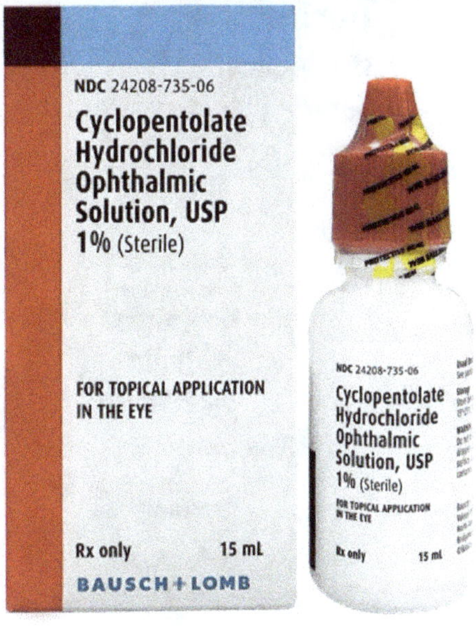

Figure 8. Tropicamide 0.5%

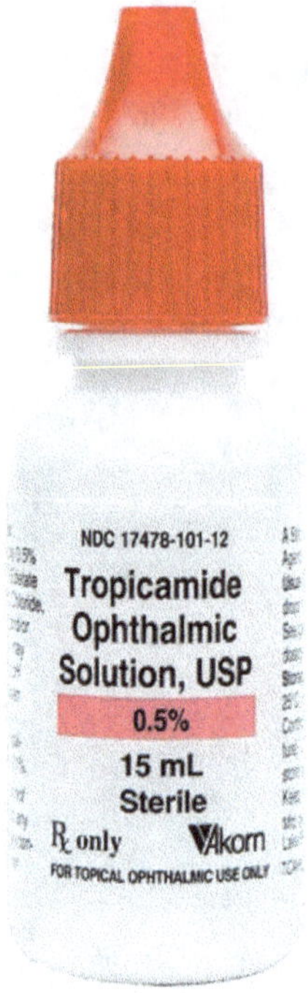

Figure 9. Tropicamide 1%

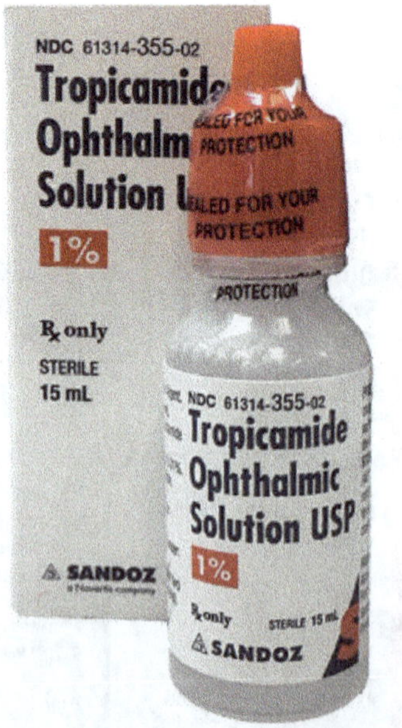

Figure 10. Phenylephrine 2.5%
Courtesy of Manufacturers Bausch & Lomb (Figure 8, Figure 9), and Akorn (Figure 10)

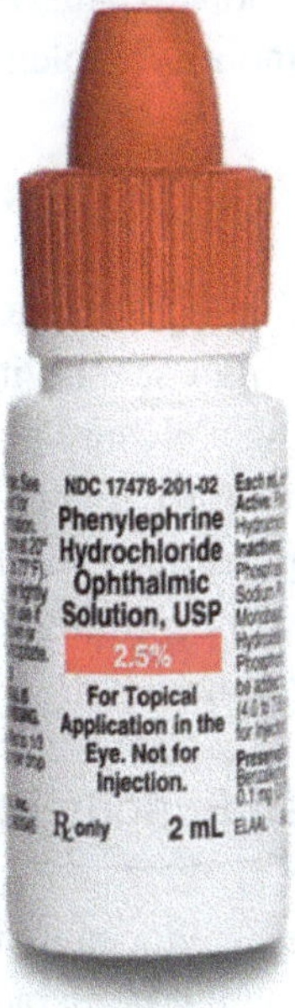

All-in-One Single Bottle Combination Drop

A clinician can make a single bottle combination drop consisting of 0.5% Cyclopentolate, 0.5% Tropicamide, and 2.5% Phenylephrine from mixing 3.75 ml of 2% Cyclopentolate, 7.5 ml of 1% Tropicamide and 3.75 ml of 10% Phenylephrine. This is a 1:2:1 ratio of Cyclopentolate, Tropicamide and Phenylephrine combination, respectively.

To create the all-in-one single bottle combination drop, add one drop of 2% Cyclopentolate, two drops of 1% Tropicamide and one drop of 10% Phenylephrine into a new bottle and shake bottle to mix. Final concentration will contain 0.5% Cyclopentolate, 0.5% Tropicamide, and 2.5% Phenylephrine. An all-in-one single bottle combination for cycloplegia and dilation helps the ease of instilling eye drops in infants and young children, especially for those who show an aversion to drops.

Table 3 shows a summary of the concentration and bottle size needed to create an all-in-one single bottle combination cycloplegic and dilation spray for young children.

Table 3. The concentration and bottle size needed to create an all-in-one single bottle combination cycloplegic and dilation drop for infants and young children

Add the following drops together	Final solution product
3.75 ml Cyclopentolate 2% (1 drop) 7.5 ml Tropicamide 1% (2 drops) 3.75 ml Phenylephrine 10% (1 drop)	0.5% Cyclopentolate 0.5% Tropicamide 2.5% Phenylephrine

Advantages of Diagnostic Drops

Dilating agents open the pupil for easier and more expansive viewing of the retina. When cyclopentolate is used, accommodation will be decreased and a cycloplegic refraction can be performed.

Side Effects of Diagnostic Drops

Anesthetic drops can cause burning and stinging sensations, making it difficult to instill drops into young children. Mydriatic drugs can cause light sensitivity and a temporary decrease in near vision. Although rare, it can also induce an acute angle closure glaucoma in narrow angles. Clinicians should be careful with the use of cycloplegic agents for patients with central nervous system disorders such as Down syndrome. Atropine may cause a potential risk of systemic toxicity in these patients. Risk of toxicity will increase with higher doses and concentration. Since atropine is not typically used in clinic as a diagnostic agent, this agent is not covered in detail.

Supplies Needed to Perform a Dilated Fundus Examination

1. Topical anesthesia such as Proparacaine (reduces irritation and enhance corneal penetration) and sodium fluorescein paper strip or combination Proparacaine-sodium fluorescein agent for tonometry procedure
2. 0.5% to 1.0% Tropicamide (depending on age)
3. 2.5% Phenylephrine
4. 0.5% to 1.0% Cyclopentolate depending on age (add to dilation exam for cycloplegic refraction)
5. Facial tissue

Procedure for Dilating a Patient

Step 1: Obtain permission from child's parent or legal guardian to dilate. Educate the patient regarding side effects of decreased accommodation at near and light sensitivity outdoors

Step 2: Dilate the patient's pupils after performing pupil testing, refraction, angle assessment and IOPs

Step 3: Recline the child halfway in the examination chair and ask an adult to hold the child's hands for support. If the child is combative, ask the adult to use their forearms or a free arm to firmly hold the child's leg

Step 4: With one hand, hold the child's forehead steady and lift the upper lid against the superior orbital rim. Use the other hand to lower the inferior eyelid and insert the drop into the palpebral conjunctiva

Step 5: If you have difficulty keeping the child's eyes open, instill the drops into the medial canthus

Step 6: If the child is extremely resistance and combative, have an assistant firmly hold the child's head

Step 7: The clinician can also use a spray instillation to the closed eyelids, and it will produce mydriasis and cycloplegia comparable to that provided by the same combination of mydriatics administered as drops to the open eyes

Figure 11 shows the instillation of eye drops into a child's eye with holding the eyelids.

Figure 11. Installation of drops into a child's eye with holding the eyelid

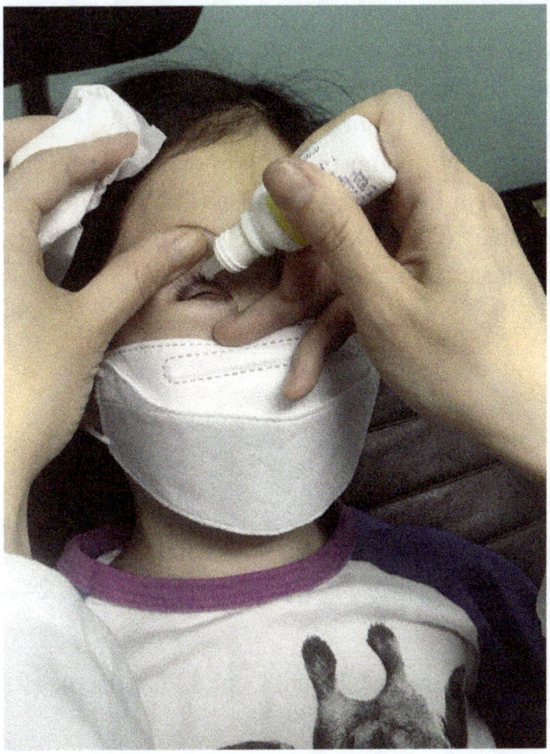

Clinical Pearls for Diagnostic Agents

Clinical Pearl: *It is important to perform punctal occlusion in infants to reduce systemic absorption.*

Clinical Pearl: *Use three drops of Cyclomydril, 5 minutes apart to achieve maximum dilation in premature infants.*

Clinical Pearl: *Use two drops of 1% Cyclopentolate, 5 minutes apart for cycloplegic refraction in children one year and older.*

Clinical Pearl: *Healthy infants and young children can use the age-appropriate individual drops or use a spray bottle combination.*

Clinical Pearl: *Many children are resistant and apprehensive to topical drop instillation. First attempt reassurance and persuasion. Try placing a drop on their finger to persuade them. If the child becomes combative, the clinician may need to use mild restraint with the help from family members.*

Clinical Pearl: *Have an adult family member hold the feet and legs to prevent the child from kicking if necessary.*

CONCLUSION

Diagnostic ophthalmic drops have become an integral part of clinical eye care in the pediatric population. Dilating agents are needed to examine the health of the eye in all children. This is especially crucial in examining premature infants to rule out retinopathy of prematurity.

Cycloplegic agents are important diagnostic tools in children who have a strong accommodative system, pseudomyopia and/or latent hyperopia. It is also useful in children who are malingering, non-communicative and uncooperative. At times it can be challenging to instill drops. However, with patience and experience, drops can be successfully instilled.

REFERENCES

Amos, J. F. (2001). Chapter 21 Cycloplegic Refraction. In Clinical Ocular Pharmacology (pp. 425-431). Butterworth-Heinemann.

Bartolone, A., & Rutner, D. (2006). Quantification of Refractive Error. In R. H. Duckman (Ed.), *Visual Development, Diagnosis, and Treatment of the Pediatric Patient* (pp. 244–258). Lippincott Williams and Wilkins.

Blansett, D. K. (2001). Dilation of pupil. In Clinical Ocular Pharmacology (pp. 405-421). Butterworth-Heinemann.

Gulden Ophthalmics. (2021). *Disposable spray caps (12 pack).* https://guldenophthalmics.com/product/disposable-spray-cap/

Gulden Ophthalmics. (2021). *Disposable spray caps video.* https://guldenophthalmics.com/video/disposable-spray-caps/

Ismail, E. E., Rouse, M. W., & De Land, P. N. (1994, April). A Comparison of drop instillation and spray application of 1% cyclopentolate hydrochloride. *Optometry and Vision Science*, *71*(4), 235–241. doi:10.1097/00006324-199404000-00001 PMID:8047334

KEY TERMS AND DEFINITIONS

Accommodation: The adjustment of the eye to keep things in focus on the retina as the distance changes.

Anesthetic: A drug used to cause insensitivity to pain.

Anticholinergic Drug: An agent that blocks the action of acetylcholine, specifically the sphincter muscle of the iris and the ciliary muscle of the lens causing dilation of the pupil and paralysis of accommodation.

Cycloplegic Agent: A drug that causes paralysis of the ciliary muscle of the eye, resulting in loss of accommodation.

Diagnostic Agents: A drug such as an eye drop used to help the doctor make conclusions on a medical condition.

Intraocular Pressure: The fluid pressure inside the eye.

Mydriatic Agent: A drug that dilates the pupil.

Tonometry: A test that measures intraocular pressure.

Chapter 12
Slit Lamp Examination on Pediatric Patients

Alanna Khattar
BronxCare Health System, USA

ABSTRACT

Slit lamp examination is an important component of a pediatric eye exam. The slit lamp instrument, also known as a biomicroscope, is used to provide a stereoscopic magnified view of the ocular structures. The slit lamp facilitates the examination of both the anterior segment as well as the posterior segment of the eyes. For posterior segment examination, handheld lenses are used in conjunction with the slit lamp. Different tools and examination techniques are often needed to examine infants, toddlers, and other pediatric patients who cannot be positioned in the slit lamp. This chapter discusses the techniques and equipment used to facilitate the ocular health examination, including anterior segment structures, posterior segment structures, and intraocular pressure measurements in the pediatric population.

INTRODUCTION

Performing a thorough ocular health examination on pediatric patients is critical for the appropriate diagnosis, treatment and management of any ocular findings they may have. While slit lamp examination, also known as biomicroscopy, is one of the most used tools for ocular health examination, it is not always possible to examine pediatric patients with this piece of equipment. Different tools and examination techniques are often needed to examine infants, toddlers and other pediatric patients who can not be positioned in the slit lamp.

For pediatric patients who can be positioned in the slit lamp, using this piece of equipment allows the clinician to examine all anterior segment structures with a magnified view. Hand held lenses are used in conjunction with the slit lamp to examine the posterior pole of the eye as well as the mid-periphery.

Tonometry is another important exam component that will be discussed in this chapter. There are a number of different methods available for obtaining an intraocular pressure reading whether it is using a Goldmann applanation tonometer or one of the many handheld device options available.

DOI: 10.4018/978-1-7998-8044-8.ch012

The goal of this chapter is to educate the reader on how to evaluate the ocular health of a pediatric patient, encompassing the anterior segment structures of the eye, portions of the posterior segment and intraocular pressure measurement.

+20D LENS WITH TRANSILLUMINATOR

Indication

A +20D lens normally used for binocular indirect ophthalmoscopy (BIO) can be used in conjunction with a transilluminator to examine the anterior segment of young patients, particularly infants and toddlers. This technique is indicated for children who are not able to have their anterior segment examination performed using a slit lamp. The +20D lens is used as the magnification source, while the transilluminator provides the light source (Figure 1).

This technique is also very useful for children of any age with special needs who are unable to be examined in the slit lamp as well as when performing bedside examinations in hospital settings.

Background

This technique allows for gross examination of the adnexa, eyelids, eyelashes, sclera, conjunctiva, lacrimal lake, cornea, iris, anterior chamber angle and lens. The +20D lens is held in front of the child's eye at a distance of less than five centimetres and the light is projected through the magnifying lens (Figure 2). Due to the close distance between the child and the +20D lens a magnified, upright, and virtual image is produced.

Clinical Pearl: *If an extra hand is needed to examine the patient for manipulation or fixation purposes, a binocular indirect ophthalmoscope (BIO) can be used as the light source instead of a transilluminator. This allows the examiner to hold the condensing lens in one hand, and have the other hand free to hold eyelids, direct fixation, or hold a toy as necessary while the BIO is worn on the examiner's head to provide the light source.*

Clinical Pearl: *A drop of sodium fluorescein can be instilled in the patient's eye to allow for further examination of the cornea and conjunctiva. Using a BIO or a direct ophthalmoscope with the cobalt filter and the +20D lens allows for examination of corneal and/or conjunctival staining patterns.*

Advantages

This technique allows the examiner to obtain a gross idea of the health of the anterior segment structures of the eye. It is beneficial to be able to look for any pathology that may need to be treated or further examined. Using the +20D lens with a transilluminator can easily and quickly detect an abnormality of the ocular adnexa, eyelids, eyelashes, sclera, conjunctiva, cornea or lens. No further equipment is needed as most clinicians will have a +20D lens for BIO examination.

Disadvantages

The main disadvantage of this technique is that it is not possible to change magnifications. Given the lower magnification compared to a slit lamp, it is often not possible to discern at what layers of tissue there may be an abnormality. Most notably it does not allow for distinctions of the different layers of the cornea or lens in a manner that a slit lamp would. It is more difficult to grade the depth of the anterior chamber angle compared to using a slit lamp. Subtle findings are difficult to appreciate with this method. Examining the anterior chamber for cells and flare is very difficult because the magnification is not strong enough.

Equipment

1. +20D condensing lens
2. Transilluminator

Figure 1. A +20D condensing lens and transilluminator can be used to examine the anterior segment of pediatric patients when they cannot be positioned in the slit lamp

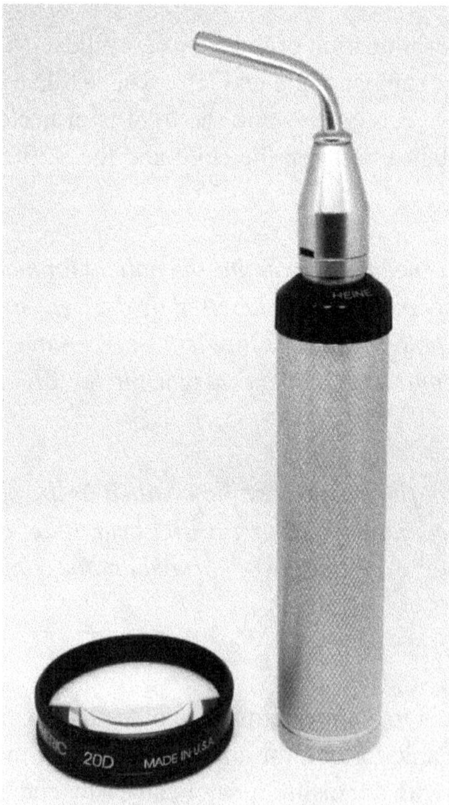

Procedure

Step 1: Proper patient placement must be first achieved

1. If the child is an infant, have the guardian hold them with the child's back to the guardian so they are facing the examiner. Alternatively, the infant can also be cradled in the guardian's arms. However, this may make it more difficult to examine if the child buries her/his head into the guardian's body
2. For toddlers and older children if they are not sitting on their own, have them sit in their guardian's lap facing forward
3. If the child is old enough to sit alone in the exam chair, raise the exam chair so you and the child are on eye level

Step 2: Starting with the right eye, hold the +20D lens in front of the child's eye, less than 5 cm away from the child, and shine the light towards the lens. If the child is old enough to follow directions, you can ask them to close the eyes to examine eyelids and eyelashes. If child is very young, it will not be possible for them to follow any specific directions

Step 3: After examining the eyelids and eyelashes, pull down the lower eyelid to examine the inferior palpebral conjunctiva. Note any signs of redness or papillae and follicles

Step 4: The inferior bulbar conjunctiva and sclera can be examined concurrently with the inferior palpebral conjunctiva. Direct the child's gaze upwards. You can move yourself upwards to give them a target. A similar action can be employed to have the child look left, right and down to allow for examination of the nasal, temporal and superior bulbar conjunctiva and sclera

Step 5: Shine the light towards the cornea to look for any opacities

Step 6: Next examine the iris and what is visible of the lens when child is undilated

Step 7: To check if the anterior chamber angles are grossly open use the shadow test. This is done using only the transilluminator. Shine the transilluminator from the temporal side of the cornea, and examine the nasal aspect of the iris. If the entire iris is illuminated the anterior chamber angle is wide open. The angle is deemed to be narrower if part of the iris is illuminated while some parts of it remain in the shadow because of the iris laying forward and blocking the light. The less illumination of the iris present, the narrower the angle (see section on shadow test angle estimation for further details)

Step 8: Repeat the examination for the left eye.

Clinical Pearl: *It is essential to keep the child's attention while performing this procedure. The examiner can move with the child as the eyes move, so minimal cooperation is necessary.*

Clinical Pearl: *If necessary, the hand that is holding the lens can also hold the child's eyelids open. The examiner holds the lens with the thumb and index fingers while holding the eyelids open with the middle finger.*

Figure 2. Anterior segment examination of a pediatric patient using a +20D condensing lens and a transilluminator. The left eye temporal conjunctiva is being examined

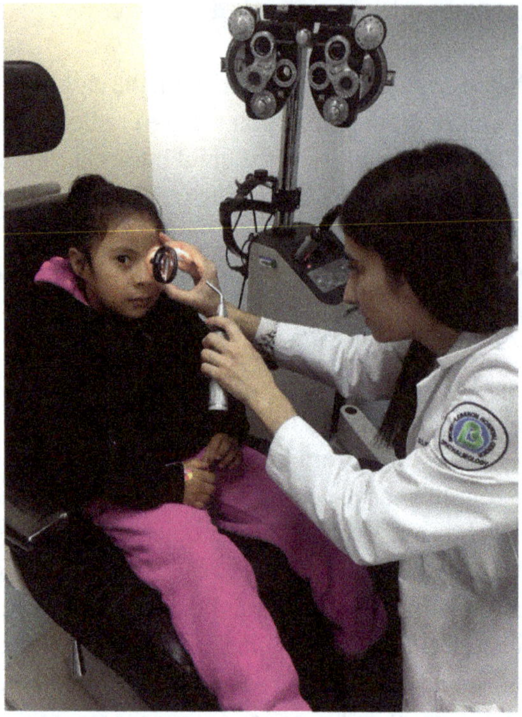

SLIT LAMP ANTERIOR SEGMENT EXAMINATION

Indications

A traditional stationary slit lamp can be used to examine all of the structures of the anterior segment. This is a component of all eye exams for any pediatric patient that is able to be positioned in this piece of equipment.

Background

Traditional slit lamps are typically attached to a stand that provides power. The slit lamp is placed on a table that can be moved both forward and backwards, as well as up and down. The table can be adjusted so both the child and the examiner are comfortable while the piece of equipment is being used.

While specific parameters vary between slit lamps, all slit lamps have the same core components. These components are the slit lamp base, patient support frame, viewing arm and illumination arm. Slit lamps typically have at least two different levels of magnification if not more, as well as a rheostat that allows for adjustment of the brightness of the light. The height and the width of the slit lamp beam can be adjusted, and different filters such as red-free and cobalt blue are available. The slit lamp beam is focused at the plane of the eye pieces.

Advantages

Both the child and the examiner have stability during the exam when positioned properly. The examiner does not need to balance or hold the equipment, and just uses the joy sticks and different dials to adjust the light beam when examining patients. This piece of equipment typically allows for the most magnified and best quality views of the anterior segment.

Disadvantages

Young children such as infants and toddlers cannot be positioned in the slit lamp. Also, the child must keep their head forward for the examiner's views to be in focus which may be difficult for younger patients. Traditional slit lamps are predominantly located in eye clinics, and are not easily portable to be set up in different settings for events such as vision screenings.

Equipment

1. Slit lamp

Procedure

Step 1: Disinfect the slit lamp prior to use

Step 2: Position the child comfortably in the slit lamp, lining up their lateral canthi with the canthus height markers on the patient support frame. Ensure that the slit lamp is at a comfortable height for the examiner as well

Step 3: Turn on the slit lamp power

Step 4: Begin the anterior segment examination on low magnification with a wide beam, and have the child close the eyes. Examine the eyelids and eyelashes of the right eye, and then move to the left eye and do the same

Step 5: Moving back to the right eye, have the child look up and pull down the lower lid to examine the inferior palpebral conjunctiva, inferior bulbar conjunctiva and inferior sclera. Have the child look down, to the right and left to examine the rest of the bulbar conjunctiva and sclera. Repeat for the left eye.

Step 6: Switch to higher magnification and shift the light source to 60 degrees and grade the temporal anterior chamber angle using the Van Herick technique (discussed in the Van Herick Angle Evaluation section)

Step 7: Next, adjust the light source angle to examine all layers of the cornea with a parallelepiped. A parallelepiped has a beam width of approximately 2mm, with the light source at an angle of about 45 degrees

Step 8: When the cornea has been scanned from limbus to limbus, then switch the light source back to 60 degrees to check the nasal anterior chamber angle again using the Van Herick technique (discussed in the Van Herick Angle Evaluation Section). The beam width can be adjusted to examine the cornea using both a parallelepiped and an optic section. Repeat for the left eye

Step 9: The iris can be examined after the cornea with the light source in the click (straight ahead) position. If you are not dilating the eye, you can also examine the lens at this time, evaluating the different layers of the lens that are visible through the pupil. If you are dilating the eye, a better view will be achieved post dilation. Repeat for the left eye

Step 10: To assess for cells and flare in the anterior chamber, ensure that the room illumination is as dim as possible. Increase the slit lamp magnification to the highest available magnification, and decrease the beam height to the shortest height. The beam width should be about that of a narrow parallelepiped. Increase the illumination level of the slit lamp as well. Position the light beam over the pupil, and then first shift the light beam to bring the iris in focus, and then shift the beam to bring the cornea in focus, and it is when the slit lamp is focused between these two structures that the anterior chamber can be assessed for cells and flare

Step 11: A drop of sodium fluorescein or a fluorescein strip hydrated with saline solution or proparacaine can be placed in the eye to examine for papillae, follicles or any corneal/conjunctival staining abnormalities. Use the cobalt filter to look for any staining or other pathology

PORTABLE SLIT LAMP

Indications

A portable slit lamp allows for examination of the anterior segment of pediatric patients when they are unable to sit in a traditional slit lamp on their own. This is another very useful piece of equipment for bedside examinations in hospital settings.

Portable slit lamps are lightweight, and you can manipulate different parameters such as the width, length and brightness of the light beam as well as change magnifications. Different filters can also be used. More modern portable slit lamps are cordless allowing the provider to be mobile and move with the patient if necessary, during examination.

The use of a portable slit lamp is advantageous for getting an in-depth look at the cornea, iris, lens and anterior chamber as well as retaining the ability to perform a thorough exam of all other anterior segment structures.

Background

Portable slit lamps are lightweight, usually weighing less than 2 pounds, allowing for easy maneuverability. These slit lamps typically offer 10X and 16X magnification. Portable slit lamps have different adjustable slit widths as well as controllable illumination levels. The slit length is usually a standard size. The light source can typically be rotated to 30 or 60 degrees in either direction. Most portable slit lamps have at least a cobalt blue filter, and may have other filters such as a red free filter. The eyepieces can be adjusted to correct for the examiner's refractive error or accommodative needs when necessary.

A recent feature of more modern portable slit lamps is that they have imaging adaptors allowing for smartphones, digital or video cameras to be used with the device. Most portable slit lamps on the market are now cordless and have a carrying case, allowing them to be easily taken to untraditional locations to help with exams, and can easily be carried between rooms in an office setting. This also allows easy maneuverability for a clinician when examining a pediatric patient who may be moving the head/eyes significantly during the exam.

There are a wide variety of portable slit lamps available. Some look like a miniature slit lamp while others are deemed “ultra-portable” composed of a magnifying bracket and lamp body. These systems may have halogen or LED lighting. The average working distance is 3 to 4 inches.

Equipment

1. Portable slit lamp (Figure 3)

Figure 3. Example of Kowa portable slit lamp

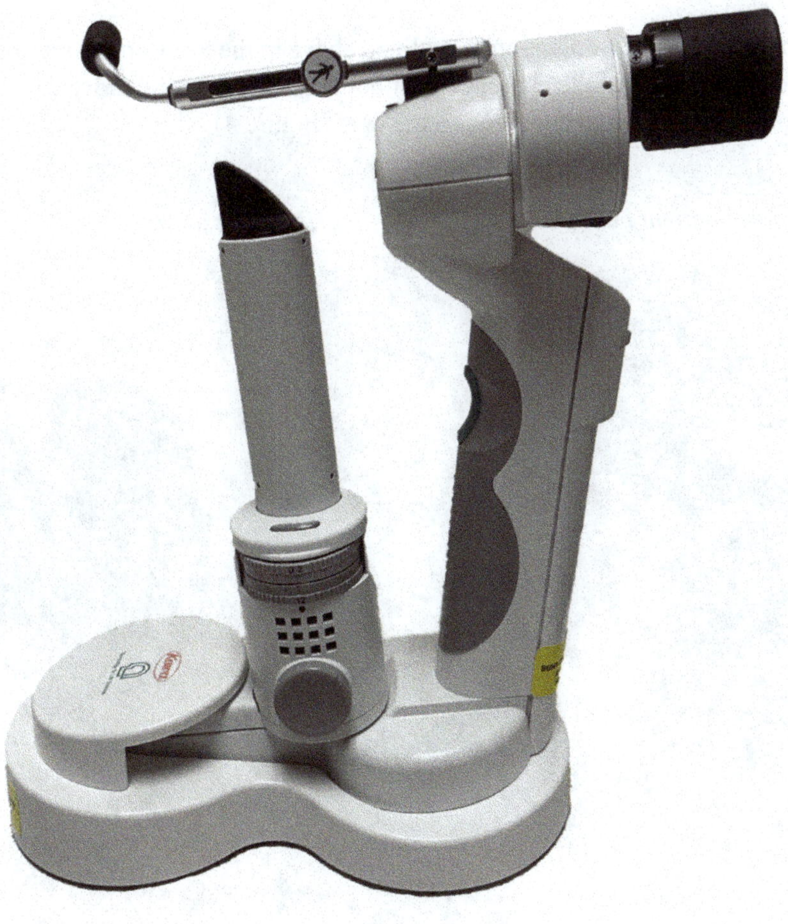

Advantages

With this technique, you have the ability to examine structures such as the cornea, iris, lens and anterior chamber to a much more magnified and detailed extent. It also allows for measurements to be taken of anterior segment findings. A portable slit lamp examination can be performed in any setting, in or out of an office, on patients of any age.

Disadvantages

A portable slit lamp is an expensive piece of equipment to purchase. The clinician must keep steady and balance the slit lamp while examining the patient which is more challenging than using a stationary slit lamp.

Procedure

Step 1: Remove the slit lamp from the base, and turn it on. Become familiar with the features, and how to manipulate them before beginning the exam

Step 2: Have the child sit in their guardian's lap facing forward, or if old enough, child can sit in the exam chair alone

Step 3: Perform the slit lamp examination as outlined above in the Slit Lamp Anterior Segment section. The main difference is that the clinician must hold the slit lamp and move with the slit lamp when examining the child and moving between the eyes (Figure 4)

Figure 4. A pediatric patient being examined using a portable slit lamp

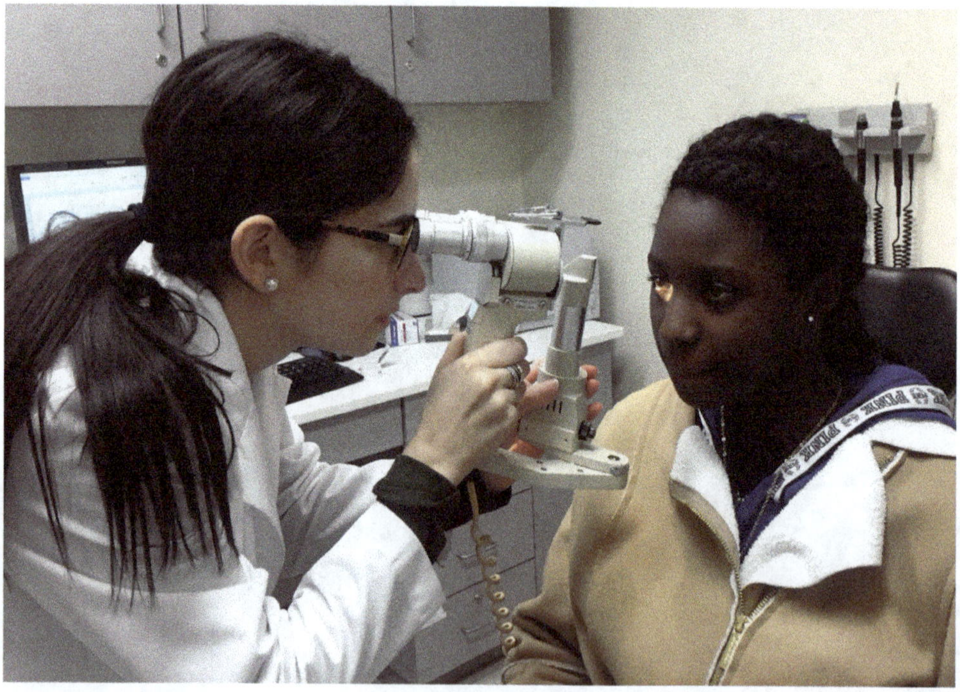

Clinical Pearl: *Having fun or interesting targets such as stickers for the pediatric patient to look at are helpful during anterior segment examination. The provider can ask the child details about the stickers, and this helps with achieving the desired fixation of gaze for examination.*

VAN HERICK ANGLE EVALUATION TECHNIQUE

Table 1. Van Herick grading scale used to assess the angle of the anterior chamber of the eye when using a slit lamp

Van Herick grade	Width of empty space compared to width of limbal corneal section
Grade 1	<1/4
Grade 2	1/4
Grade 3	1/2 to 1/4
Grade 4	≥1

(Van Herick et al., 1969)

Indication

The Van Herick technique is used to evaluate the anterior chamber angle with slit lamp biomicroscopy. If the anterior chamber angles appear narrow using this technique, this indicates that gonioscopy should be performed prior to dilation to further assess the structures of the angle.

Background

As part of a routine eye exam, the clinician must examine the contents of the anterior chamber (AC) for its clarity, signs of inflammation, and to ensure that the AC is open and the patient is not at risk for angle closure. In children the anterior chamber angles are usually wide open. With age, the lens will thicken, pushing the iris forward and narrowing the anterior chamber angle and shortening the anterior chamber depth. In addition to age, there are other risk factors that may cause a narrower angle. These includes female sex, family history, hyperopia, shorter axial length and East Asian descent (Kanski et al., 2011).

This section focuses on the most common techniques used to assess the anterior chamber angle in pediatric patients. However, if a pediatric patient is a glaucoma suspect or there is concern for a condition such as Axenfeld-Rieger syndrome where developmental abnormalities of the AC angle may exist, gonioscopy should be performed. If a pediatric patient is unable to tolerate the procedure of gonioscopy, another option for evaluation of the AC angle is to perform an optical coherence tomography (OCT) of the angle (Figure 5). OCT is a powerful tool used to exam both the posterior and anterior segment of the eye. An OCT of the AC angle captures cross-sectional images of the iridocorneal angle. The angle is assessed by comparing the position of the iris in relation to the structures of the AC angle. It is a non-contact technique that can help determine if an eye is at risk for angle closure.

The anterior chamber angle should be examined prior to the instillation of dilation drops.

Advantages

This technique is fast, easy, non-invasive and accurate. It correlates well with gonioscopic findings.

Disadvantages

This method requires the child to be cooperative and to be able to sit behind the slit lamp for examination.

Equipment

1. Slit lamp with the light beam as an optic section

Procedure

Step 1: Decrease the width of the vertical slit lamp beam to as narrow as possible (known as an optic section). Then place the optic section at the temporal limbus just inside the corneal-scleral junction and directed at a 60 degree angle

Step 2: The depth of the anterior chamber (AC) at the temporal limbus is compared with the width of the optic section (which represents the thickness of the cornea) (Figure 6). The depth of the anterior chamber is represented by the width of the non illuminated part of the iris located between the optic section and the reflection of the slit beam on the iris

Step 3: Assess the depth of the anterior chamber angle at both the temporal and nasal limbus. This serves as a reliable average for the entire angle (Table 1)

1. If the depth of the anterior chamber is equal to or greater than the thickness of the cornea then the angle is considered to be wide open, a grade 4 angle (Figure 7)
2. If the depth of the AC is equal to half the thickness of the cornea the angle is classified as a grade 3 angle
3. If the depth of the AC is ¼ the corneal thickness the angle is classified as a grade 2 angle
4. If the depth of the AC is < 1/4 the corneal thickness the angle would be classified as a grade 1 angle
5. If the depth of the AC is grade 2 or less, gonioscopy should be performed prior to dilation to further assess the structures of the angle

Figure 5. OCT of the anterior chamber angle of the eye. This image demonstrates an open anterior chamber angle. This is an alternative way to assess the anterior chamber of the eye in a pediatric patient if other methods are unattainable

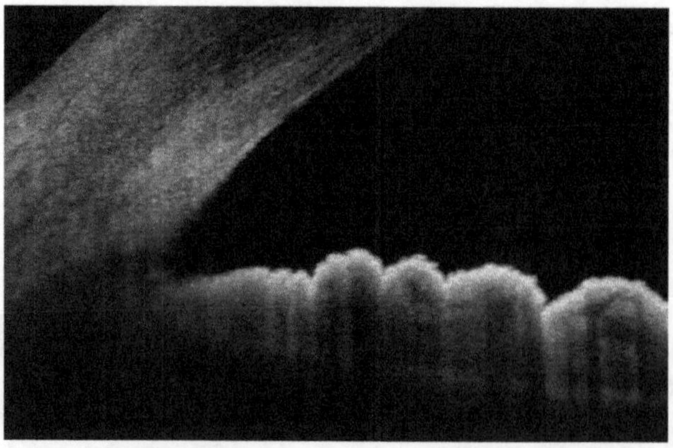

Figure 6. Schematic demonstrating the use of the Van Herick technique to assess anterior chamber angles of different depths
Source: Tak-Man Kimberly Fung OD, 2021

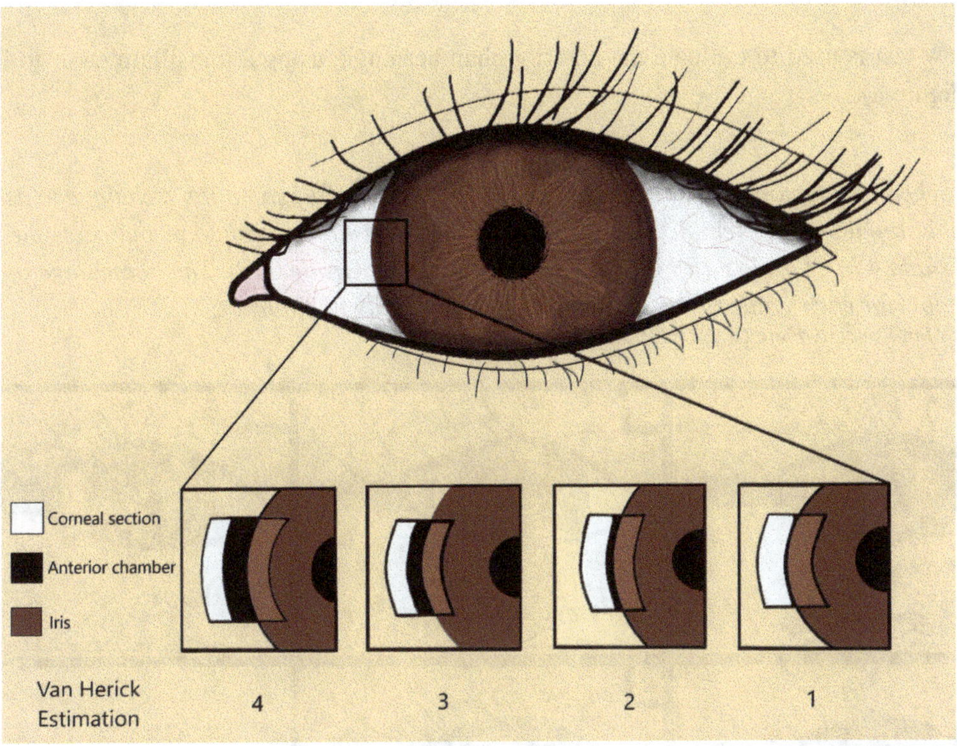

Figure 7. Slit lamp photo demonstrating checking of the anterior chamber angle using the Van Herick technique. The Van Herick grading in this image would be a grade 4 with the non-illuminated area formed between the optic section and the reflection of the slit lamp beam on the iris being larger than the thickness of the beam of the optic section

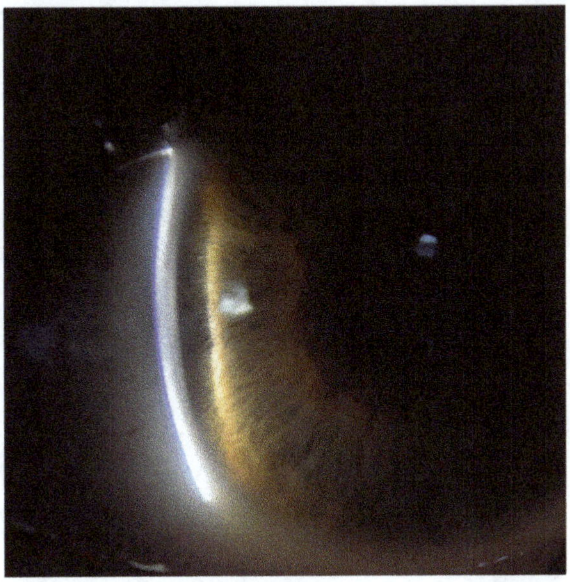

SHADOW TEST ANGLE ESTIMATION

Indication

The shadow test is used to evaluate the anterior chamber angle using a transilluminator to illuminate the iris (Figure 8).

Figure 8. Schematic demonstrating the use of the shadow test angle estimation technique to assess anterior chamber angles of different depths. The percentage of nasal iris in shadow indicates the following grades - Grade 4 (a), Grade 3 (b), Grade 2 (c), Grade 1 (d), Grade 0 (e). The percentage of the nasal iris in shadow for each grade is further described numerically in Table 2
Source: Tak-Man Kimberly Fung OD, 2021. (Adapted from [Elliot, 2007])

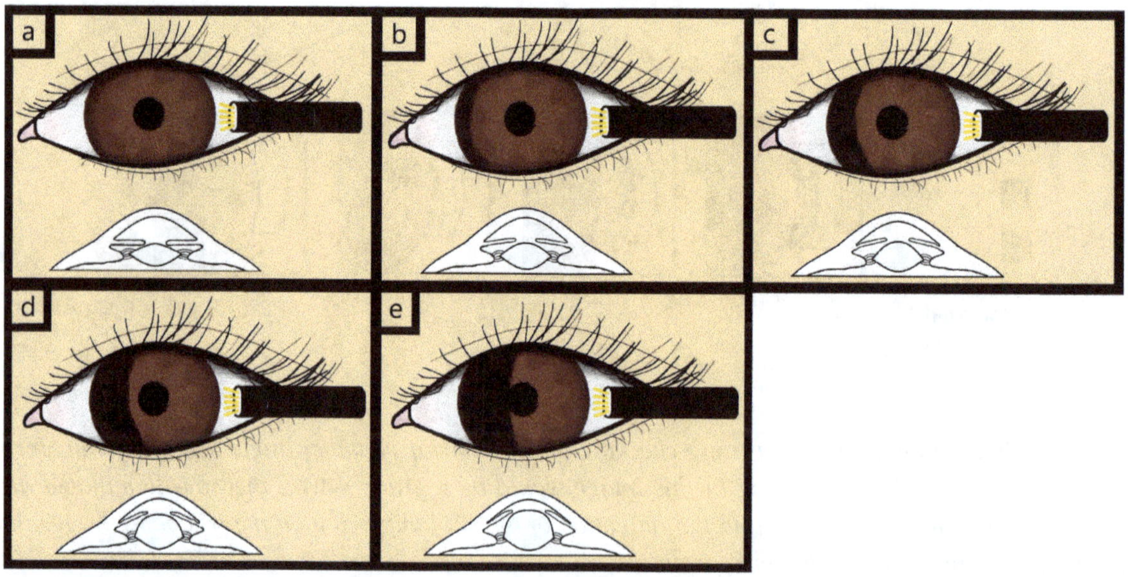

Background

The shadow test is a technique that can be used to assess if the anterior chamber angle is open or narrow. It is often used when a patient is unable to be positioned in the slit lamp to have the anterior chamber angle assessed using the Van Herick angle estimation technique. Narrow anterior chamber angles have a bowed iris, so the narrower an angle is, the more of the nasal iris that will be in shadow when the light is directed at the temporal limbus.

Advantages

This is a quick and reliable technique to identify a critically narrow angle that might be predisposed to angle closure.

Disadvantages

The technique is a less accurate method compared to the Van Herrick estimate in the slit lamp or gonioscopy.

Equipment

1. Transilluminator

Procedure

Step 1: Dim the room lights and have child look straight ahead
Step 2: Direct the transilluminator light beam at the temporal limbus (Figure 9)
Step 3: The entire iris will illuminate if the iris lies in a flat plane with a deep anterior chamber, indicating the angle is wide open, with a 45 degree angle between the iris and cornea. This represents a grade 4 angle
Step 4: If the light beam illuminates the temporal iris with a shadow on the nasal iris, the angle is shallow. The angle between the iris and cornea may be 20 degrees or less (grade 2 to 0). See table 2 for a detailed grading scale

Clinical Pearl: *If the light is positioned too far anteriorly or if the eye is deviated temporally, the penlight may illuminate the nasal aspect of the iris directly, giving a false-negative result.*

Figure 9. The shadow test angle estimation technique being used to evaluate two different patients. Figure 9A demonstrates a wide-open angle using the shadow test, while Figure 9B demonstrates a more narrow angle with about 75% of the nasal iris in shadow

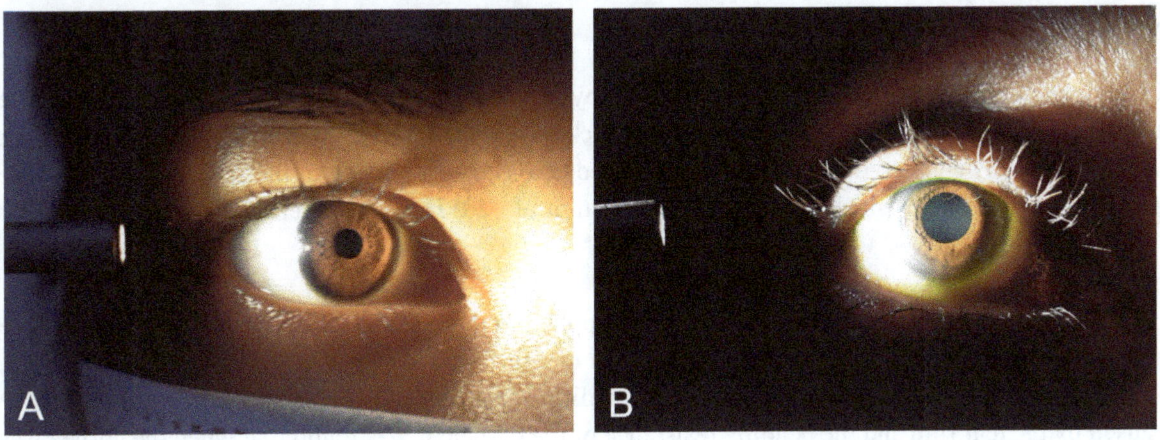

Table 2. Estimation of anterior chamber angle depth using the shadow test angle estimation technique

Shadow Test Grade	Percent of nasal iris in shadow
Grade 0	100%
Grade 1	75%
Grade 2	50%
Grade 3	25%
Grade 4	0%

(Elliott, 2007)

MEASURING INTRAOCULAR PRESSURE

Goldmann Applanation Tonometry

Indications

Checking the intraocular pressure (IOP) of patients is very important, regardless of their age. While measuring the intraocular pressure of pediatric patients can be difficult at times, a number of methods are available to allow the examiner to get a reliable measurement. The standard of care when it comes to intraocular pressure (IOP) measurements is Goldmann applanation tonometry (GAT).

There are a number of different ocular conditions that can cause an elevated IOP in a pediatric patient, such as congenital glaucoma, uveitis and sequelae of ocular trauma such as a hyphema. IOP must be measured reliably in these patients to monitor their conditions.

There is no age at which it is expected that a pediatric patient can successfully have GAT performed on them. The ability of each pediatric patient to sit still and fixate differs, and this must be assessed on a child-by-child basis.

Background

Goldmann applanation tonometry measures IOP by providing a force which flattens the cornea. The theory behind this technique is based on Imbert-Fick law. This law states that the pressure (P) within a sphere is roughly equal to the external force (f) needed to flatten a portion of the sphere, divided by the area (A) of the sphere which is flattened (Kirstein et al., 2011). The law can be expressed as such:

$$Pressure = \frac{force}{area}$$

However, Imbert-Fick law cannot be directly applied to the cornea because it is working under the assumption that the cornea is infinitely thin, has a dry surface and is perfectly elastic (Kirstein et al., 2011). To account for these factors, the law is modified to take into account the surface tension force caused by the tear film and the bending resistance of the cornea. It was found that when the cornea was applanated with an applanation diameter of 3.06 mm, which leads to an applanation area of 7.35 mm^2, the effects of surface tension and bending resistance become equal and cancel each other out (Kirstein et al., 2011).

A disinfected cylindrically shaped truncated probe is used to applanate on the cornea after an anesthetic and dye has been introduced into the precorneal tear film of the eye. The tonometer tip is a plastic biprism that creates two semi-circles when it applanates the cornea. To alter the force applied to the cornea the practitioner turns the tension knob. It is crucial that a Goldmann tonometer is calibrated properly, or all IOP readings will be incorrect. The correct measurement is obtained when the internal aspects of the two semi circles are just in contact with each other. The semi circles touch when 3.06 mm of the cornea is applanated. The unit of measurement for IOP is millimeters of mercury (mmHg).

Advantages

Goldmann applanation tonometry is the gold standard measurement against which measurements from all other IOP measuring devices are compared. It is considered to be the most accurate form of measuring IOP. It is a low-cost form of IOP measurement.

Disadvantages

Goldmann applanation tonometry method involves using an anesthetic agent and is the most invasive form of IOP measurement that needs a child's cooperation. It can frighten children to have something coming directly towards their eye. If there is too much or too little fluorescein dye in the eye it can lead to overestimation and underestimation respectively of IOP. Corneal thickness can affect IOP readings with this method as well. Thick corneas produce an overestimation of IOP while thin corneas produce an underestimation. When a patient has corneal scarring or other corneal irregularities the accuracy of the measurement is decreased.

With this technique there is an increased risk for a spread of infection since the same probe historically was being used on multiple patients. The probe must be cleaned between each encounter. Disposable tonometer tips are now available, which eliminates the risk of infection from a reusable tonometer probe. There is also a risk of a corneal abrasion if the child suddenly moves while their IOP is being checked.

Equipment (Figure 10)

1. Slit lamp
2. Goldmann tonometer probe
3. 0.5% proparacaine ophthalmic solution and sodium fluorescein dye strips or a combination eye drop containing both the anesthetic and dye

Procedure

Step 1: Disinfect the reusable tonometer tip in accordance with current Center for Disease Control (CDC) guidelines and ensure no residual cleaning agent remains on the probe to come in contact with the cornea. If using a disposable tonometer tip, remove from packaging and attach to Goldmann apparatus

Step 2: Instill either one drop of 0.5% proparacaine ophthalmic solution in each eye and then instill dye from a sodium fluorescein strip that is moistened with saline solution or a drop of 0.5% proparacaine ophthalmic solution in each eye, or instill one drop of an anesthetic/dye combination drop into each eye

Step 3: Position child comfortably in the slit lamp
Step 4: Move the tonometer tip apparatus into place, in the click position for the right eye
Step 5: Move the light source (illumination arm) to the left, and turn on the cobalt blue filter. Make the beam as tall and wide as possible, and turn the light source up to full brightness
Step 6: Instruct child to fixate on the proper target, and to take a large blink and hold the eyes open as wide as possible without blinking
Step 7: Move the tonometer tip forward and applanate the cornea
Step 8: Make sure that the semi-circle mires are centered on the cornea both vertically and horizontally. If one of the mires is larger than the other, move the probe towards the larger semi-circle to correct for this. If the top mire is larger than the bottom mire, the applanator position is misaligned vertically on the cornea
Step 9: Adjust the tension knob until the inner portion of the semi-circles are just in contact, and are not over-shooting or under-shooting alignment. If the mires are overlapped too far, it means that the pressure from the applanator is too high. If the mires are not yet overlapped, it means that the pressure from the applanator is too low (Figure 11)
Step 10: When the semi-circle mires are aligned appropriately, the reading on the dial is the IOP measurement for the right eye
Step 11: To repeat the procedure for the left eye, move the light source to the opposite side. Otherwise, the set up and procedure are the same.

Figure 10. A: Goldmann tonometer. B: Goldmann tonometer with cobalt blue filter, prepared for applanation

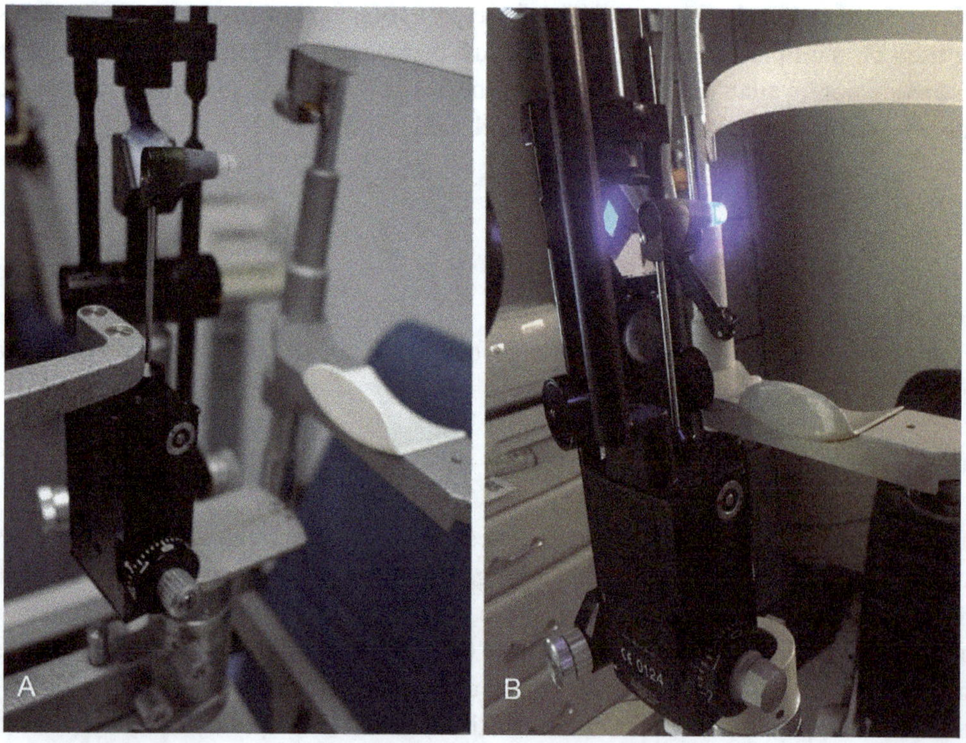

Clinical Pearl: *When performing Goldmann tonometry on pediatric patients, instruct them to open the eyes as if they saw a ghost, and pretend they are having a staring contest and count to 20 with them.*

Clinical Pearl: *For pediatric patients, have them hold on to the side bars of the slit lamp "like they're riding a motorcycle" for stability.*

Clinical Pearl: *Make sure child is not trying to also open the mouth when you ask them to open the eyes. Additionally, you must ensure child is breathing normally and not holding the breath.*

Clinical Pearl: *If the child will not keep the eyes open, the examiner can hold the eyelids open. Care must be taken to hold the upper eyelid up against the orbital bone, not against the globe. Holding the globe will artificially increase the eye pressure.*

Clinical Pearl: *If the child is nervous, ask them to focus on keeping the chin in the slit lamp cup, forehead pressed up against the bar and keeping the other eye open, and inform the child you will take care of the rest.*

Clinical Pearl: *Inform the child they may feel a tickle on the eyelashes, and that is all they will feel.*

Clinical Pearl: *Have the child's guardian help with holding the child's head forward in the slit lamp if she/he is continually backing away.*

Figure 11. Examples of different alignments of Goldmann applanation tonometry semi-circle mires. A) Appropriately aligned to take the IOP measurement with the semi-circles just touching. This indicates the reading of the applanator equals the pressure of the globe. B) The semi-circular mires are overlapped too much, indicating the pressure from the applanator is too high. C)The semi-circular mires are not yet overlapped, indicating the pressure from the applanator is too low. D) Inadequate dye remains in the eye which will lead to an incorrect IOP recording. E. There is excess dye in the eye, which will also lead to an incorrect IOP reading
Source: Tak-Man Kimberly Fung OD, 2021

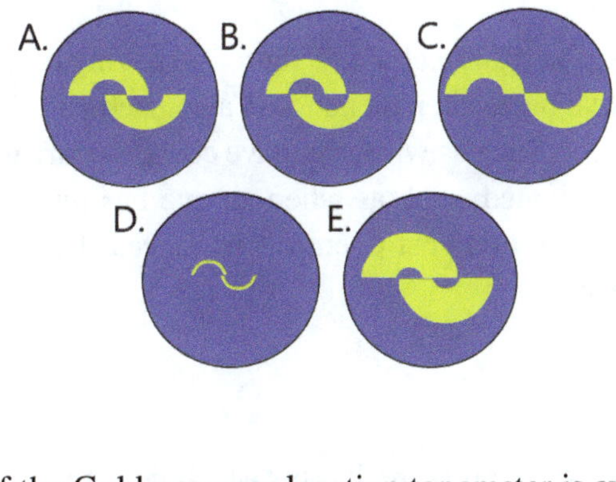

A hand-held adaptation of the Goldmann applanation tonometer is available, known as the Perkins hand-held applanation tonometry. This tonometer also employs Imbert-Fick's law and uses tonometer tips in the same fashion as a Goldmann applanation tonometer. The Perkins Mk3 (Haag Strait) is compatible with disposable tonometer tips to decrease the risk of infection when using the device. The Perkins tonometer can be used if a patient is seated or in a supine position, which is very useful when examining a pediatric patient in either a traditional or non-traditional exam setting (Haag-Strait UK, 2020).

The use of Perkins applanation tonometry has been well established in animals, but there have been fewer studies in humans. Arora et al. (2014) compared Perkins applanation with Goldmann applanation in 100 eyes of 100 patients and found the IOP measurements to be closely comparable with a clear correlation between the two types of readings. The mean difference between Perkins and Goldmann readings was found to be 0.22 mmHg.

DIGITAL INTRAOCULAR PRESSURE MEASUREMENTS

Indications

To obtain an estimated intraocular pressure (IOP). Digital IOP measurements are simple, quick and a useful technique for obtaining a gross IOP when examining infants and toddlers.

Background

Digital palpation is used for a gross measurement of IOP. It is an old method of IOP measurement and this technique has been used for many centuries. An examiner's sense of touch can be trained to a certain extent to allow for translation of the tactile measurement into an approximate IOP measurement. When an increase in tension is felt this correlates with a higher IOP reading, and the opposite correlates with a lower IOP reading. This method is most useful to screen for a considerable increase in IOP. Studies have shown success with examiners being able to correctly identify IOP higher than 30 mmHg the majority of the time using this technique (Baum et al., 1995). Another study that compared digital palpation with non-contact tonometry measurements found a statistically significant correlation for the digital tension measurement compared with the non-contact tonometry reading (Ficarra et al., 2002).

Advantages

No equipment is necessary to perform this technique, therefore having no cost to the clinician. It is useful for very young and uncooperative pediatric patients. It is also useful in situations where other forms of IOP measurements cannot be done, such as with extensive corneal scarring. There are certain instances when the globe should not be palpated, such as when an eye has undergone significant trauma with concern for a globe rupture, or in certain post-operative instances. There is no anesthetic that needs to be introduced to the patient's eyes.

Disadvantages

It is a gross measurement of intraocular pressure. It is not a technique that is useful for monitoring patients with glaucoma or other pathological conditions with elevated IOP. Performing this properly requires some training to learn the tactile difference between a soft and hard eye to the touch with respect to IOP.

Equipment

None

Procedure

Step 1: Ask child to close eyes and look down
Step 2: Move any redundant skin superiorly with the examiner's index fingers
Step 3: Using the index fingers of both hands gently apply pressure to the superior part of the closed eyelids in the 12 o'clock meridian. Alternate between each eye
Step 4: Estimate the force necessary to indent the globe
Step 5: Record whether the eyes are soft to touch, medium to touch or hard to touch. It is also important to note if the digital palpation felt equal between the two eyes, or if there is a difference in pressure between both eyes based on digital palpation

Clinical Pearl: *The clinician can learn to quantify digital IOP more precisely by practicing digital pressures after Goldmann applanation tonometry (GAT) and learning the tactile feeling of an eye with a known quantitative IOP.*

TONOPEN

Indications

Obtaining an accurate IOP measurement is important for patients of all ages. When patients are young they are often not able to sit in the slit lamp, or are apprehensive to do so. A Tonopen provides an alternative method that gives the clinician a numerical value of IOP measurement.

Background

A Tonopen is a handheld IOP measuring device (Figure 12). It must be calibrated before usage. A plunger is attached to a strain gauge in the apparatus. As the plunger of the Tonopen indents the cornea, the gauge reads an increase in pressure. When the pressure reaches the point at which it flattens the cornea, the strain is momentarily alleviated from the plunger. The applanation point is considered to be at the point of reduced strain (Kirstein et al, 2011).

The cornea is applanated multiple times before an average resulting measurement is displayed. This point is automatically read by the device and an average of all the readings obtained is displayed, as well as the statistical confidence indicator. Each Tonopen may have a different way of expressing the confidence of the measurements, so it is important to know how to interpret the readings. If the final reading is noted with a high confidence level then the measurement is acceptable. If the confidence level of the readings is low, repeat measurements should be taken.

Advantages

Advantages of the Tonopen are that it is portable and can be used in any setting on a patient of any age. It is especially convenient to get an IOP reading on young children and infants when necessary. A new plastic cover is placed on the tip of the Tonopen each time it is used, which significantly decreases the risk of infection. The Tonopen applanates a smaller area of the cornea, making it more useful when corneal surface irregularities are present to obtain a reading.

Disadvantages

Use of anesthetic is necessary with this method of IOP measurement. The patient will see the Tonopen coming towards their eye which can be alarming. If a child is constantly moving their head to avoid it there is an increased risk of corneal abrasion. Tonopens are also expensive. It is also necessary to take multiple readings for each eye which prolongs the procedure for the patient.

Equipment

1. 0.5% proparacaine ophthalmic solution
2. Tonopen
3. Tonopen tip covers

Figure 12. Tono-pen AVIA® prepared for use with tip cover in place

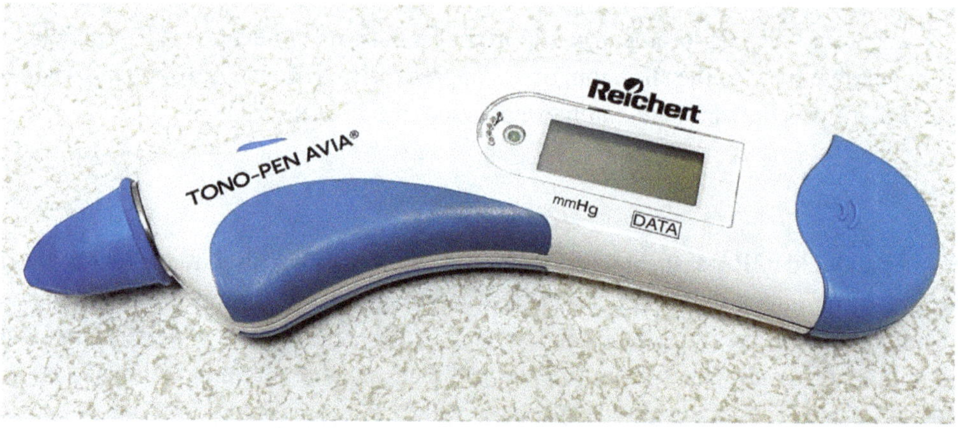

Procedure

Step 1: Place one drop of 0.5% proparacaine ophthalmic solution in each eye
Step 2: Press the power button to turn on the Tonopen
Step 3: Make sure to calibrate the Tonopen per the instructions for the specific model being used
Step 4: Place the tip cover on the device, making sure that it is not applied too tightly or loosely. The rubber cover should be flat across the tip but not taut

Step 5: If the child is old enough to sit on alone, have child sit facing straight ahead in the exam chair. If the child is too young to sit in the chair on own but can sit up, they can sit in the guardian's lap facing you. If the child is an infant, you can have the guardian cradle them and hold the arms down
Step 6: Select a target for the child to look towards, located straight across the room
Step 7: Align the Tonopen so that the probe is perpendicular to the cornea. Hold it as if holding a pencil. One hand may be needed to hold the eyelids open. If necessary the examiner can also brace the hand holding the Tonopen on the child's bridge of the nose or cheek – this provides increased control over any small movements needed to align the Tonopen with the cornea
Step 8: Ask child to open both eyes as wide as possible and look at the target
Step 9: Press the activation button to initiate applanation mode
Step 10: Starting with the right eye, very briefly and lightly tap the center of the corneal surface. When a reading has been taken the Tonopen will make a "chirp" sound indicating a successful measurement
Step 11: When the entire group of measurements has been collected a different beep tone will indicate the readings are complete and the IOP measurement will appear on the LCD screen along with the statistical confidence indicator of the measurement
Step 12: Repeat the same procedure for the left eye. If the examiner is more stable with one hand compared to the other, that hand can continue to hold the Tonopen and stay positioned on that side of the child even when the left eye is being measured

NON-CONTACT TONOMETRY

Indications

Non-contact tonometry (NCT) is used to measure intraocular pressures. It is a non-invasive technique that has an appeal in many different settings, and for different patient populations one of which being the pediatric patient population.

Background

Non-contact tonometers use a forceful stream of air to flatten the cornea. The cornea is "applanated" by the air. The force of the air puff increases until the cornea is applanated over a predetermined area (Kirstein et al., 2011). The force increases steadily and in a linear fashion. The applanation force is then translated into a measure of intraocular pressure.

The IOP is measured through a light source. The patient looks at the target light, and this light reflects off the cornea and travels towards a sensor in the tonometer at a specific angle. As the cornea is being flattened by the stream of air, the angle of the light reflection off the cornea is changed. When the cornea is flattened, the light is reflected off the cornea in such a way that the sensor will absorb the maximal amount of light. The amount of time that is necessary for this maximal amount of light to be absorbed is recorded and then converted by the instrument into an IOP reading in mmHg (Kempf et al., 2006).

If the IOP in an eye is high, a higher force will be needed to flatten the cornea. The point in time at which the cornea is flattened occurs later during the air pulse in an eye with a higher IOP since more force will need to be applied to reach the desired end point. The softer the eye is, the less time it will take to be flattened by the stream of air, resulting in a lower IOP reading. The stream of air that the patient feels is extremely brief.

Advantages

No anesthetic eye drop is required because the cornea is not contacted. It is easy to use with children since they don't see a device physically coming towards their eye. This method is particularly useful for children who have an allergy to anesthetics or fluorescein dye.

If a child is presenting for a contact lens exam, this method allows IOP to be checked without the use of fluorescein dye that would otherwise need to be washed out of the eye or the child would need to wait until the dye fully drained for it to not be soaked up by the contact lens.

The measurement from the apparatus is objective, and not dependent on the subjective reading of the examiner so there is no inter-observer variation. There is also reduced risk of infection spread between patients since a probe is not coming in contact with the cornea itself.

Disadvantages

Children are very apprehensive about the "air puff" test, and get very squeamish and tend to move away, which can make obtaining a measurement difficult.

Measurement errors are induced by variations in corneal properties such as corneal thickness and corneal surface irregularities. The NCT measurements are only a measurement at a brief instant in time, which does not consider the cycling of IOP as the choroid fills and empties with blood with the cardiac cycle (Kirstein et al., 2011).

Equipment

1. Non-contact tonometer

Procedure (Stationary Non-Contact Tonometer)

Step 1: Clean off the chin and forehead rests of the non-contact tonometer
Step 2: Position and align the patient comfortably in the machine
Step 3: Align the machine with the child's right eye
Step 4: Ask the child to find the target light source inside of the machine, and to look directly towards it
Step 5: Instruct the child to take a large blink and open their eyes as wide as possible
Step 6: The examiner presses the button to release the stream of air and the measurement is taken by the machine
Step 7: Move the non-contact tonometer over so it is now aligned with the left eye
Step 8: Repeat the same procedure on the left eye

Clinical Pearl: *Make sure the pediatric patient has their eyes open wide so that their eyelashes are not in the way and will not interfere with the IOP measurement.*

While stationary non-contact tonometers are more commonly found in ophthalmic offices, hand held non-contact tonometers are available as well. The hand-held non contact tonometer offers significant advantages especially when working with the pediatric population. The hand-held equipment no longer requires the child be positioned in a chin rest. These devices can be used for a pediatric patient of any age, whether the child is sitting on their own or in their guardian's lap. Hand held non-contact tonometers also occupy less space in the office setting compared to a stationary or desktop non-contact tonometer.

REBOUND TONOMETRY

Indications

This method of tonometry is one of the newer handheld devices available. It is very useful for pediatric patients of all ages, especially when they are unable to be positioned in the slit lamp. It is user friendly, and able to be employed in any setting where it may be necessary to obtain an IOP reading without the use of a slit lamp.

Background

The theory behind this type of tonometry is that a harder eye (with a higher IOP) will cause a faster deceleration of a probe that is introduced towards it compared to a softer eye (with a lower IOP).

A rod probe is what contacts the eye. The probes are disposable, and are made of a magnetized steel wire shaft that is covered with a round plastic tip at the end (Cervino, 2006). The plastic tip minimizes the risk of corneal injury when the probe touches the cornea. When the button is initiated for a pressure reading, the probe hits the cornea and bounces back. The maximum deceleration or impact duration is measured (Kontiola, 1997). The probe bounces back faster as the IOP increases, so the shorter duration of impact the higher the IOP is (Cervino, 2006). Measurements are taken very quickly, faster than the corneal reflex.

The software is typically programmed to take six measurements, where the highest and lowest are deleted and the rest are averaged to get the final read out (Cervino, 2006).

Grigorian et al. (2015) compared the use of the iCare rebound tonometer with Goldmann applanation tonometry in a pediatric population. The study found that readings from the two instruments were consistently correlated. IOP readings by iCare were found to be consistently higher than GAT by an average of 1.38 mmHg. Clinically, this translated to an insignificant difference with measurements being within 3 mmHg in 72.42% of eyes (Grigorian et al., 2015). Feng et al. (2015) compared IOP measurements obtained by rebound, non-contact and GAT in healthy pediatric patients who did not have glaucoma. This study compared IOP measurements as well as tolerability in a pediatric population with patients aged 3 to 15 years old. The mean difference between rebound and Goldmann applanation tonometry was found to be 1.81 ± 2.43 mmHg. Rebound tonometry was found to overestimate IOP compared to non-contact tonometry by 0.81 ± 2.74 mmHg. Non-contact tonometry was found to be tolerated best by children of all ages, with all three methods having a higher success rate in obtaining readings with children above the age of 10 years old. Gandhi et al. (2011) compared the iCare ONE rebound tonometer to Goldmann applanation tonometry in pediatric glaucoma or glaucoma suspect patients and found that the absolute value of mean IOP difference was 3.3 ± 4.0 mmHg higher with iCare ONE.

Advantages

Rebound tonometry is well tolerated by pediatric patients. It is a handheld tonometer and does not require anesthesia. It is tolerated better than GAT. Readings generally correlate with GAT as well. There is minimal sensation associated with performing this procedure. The probe is disposable, which reduces the risk of spreading infection. A very small region of the cornea is applanated, which is helpful with cases of corneal pathology that may otherwise lead to less reliable readings.

Disadvantages

Corneal thickness has been reported to affect IOP readings with rebound tonometers. IOP readings tend to be higher with rebound tonometry compared to GAT, however in healthy populations it is not clinically significant (Feng et al., 2015). The repeatability of readings is not as consistent when compared to GAT, but is more consistent when compared to other portable tonometers (Davies et al., 2006).

Equipment

1. Rebound tonometer (Figure 13)
2. Disposable rebound tonometer probes

Procedure

Step 1: Insert a disposable probe into the rebound tonometer
Step 2: Turn on the tonometer, with the probe held up towards the ceiling so it gets properly secured in place by the device
Step 3: Have the child sitting facing forward if they are able to sit on their own, or have them sit facing forward in their guardian's lap
Step 4: Have the child look straight ahead at a target
Step 5: Adjust the forehead support as needed to steady the tonometer against the child's forehead
Step 6: Move the rebound tonometer within 4 to 8 mm of the child's eye, so the probe has room to move forward to strike the cornea and then bounce back
Step 7: To initiate a reading press the main button on the back of the rebound tonometer, and ensure the tonometer is aligned so the probe strikes the central cornea. Repeat until the necessary number of readings for the device have been obtained
Step 8: After the grouping of readings have been collected, a read out of the IOP measurement and standard deviation is displayed on the screen
Step 9: Repeat the same procedure for the second eye

HAND-HELD LENSES USED IN CONJUNCTION WITH SLIT LAMP BIOMICROSCOPY

There are several different handheld lenses available to be used in conjunction with the slit lamp to examine the posterior segment of the eye. The lenses span a spectrum that provides variable magnification and field of views. The higher the dioptric power of a lens (for example a 90D lens) provides a larger field of view and less magnification, whereas a lower dioptric power of a lens (for example a 60D lens) will provide the clinician with a smaller field of view but higher magnification.

For the purpose of this book, we will focus on the most popular lenses used in clinics in conjunction with the slit lamp, the 90D and 78D lenses.

Figure 13. An Icare rebound tonometer being used on a pediatric patient to measure IOP

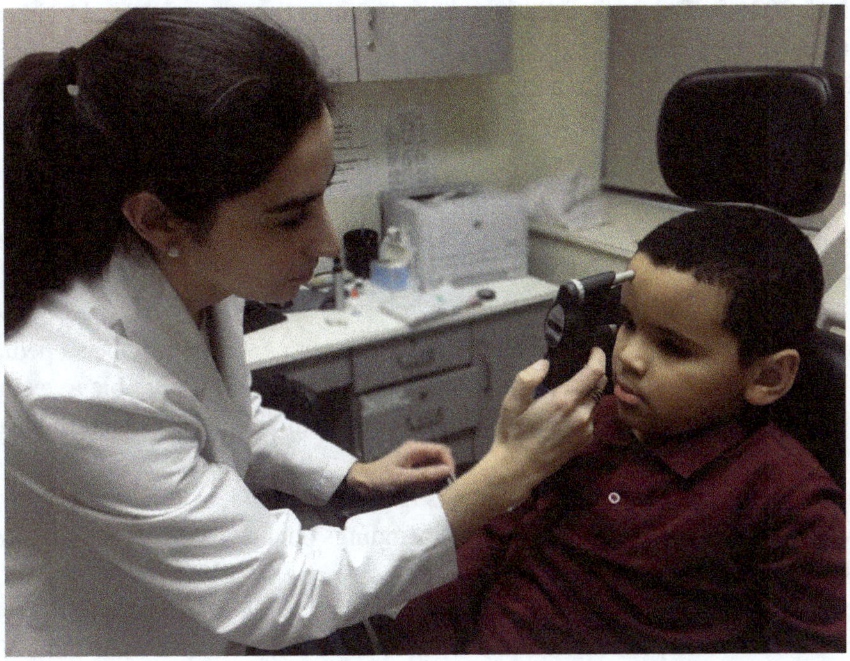

90D LENS

Indications

Being able to examine the posterior segment in detail is a very important aspect of a pediatric eye exam. If a pediatric patient can be positioned in the slit lamp and is generally able to keep fixation this is one of the preferred methods to examine the posterior pole.

A 90D lens is used in conjunction with the slit lamp to examine all the components of the posterior pole – the optic nerve, macula, retinal blood vessels and surrounding retinal tissue (Figure 14). It is very important to rule out any pathology in a pediatric patient that may be the etiology of decreased vision, or reveal systemic health issues. A 90D lens can also be used to perform extended fundoscopy. If retinal/choroidal findings are found when performing binocular indirect ophthalmoscopy, the finding can be further examined by having the patient look towards that same direction in the slit lamp to allow for a more magnified view.

Background

A 90D lens is a double aspheric, high plus powered, non-contact fundoscopy lens that provides a magnified stereoscopic view of the retina when used with a slit lamp (Figure 15). The image is inverted and reversed.

The 90D lens provides the least magnification compared to the other non-contact fundoscopy lenses available, but provides the greatest field of view. For example, with a Volk 90D lens, the magnification provided with a 90D lens is 0.76X. The static field of view is 74° while the dynamic field of view is 89° (Volk Optical, 2021a). The static field of view represents the amount of field viewable when the fundoscopy lens is centered over the pupil but is kept stationary. The dynamic field of view represents the extent of the field that can be examined by moving the fundus lens across the patient's entire pupil. The working distance with this lens is 7mm (Volk Optical, 2021a).

Fundoscopy lenses from different companies have slightly different parameters. All parameters for different lenses are outlined by their manufacturer and easily accessible.

Advantages

A patient does not need to be dilated to examine the fundus with a 90D lens. Once a pediatric patient is old enough to sit on their own and can be positioned in the slit lamp it is possible to examine the entire posterior pole un-dilated. This is facilitated by the fact that pediatric patients tend to have larger pupils than adults.

This technique can be used with dilated patients as well. A 90D lens can be used for extended fundoscopy, allowing a more magnified view of ocular findings outside of the posterior pole compared to the view on BIO.

In pediatric patients with poor fixation, a 90D lens is a good choice because it allows you to examine more of the retina at one time, so the examiner is able to observe more in their field of view at once while the opportunity is available.

Due to the decreased magnification of a 90D lens, it facilitates viewing around a media opacity that may be obstructing part of the view into the retina.

Due to the small size of the 90D lens, it can be easier to manipulate with deep set eyes to achieve the desired working distance.

Disadvantages

A 90D lens has decreased magnification compared to other fundoscopy lenses, so subtle findings on examination of the posterior pole may be less obvious or missed. This lens has a smaller diameter, so it is more difficult for some practitioners to manipulate.

Clinical Pearl: *It may be easiest to position a pediatric patient in the slit lamp if they sit at the edge of the exam chair instead of further back.*

Clinical Pearl: *For children who are not tall enough to comfortably fit in the slit lamp while sitting, they can stand on the foot rest of the exam chair to facilitate positioning. Lower the exam chair all the* *way down to the ground, and have the child stand on the foot rest. You can then position the slit lamp so the child is comfortable. Have the child hold on to the bars of the slit lamp with their hands for support.*

Clinical Pearl: *Do not make the decision if a child can or cannot be examined in the slit lamp based purely on their age. Some younger children can easily be examined in the slit lamp. This decision should be made based on the maturity of the child.*

Clinical Pearl: *Placing stickers on the slit lamp magnification dials on the side of the slit lamp provides targets for pediatric patients to look at during examination.*

Equipment – Undilated 90D

1. 90D lens
2. Slit lamp

Procedure

Undilated 90D examination of the posterior segment:

Step 1: Position the child in the slit lamp

Step 2: Start by examining the right eye. Have them look at the desired target – whether that be the provider's right ear, an earring, sticker or another target. Alignment of the child's gaze is especially important with undilated 90D

Step 3: Begin with the slit lamp pulled back, and the lens held at the appropriate working distance from the eye (about 7mm), and in line with the pupil so that the light is travelling from the slit lamp through the 90D lens and into the child's pupil. Move the slit lamp forward until the retina comes into focus

Step 4: Alternatively, the examiner can opt to begin with the lens positioned as above, but with the slit lamp forward. The slit lamp can then be pulled back to bring the retina into focus. This method is easier to use for a dilated 90D exam, but can work for undilated 90D examination as well

Step 5: Examine the retina in a systematic pattern

Step 6: Start with the optic nerve, and make note of the size of the optic disc, blood vessels, disc margins, color, peripapillary atrophy and cup to disc ratio

Step 7: Examine the retinal vascular arcades in the posterior pole. Move the light source to scan the inferior and superior temporal arcades, as well as the superior and inferior nasal arcades to the extent possible depending on the patient's pupil size. Note any vessel changes or abnormalities

Step 8: Move the light beam temporally in the retina from the optic nerve to travel to the macula. Make note of the foveal contour, presence or absence of a foveal light reflex, any pigmentary changes or other signs of pathology

Step 9: If the child's eye is not dilated, it is more challenging to continuously have a view. Move the lens in very small circular movements to re-align the lens with the slit lamp and patient's pupil when necessary

Step 10: Repeat to examine the left eye. Switch the child's fixation target to the examiner's left ear or earring, sticker or desired target

Clinical Pearl: *When the child's pupils are not dilated and the examiner is experiencing difficulty obtaining a clear view, adjust the beam and light source to a smaller beam and decrease the light source.*

Equipment – Dilated 90D

1. 90D lens
2. Slit lamp
3. 0.5% proparacaine ophthalmic solution
4. 1% tropicamide ophthalmic solution
5. 2.5% phenylephrine ophthalmic solution

Procedure

Dilated 90D

Step 1: To perform a dilated 90D examination, child's pupils must first be dilated. Place one drop of 0.5% proparacaine ophthalmic solution in each eye. Then place one drop of 1% tropicamide ophthalmic solution and one drop of 2.5% phenylephrine ophthalmic solution in each eye to dilate the eyes
Step 2: After the pupils have had sufficient time to dilate, position the child in the slit lamp
Step 3: Examine the retina using the same procedure as described in the undilated 90D section
Step 4: To perform extended fundoscopy using the 90D lens to examine more mid-peripheral and peripheral views, have the child begin by looking in the desired direction. For example: If you want to examine the superior quadrant, have the child look up. Hold the lens slightly inferior but parallel with the child's pupil. Move the light beam in the opposite direction of the child's direction of gaze. In this case move the light source inferiorly to obtain a view further and further out into the superior mid-periphery and periphery. This technique is extremely helpful for examining retinal findings outside of the posterior pole with increased magnification compared to BIO

78D LENS

Indications

There are different methods and lenses that can be employed to examine the posterior segment in pediatric patients. For a view of the posterior pole with increased magnification, a 78D lens is an excellent option. The 78D lens is used in conjunction with the slit lamp to examine the optic nerve, macula, retinal blood vessels as well as the surrounding retina/choroid in the posterior pole (Figure 14).

A 78D lens allows for more subtle findings to be noted on examination compared to a lens with less magnification.

Figure 14. A pediatric patient positioned in the slit lamp having their posterior segment examined using a (A): 90D lens and (B): 78D lens

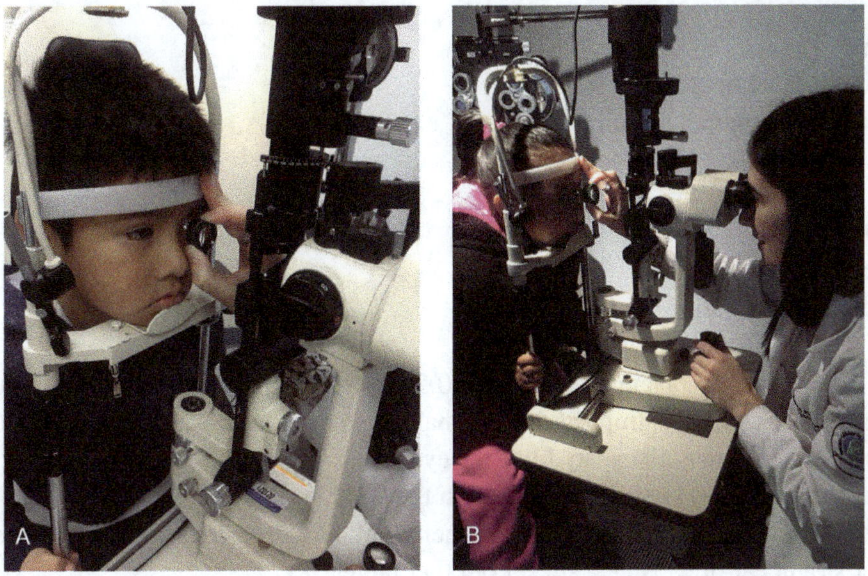

Background

A 78D lens is a double aspheric, high plus powered, non-contact fundoscopy lens that provides a magnified stereoscopic view of the retina when used with a slit lamp (Figure 15). The image is inverted and reversed.

The 78D lens is a good all-around lens providing a balance with more magnification than a 90D lens and more field of view compared to a 60D lens. With a Volk 78D lens, the magnification the lens provides is 0.93X. The static field of view is 81°. The dynamic field of view which describes how much of the field can be viewed when moving the fundus lens from one edge of the pupil to the other is 97°. The working distance with this lens is 8mm (Volk Optical, 2021b).

Fundoscopy lenses from different companies have slightly different parameters. All parameters for different lenses are outlined by their manufacturer and are easily accessible.

Advantages

The 78D lens provides increased magnification, while retaining a field of view that allows for easy navigation of the posterior pole. This lens has a larger diameter than a 90D, making it easier to manipulate for certain providers.

Disadvantages

The patient typically must be dilated to use this lens. While a 78D lens can be used with an undilated pupil, it is much more challenging. It can be more difficult to manipulate the lens with patients with deep set eyes to achieve the desired working distance due to the larger diameter of the lens.

Equipment

1. 78 D lens
2. Slit lamp
3. 0.5% proparacaine ophthalmic solution
4. 1% tropicamide ophthalmic solution
5. 2.5% phenylephrine ophthalmic solution

Procedure

Dilated 78D lens examination

Step 1: Dilate the pupils by placing one drop of 0.5% proparacaine ophthalmic solution in each eye. Then place one drop of 1% tropicamide ophthalmic solution and one drop of 2.5% phenylephrine ophthalmic solution in each eye to dilate the eyes
Step 2: After the pupils have been dilated, position the child in the slit lamp
Step 3: Start by examining the right eye. Have them look at the desired target – whether that be the examiner's right ear or earring, a sticker or other target
Step 4: Begin with the slit lamp pulled back, and the lens held at the appropriate working distance from the eye (about 8 mm), and in line with the pupil so that the light is travelling through the 78D lens and into the child's pupil. Move the slit lamp forward until the retina comes into focus
Step 5: Alternatively, the examiner can opt to begin with the lens positioned as above, but with the slit lamp forward. The slit lamp can then be pulled back to bring the retina into focus
Step 6: Examine the retina using the same procedure as described in the undilated 90D section
Step 7: Extended fundoscopy can be performed with a 78D lens the same way as described using a 90D lens

Figure 15. Volk 90D and 78D double aspheric lenses that can be used for examining the posterior segment

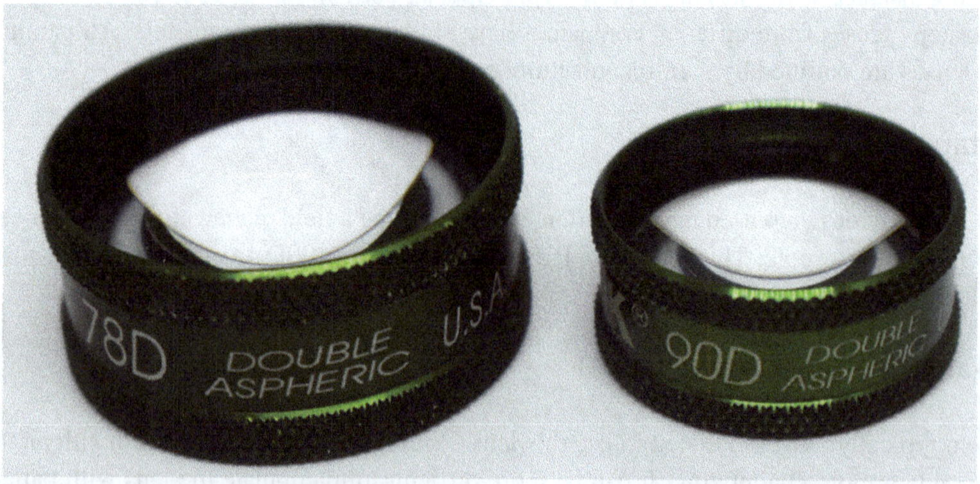

CONCLUSION

There are many techniques and tools at the clinician's disposal to perform a thorough ocular health examination on a pediatric patient of all ages. Slit lamp examination of both the anterior and posterior segment, along with tonometry are core components of a pediatric ocular health exam that provide valuable information to ensure pediatric patients receive the highest quality of eyecare.

ACKNOWLEDGMENT

The author would like to thank Tak-Man Kimberly Fung, OD for her illustration contributions to this chapter.

REFERENCES

Arora, R., Austin, M., & Bellamy, H. (2014). Applanation tonometry: A comparison of the Perkins handheld and Goldmann slit lamp-mounted methods. *Clinical Ophthalmology*, 605–610. doi:10.2147/OPTH.S53544 PMID:24707165

Baum, J., Chaturvedi, N., Netland, P. A., & Dreyer, E. B. (1995). Assessment of Intraocular Pressure by Palpation. *American Journal of Ophthalmology*, *119*(5), 650–651. doi:10.1016/S0002-9394(14)70227-2 PMID:7733191

Cervino, A. (2006). Rebound tonometry: New opportunities and limitations of non-invasive determination of intraocular pressure. *The British Journal of Ophthalmology*, *90*(12), 1444–1446. doi:10.1136/bjo.2006.102970 PMID:17114589

Davies, L. N., Bartlett, H., Mallen, E. A. H., & Wolffsohn, J. S. (2006). Clinical evaluation of rebound tonometer. *Acta Ophthalmologica Scandinavica*, *84*(2), 206–209. doi:10.1111/j.1600-0420.2005.00610.x PMID:16637838

Elliott, D. B. (2007). *Clinical Procedures in Primary Eye Care: Expert Consult: Online and Print* (3rd ed.). Butterworth-Heinemann.

Feng, C. S., Jin, K. W., Yi, K., & Choi, D. G. (2015). Comparison of Intraocular Pressure Measurements Obtained by Rebound, Noncontact, and Goldmann Applanation Tonometry in Children. *American Journal of Ophthalmology*, *160*(5), 937–943.e1. doi:10.1016/j.ajo.2015.07.029 PMID:26210864

Ficarra, A. P., Sorkin, R., & Morrison, C. (2002). Assessment of intraocular pressure in children by digital tension. *Optometry (St. Louis, Mo.)*, *73*(8), 499–506. PMID:12365673

Gandhi, N. G., Jones, S., Prakalapakorn, S. G., & Freedman, S. F. (2011). Icare ONE handheld rebound tonometry versus Goldmann applanation in children with known and suspected glaucoma. *American Journal of Ophthalmology*, *15*(1), 843–849.e1. doi:10.1016/j.ajo.2012.05.003 PMID:22840485

Grigorian, F., Grigorian, A. P., Li, A., Sattar, A., Krishna, R., & Olitsky, S. E. (2015). Comparison of the Icare rebound tonometry with the Goldmann applanation tonometry in a pediatric population. *Journal of American Association for Pediatric Ophthalmology and Strabismus, 19*(6), 572–574. doi:10.1016/j.jaapos.2015.08.009 PMID:26691047

Haag-Strait, U. K. (2020). *Perkins Mk3 Tonometer Brochure.* https://www.haag-streit.com/fileadmin/Haag-Streit_UK/Downloads/CCO_downloads/Perkins_downloads/Perkins_brochure.pdf

Kanski, J. J., Bowling, B., Nischal, K. K., & Pearson, A. (2011). *Clinical Ophthalmology* (7th ed.). Elsevier Saunders.

Kempf, R., Kurita, Y., Iida, Y., Kaneko, M., Mishima, H. K., Tsukamoto, H., & Sugimoto, E. (2006, August). Understanding eye deformation in non-contact tonometry. In *2006 International Conference of the IEEE Engineering in Medicine and Biology Society*. EMBS Annual International Conference. 10.1109/IEMBS.2006.259905

Kirstein, E. M., Lsheikh, A., & Gunvant, P. (2011). Tonometry – Past, Present and Future. In Glaucoma - Current Clinical and Research Aspects (pp. 85–108). Intech. doi:10.5772/37393

Kontiola, A. (1997). A new electromechanical method for measuring intraocular pressure. *Documenta Ophthalmologica, 93*(3), 265–276. doi:10.1007/BF02569066 PMID:9550354

Van Herick, W., Shaffer, R. N., & Schwartz, A. (1969). Estimation of width of angle of anterior chamber. Incidence and significance of the narrow angle. *American Journal of Ophthalmology, 68*(4), 626–629. doi:10.1016/0002-9394(69)91241-0 PMID:5344324

Volk Optical. (2021a). *90D.* https://www.volk.com/collections/slit-lamp-lens/products/slit-lamp-lens-non-contact-90d

Volk Optical. (2021b). *78D.* https://www.volk.com/collections/slit-lamp-lens/products/slit-lamp-non-contact-78d

KEY TERMS AND DEFINITIONS

78D Lenses: Hand-held lenses used to examine the retina in conjunction with a slit lamp, provides a larger magnification and smaller field of view compared to the 90D lenses.

90D Lenses: Hand-held lenses used to examine the retina in conjunction with a slit lamp, provides a smaller magnification and larger field of view compared to the 90D lenses.

Anterior Segment Examination: Examination of the adnexa, eyelids, eyelashes, sclera, conjunctiva, tear film, cornea, iris, anterior chamber angle and lens of the eye.

Goldmann Applanation Tonometry (GAT): The gold standard technique to measure intraocular pressure of the eye.

Posterior Pole Examination: Examination of the optic nerve, retinal vessels, and macula in the posterior pole of the eye.

Slit Lamp: Equipment used to examine both the anterior segment and posterior segment of the eye in conjunction with handheld lenses.

Tonometry: Measuring the intraocular pressure of the eye. Can be performed using a variety of different methods/pieces of equipment.

Van Herick Angle Evaluation: Technique used to evaluate the depth of the anterior chamber angle of the eye using a slit lamp.

Chapter 13
Fundus Examination in Pediatric Patients:
Direct Ophthalmoscope and PanOptic Ophthalmoscope

Alanna Khattar
BronxCare Health System, USA

ABSTRACT

There are a number of different pieces of equipment and techniques available for examination of the fundus of a pediatric patient. Two of these tools are handheld devices, the direct ophthalmoscope and PanOptic™ ophthalmoscope. Both of these devices allow for examination of the posterior pole of the eye. This chapter will discuss the indications, advantages, and disadvantages of both of these pieces of equipment in addition to how to use the equipment to examine the posterior segment of a pediatric patient.

INTRODUCTION

The direct ophthalmoscope can be used to examine the posterior pole, macula and ocular media in both dilated and undilated fundi. The handheld direct ophthalmoscope produces an erect magnified real image. There are several different filters that can be used. The size of the illumination source can be adjusted to compensate for the size of the patient's pupil. Direct ophthalmoscopy can also be used to evaluate the eye's fixation pattern using visuoscopy. Visuoscopy testing is best performed when the patient is dilated.

Direct ophthalmoscopy can be performed on children of all ages, and is especially helpful for toddlers, pre-school and school aged children who are unable to be positioned in the slit lamp for examination of the fundus with lenses such as a 90D or 78D. It is useful as well for examining patients with undilated pupils, providing increased magnification for examination of the posterior pole. While a direct ophthalmoscope can be used on infants as well, other methods may allow for better views of the posterior pole given limited cooperation with this youngest age group.

DOI: 10.4018/978-1-7998-8044-8.ch013

BACKGROUND

The direct ophthalmoscope head connects to a handle (the power source). The head contains plus and minus power lenses used to compensate for refractive errors. There is an illumination system and a viewing system (Figure 1). The illumination system is composed of an incandescent light source, an aperture, two lenses and a small 45° mirror (Timberlake & Kennedy, 2005). It also contains a wheel that has multiple different apertures. Most direct ophthalmoscopes have two or three different size white light circles, blue and green filters, a slit and a visuoscopy target. A half circle is another type of aperture available. The viewing system is composed of condensing lenses and a viewing aperture. Condensing lenses can range in power from high plus to high minus lenses with the range varying depending on the ophthalmoscope manufacturer. The role of the condensing lenses is to allow for the image of the retina to be brought into focus if the eye is not emmetropic.

Figure 1. Image of the different systems that compose a direct ophthalmoscope. Source: Tak-Man Kimberly Fung OD, 2021
(Adapted from [Cordero, 2016])

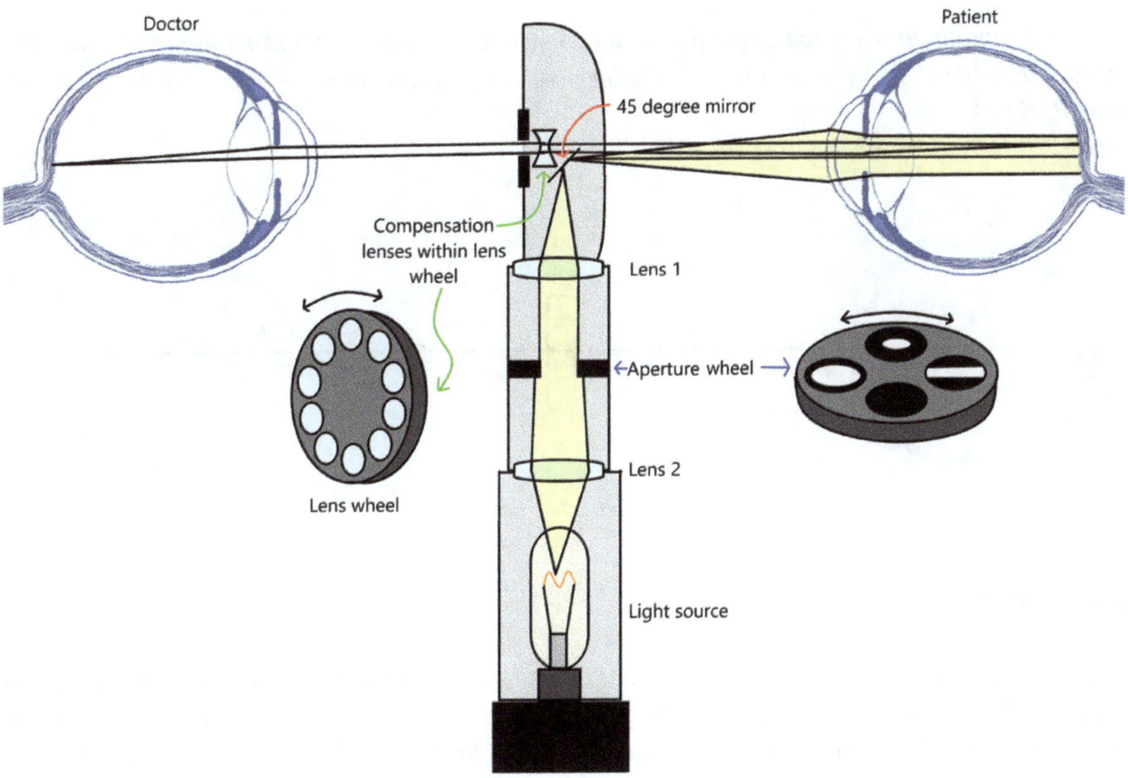

In the viewing system, the light rays are reflected off the patient's retina and exit through their pupil. The light rays then pass through the lens in the direct ophthalmoscope and enter the examiner's eye and create an image on the examiner's retina. This image the examiner sees is a virtual, upright and magnified image. The angular magnification produced by this system is approximately 15X. The standard field of view with a direct ophthalmoscope is 5° (Cordero, 2016). With an emmetropic patient, there is no need for a compensating lens to focus the image on the examiner's retina, because the rays that leave the patient's eye are parallel and ultimately the light rays comes into focus on the examiner's retina (Figure 2). This is not the case when the patient is ametropic.

With a myopic patient, the light rays converge as they exit the patient's eye, therefore the light rays will come into focus in front of the examiner's retina. To correct this, a concave lens is needed to diverge the rays to make them parallel to ultimately allow a clear image to be produced on the examiner's retina (Figure 3). The power of the concave lens needed depends on what the patient's refractive error is and the distance from the patient that this technique is being performed. With a hyperopic patient, the light rays come into focus behind the examiner's retina, therefore a convex lens is needed to converge the light rays so that they come into focus on the examiner's retina (Figure 4). The power of the lens needed for the hyperope is determined the same way as previously stated for a myope.

Figure 2. A simplified ray tracing diagram of an emmetropic observer (O) examining the retina of an emmetropic subject (S) using a direct ophthalmoscope. Fp: focal point. Source: Tak-Man Kimberly Fung OD, 2021
(Adapted from [Timberlake & Kennedy, 2005]).

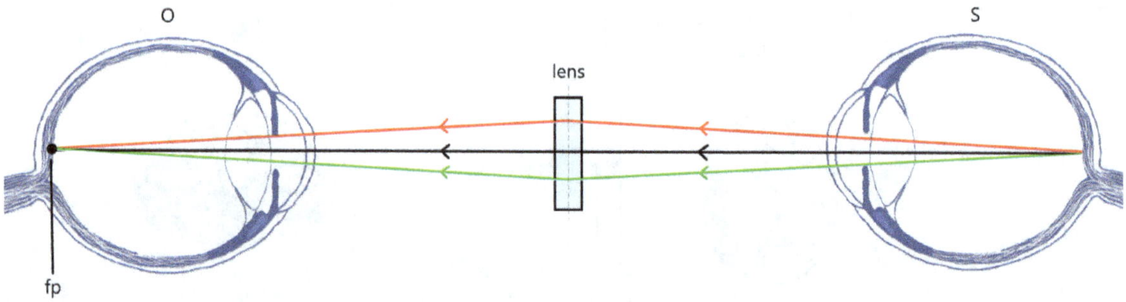

Advantages

Advantages of the direct ophthalmoscope include ease of use, good patient comfort, can be used without dilation, and can provide an estimate of the patient's visual compromise due to media opacification. It is handheld providing portability at a low cost. This technique can be performed in any clinical or screening setting, on children of almost all ages. It is especially very useful for small children who are unable to be positioned in the slit lamp. The degree of magnification facilitates the examination of the optic nerve, macula, and blood vessels in the posterior pole.

Figure 3. Top – A ray tracing diagram demonstrating the location of image formation at the focal point (fp) in front of the retina of an emmetropic observer (O) as the retina of a myopic subject (S) is examined with no lens in place. Bottom – With an appropriate concave (minus) lens in place, the rays come to a focal point located on the observer's retina, forming a clear image. Source: Tak-Man Kimberly Fung OD, 2021
(Adapted from [Timberlake & Kennedy, 2005]).

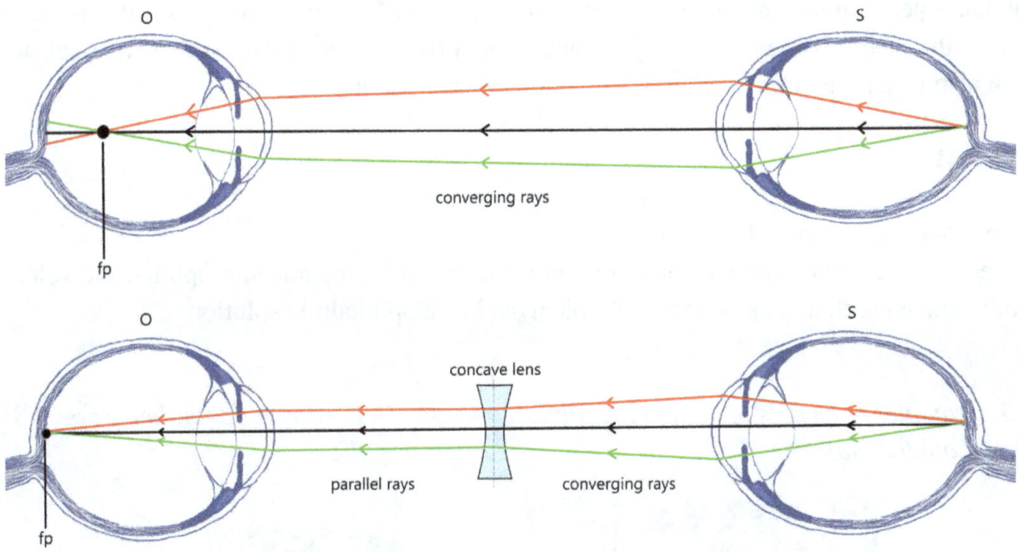

Figure 4. Top – A ray tracing diagram demonstrating the location of image formation at the focal point (fp) behind the retina of an emmetropic observer (O) as the retina of a hyperopic subject (S) is examined with no lens in place. Bottom – With an appropriate convex (plus) lens in place, the rays come to a focal point located on the observer's retina, forming a clear image. Source: Tak-Man Kimberly Fung OD, 2021
(Adapted from [Timberlake & Kennedy, 2005]).

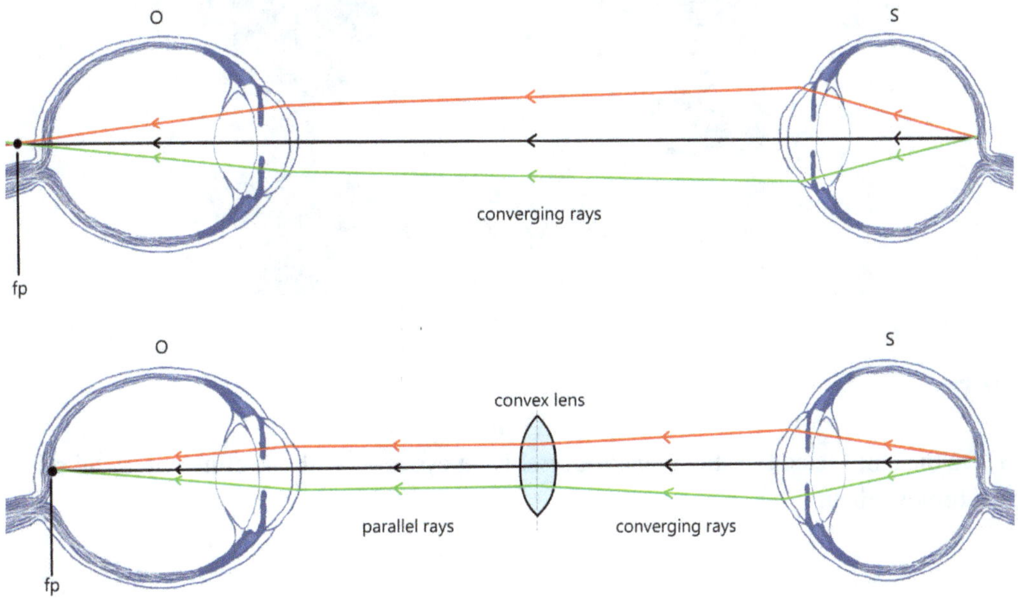

Disadvantages

The disadvantages of the direct ophthalmoscope are that it lacks stereopsis, involves a close working distance, dependence on refractive errors for clarity and magnification, and it has a small field of view (about two disc diameters). With most children, only the posterior pole can be examined, but it is optically possible to see out to the point of the equator. Stereopsis is not obtained with this technique since the clinician is performing it monocularly. Due to the amount of magnification, it is difficult to examine the retina if the media is hazy anteriorly because it is difficult to navigate around the unclear media. Glare can also be a problem, resulting in a degraded image quality.

Equipment

1. Direct ophthalmoscope (Figure 5)
2. If necessary to dilate the patient to obtain a view: 0.5% proparacaine ophthalmic solution, 1% tropicamide ophthalmic solution, 2.5% phenylephrine ophthalmic solution

Figure 5. Examples of models of direct ophthalmoscope. 5A: Heine direct ophthalmoscope. 5B: Welch Allyn direct ophthalmoscope

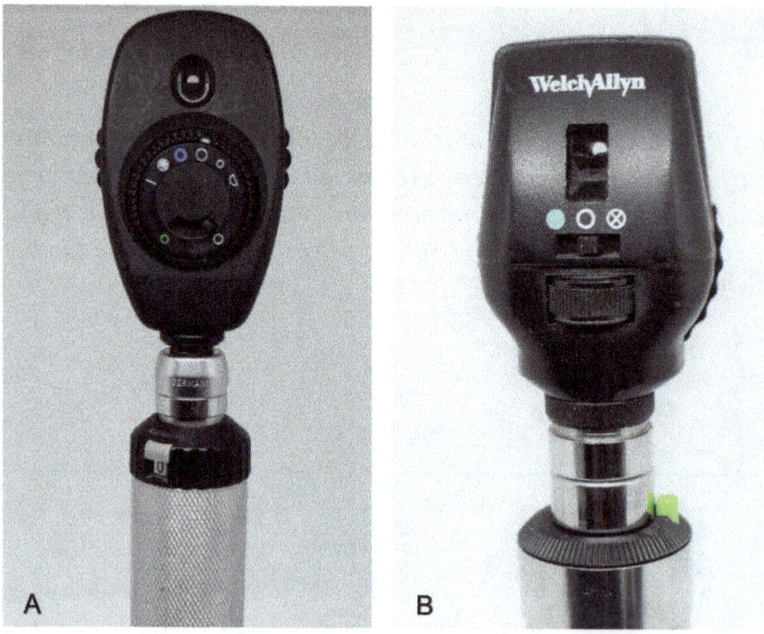

Procedure

Step 1: Have the child seated or standing comfortably, at eye level with the clinician. If child is wearing spectacles, remove them

Step 2: Inform the child and the guardian that you are going to shine a light in the eyes, and that your instrument will come close to the eyes but will not touch them

Step 3: Choose the appropriate aperture size based on the size of the patient pupil. If the pupil is very small, using a smaller aperture size will facilitate getting a view of the retina

Step 4: Have the child look at a target (e.g., guardian) across the room. The target can either be straight ahead or at an angle.

Step 5: To examine the right eye, position yourself to the right of the child. Hold the direct ophthalmoscope with the right hand and look through the direct ophthalmoscope using your right eye starting about an arm's length away from the child, and slowly move closer to the eye. Approach the eye from about a 15° angle temporal to child's line of sight (Carlson & Kurtz, 2004). As you move closer with the direct ophthalmoscope, the red reflex of the child's retina becomes visible.

Step 6: As you approach the eye, slowly adjust the condensing lenses (start with high plus power and then decrease the lens power) until you see the iris is in focus. When the retina starts to come into focus, about one or two centimeters from the eye, further adjust the lens power until the retina comes into clear focus (Figure 6)

Step 7: Once the retina is in focus, if the optic nerve is not in view initially, move your body position and the direct ophthalmoscope together to help locate the optic nerve. Since the view of the retina is direct, to find the optic nerve that is anatomically located nasally, move the light source towards the nasal aspect of the eye. The blood vessels will become larger in caliber as you approach the optic nerve

Clinical Pearl: *To locate and obtain a view of the right optic nerve, have the child focus on a target in the distance and slightly to his/her left.*

Step 8: When the optic nerve is in focus, note the C/D ratio as well as the disc color, margins, and any other notable findings

Step 9: Examine the macula by moving the direct ophthalmoscope light source temporally. Alternatively, ask the child to look directly at the light source of the direct ophthalmoscope

Step 10: Navigate throughout the posterior pole by moving the light source and your head with the light source

Step 11: To examine the left eye, hold the direct ophthalmoscope with the left hand and look through the device with your left eye. Stand on the left side of the child and approach from an angle of about 15 degrees temporal to the child's line of sight (Carlson & Kurtz, 2004)

Step 12: Repeat steps 6-10 on the left eye

Clinical Pearl: *To locate and obtain a view of the left optic nerve, have the child focus on a target in the distance and slightly to his/her right.*

Clinical Pearl: *You can place the hand that is not holding the direct ophthalmoscope on the back of the exam chair for stability.*

Clinical Pearl: *To gauge if you are examining the patient from the correct close distance, you can use your index or middle finger as a distance measure. If your knuckle of the index or middle finger is*

touching the patient's cheek, then you are sufficiently close enough to get the best view of the fundus. This also adds stability to holding the instrument while maneuvering and observing the posterior pole.

Clinical Pearl: *To minimize pupil constriction, use the small aperture size which will decrease illumination. Shining the light source slightly off axis can also decrease the extent of pupil constriction.*

Clinical Pearl: *If getting the retina in focus is proving to be difficult, back away, reset the lenses in the direct ophthalmoscope and start over.*

Clinical Pearl: *There are usually three aperture sizes in the ophthalmoscope. The middle size circle corresponds to an average sized optic nerve. If the optic nerve head is smaller than the middle size circle, this indicates a smaller than average size nerve, if the optic nerve head is larger than the middle size circle, this indicates a larger than average size nerve.*

Clinical Pearl: *The aperture with a center circle and a cross grid is used for visuoscopy. This is the only way to test for a monocular fixation pattern in a strabismic eye.*

Figure 6. A – Setting up to begin direct ophthalmoscopy with the ophthalmoscope held at a distance, and a high plus lens dialed in. B – Appropriate working distance to examine the posterior segment using a direct ophthalmoscope

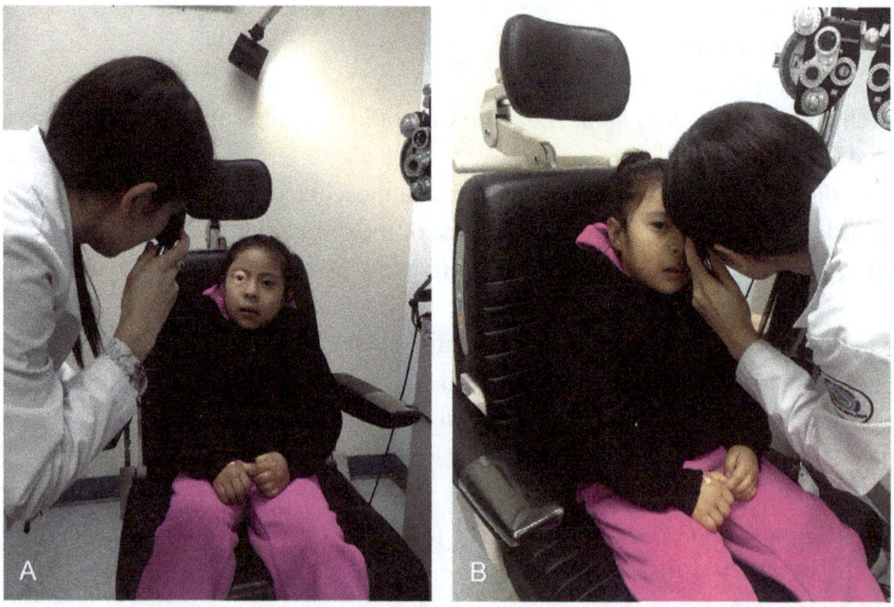

PANOPTIC™ OPHTHALMOSCOPE

Indications

The PanOptic™ ophthalmoscope (Figure 7) is used to examine the fundus, primarily the posterior pole. It can be used on both undilated and dilated eyes to look for signs of ocular pathology. It is used to obtain a magnified view of the optic nerve, macula, blood vessels and retinal tissue in the posterior pole. The PanOptic™ ophthalmoscope is a portable handheld device and can be used in any clinical setting. It is an alternative to the direct ophthalmoscope. This piece of equipment can be used on children of all ages and is especially useful for those who are unable to be positioned in the slit lamp to examine the posterior pole. While the PanOptic™ ophthalmoscope can be more challenging to use on infants than toddlers, pre-school and school aged children it is possible to use this device with all pediatric age groups. The PanOptic™ ophthalmoscope has adjustable apertures, filters and lenses.

The PanOptic™ ophthalmoscope also allows a magnified examination of the anterior segment, particularly useful for a child who cannot be examined in the slit lamp.

Figure 7. A PanOpticTM ophthalmoscope produced by Welch Allyn

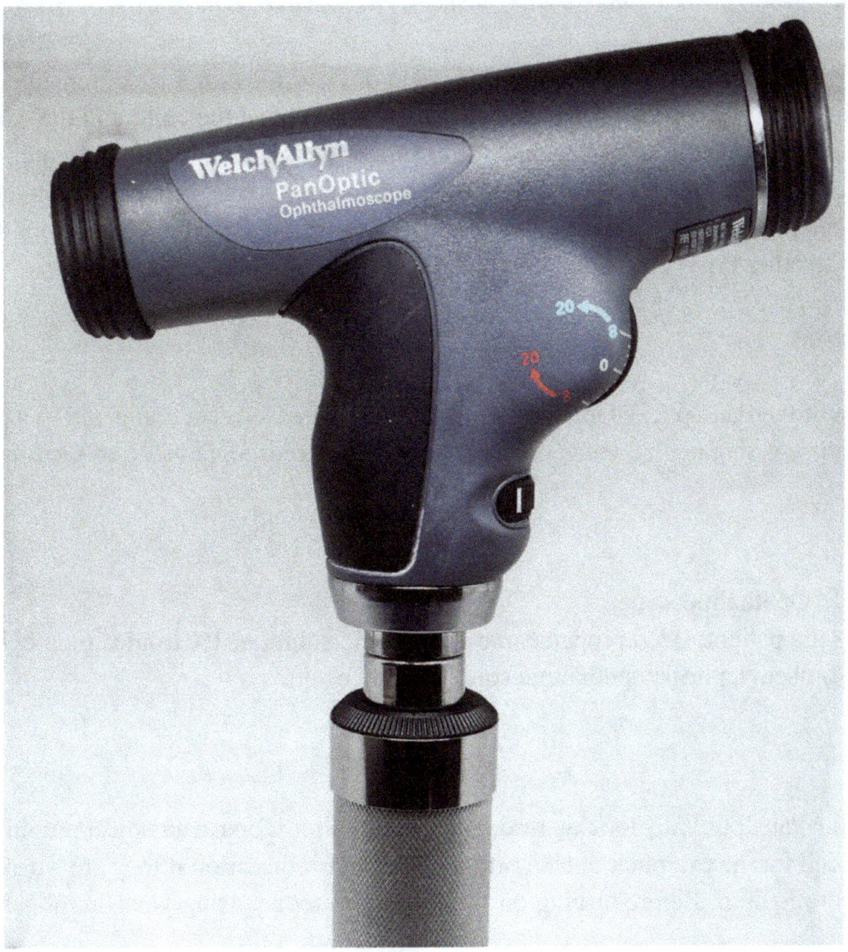

Background

The PanOptic™ ophthalmoscope employs Axial PointSource™ optics. This technology converges the illumination system to a point on the cornea that facilitates entry into small pupils for examination. The illumination pathway is then able to diverge to the retina resulting in a wide area of the fundus being illuminated. The field of view produced by this optical system is 25° (Welch Allyn, 2013). The magnification of the image produced is an increase of 26% compared to the direct ophthalmoscope (Welch Allyn, 2013). The image produced is an upright, non-inverted image. This piece of equipment is available with several different apertures. There are three different sized apertures which can be used for different pupil sizes. The micro spot pupil is used for very small undilated pupils. The small aperture is used for undilated pupils. The large aperture size is used for an examination of the optic nerve when the pupil is dilated. There is a slit aperture to help examine for elevation of retinal lesions and the optic disc. There is also a half-moon aperture. There are both red-free and cobalt blue filters. The red free filter helps distinguish and further examine retinal findings, while the cobalt blue filter can be used to examine the cornea with magnification after staining with sodium fluorescein.

The PanOptic™ ophthalmoscope has a focusing lens range from +20D to -20D to compensate for the refractive error (Welch Allyn, 2013).

Advantages

The PanOptic™ ophthalmoscope provides a wider field of view allowing for examination of more of the retina at one time. There is an increased working distance between the child and the examiner, which makes it more comfortable for the child while the examination is taking place. This equipment has technology that decreases the amount of glare to allow for a crisper image. It is possible to get views more peripherally when the child looks in different gazes. Learning to use the PanOptic™ ophthalmoscope is easy compared to other types of ophthalmoscopes.

Disadvantages

A disadvantage of the PanOptic™ Ophthalmoscope is the increased cost compared to a direct ophthalmoscope. The view is monocular which does not allow for stereoscopic views of the fundus.

Equipment

1. PanOptic™ Ophthalmoscope
2. If dilating the patient: 0.5% proparacaine ophthalmic solution, 1% tropicamide ophthalmic solutions, 2.5% phenylephrine ophthalmic solution can be added

Procedure

Step 1: Focus the PanOptic™ by looking through the ophthalmoscope at an object roughly 15 feet away. It is recommended for the examiner to take off their spectacle correction if they are wearing spectacles, however it is not required. Before turning on the ophthalmoscope, using your thumb adjust the focusing wheel until the object 15 feet away is in focus. This allows for any adjustments for the examiner's refractive error.

Step 2: Stand on the right side of the child to examine the right eye. Place your hand on the exam chair to aid with stability

Step 3: Begin with the aperture dial with the green line clicked into position. This is the small aperture. It can be adjusted based on the child's pupil size to either the micro spot or large aperture

Step 4: When the ophthalmoscope is turned on you can adjust the intensity of the light

Step 5: Position yourself approximately 15 degrees to the temporal side of the child's eye

Step 6: Instruct the child to look straight ahead at a distance target. It is helpful to use the child's guardian as the target to keep attention

Step 7: Begin approximately six inches away and slowly move towards the eye. Look for the red retinal reflex

Step 8: Continue moving towards the eye until the eye cup is in contact with the child's brow. For the largest view compress the eye cup halfway against the child's brow

Step 9: Once the fundus is in view, adjust the focusing knob until the posterior pole is in crisp focus

Step 10: When the optic nerve is in focus, note the C/D ratio as well as the disc color, margins and any other notable findings

Step 11: Examine the macula by moving the light source temporally from the optic disc. You can also ask the patient to look directly at your light

Step 12: Navigate throughout the posterior pole by moving the light source and your head with the light source

Step 13: To examine the left eye, hold the PanOptic™ ophthalmoscope in your left hand and look through the device with your left eye. Stand on the left side of the child about 15 degrees temporally, to examine the left eye.

Clinical Pearl: *Purchase the PanOptic™ head only and use the battery handle of the direct ophthalmoscope instead of buying a new set.*

CONCLUSION

Examining the fundus of pediatric patients is extremely important. Both the direct ophthalmoscope and PanOptic™ ophthalmoscope are invaluable tools when working with the pediatric population that allow for a magnified view of the optic disc, macula and posterior pole in general. Their hand-held nature allows for ease of use especially with pediatric patients who are unable to sit in a slit lamp for examination. Both pieces of equipment can also be used in non-traditional exam settings such as in an emergency room or a vision screening at a school to aid in proper diagnosis and management of pediatric patients.

ACKNOWLEDGMENT

The author would like to thank Tak-Man Kimberly Fung, OD for her illustration contributions to this chapter.

REFERENCES

Carlson, N., & Kurtz, D. (2004). *Clinical Procedures for Ocular Examination* (3rd ed.). McGraw-Hill Education.

Cordero, I. (2016). Understanding and caring for the direct ophthalmoscope. *Community Eye Health Journal, 29*(93), 17. https://www.cehjournal.org/article/understanding-and-caring-for-the-direct-ophthalmoscope/

Timberlake, G. T., & Kennedy, M. (2005). The Direct Ophthalmoscope How it Works and How to Use It. In *The Direct Ophthalmoscope How it Works and How to Use It* (pp. 1–35). University of Kansas. https://web.media.mit.edu/~raskar/Eye/TheDirectOphthalmoscope.pdf

Welch Allyn. (2013). *PanOptic Ophthalmoscope Brochure*. Retrieved September 27, 2021, from https://www.canmedhealthcare.com/parent/WelchAllyn_PanOptic_Ophthalmoscope.pdf

KEY TERMS AND DEFINITIONS

Apertures: In the context of ophthalmoscopes, this represents the different sizes and shapes of illumination along with different filters that can be used when examining a patient.

Direct Ophthalmoscope: A monocular, hand-held ophthalmic device that produces an erect, magnified, and real image primarily used to examine the posterior segment of the eye.

Field of View: In the context of ophthalmoscopes, this references the extent of the retina that is visible at one time while using this device.

Macula: A round area of the retina located in the posterior pole of the eye, inside the temporal vascular arcades, that is responsible for central vision.

Optic Nerve: Also known as cranial nerve II, this nerve carries afferent nerve fibers that originate in the retinal ganglion cells, transmitting visual information from the retina to the brain.

PanOptic™ Ophthalmoscope: A monocular, hand-held ophthalmic device that produces an upright, non-inverted image primarily used to examine the posterior segment of the eye. This device has a larger field of view compared to a direct ophthalmoscope.

Posterior Pole: The portion of the retina containing the optic nerve, macula, and part of the vessel arcades.

Chapter 14
Fundus Examination in Pediatric Patients Using Indirect Ophthalmoscopy:
Binocular Indirect Ophthalmoscopy (BIO), BIO With Scleral Indentation, BIO in Premature Infants

Danielle M. Ledoux
https://orcid.org/0000-0002-4722-2677
Specialized Pediatric Eye Care, Inc., USA

Brandon Johnson
New York Retina Center, USA

Issac Moradi
Retina Group, USA

Lily Zhu-Tam
Citywide Eye Care Optometry, USA

ABSTRACT

The goal of this chapter is to provide the clinician with an understanding of binocular indirect ophthalmoscopy (BIO) and helpful clinical techniques for success in examining the fundus of the pediatric patient, including scleral depression. The challenging technique to examine the premature infant at risk for retinopathy of prematurity will be explained in detail, including the standard classification of the disease with photos depicting the different location and stages of disease. BIO with the addition of scleral indentation helps the clinician diagnose and locate lesions that may otherwise go undetected, such as retinal holes, tears, or vitreoretinal adhesions. Complete examination of the fundus of a child is no less important than of any other patient who seeks eye care but often requires efficiency and precision (as well as many human arms). Time is a rate limiting aspect when examining children so preparation and experience will lead to success.

DOI: 10.4018/978-1-7998-8044-8.ch014

INTRODUCTION

The goal of this chapter is to provide the clinician with an understanding of binocular indirect ophthalmoscopy (BIO) and helpful clinical techniques for success in examining the fundus of the pediatric patient. The challenging technique to examine the premature infant at risk for retinopathy of prematurity will be explained in detail, including the standard classification of the disease with photos depicting the different location and stages of disease. BIO with the addition of sclera indentation, which allows for greater ease in viewing tissue layer separation and surface irregularities, will be covered as well. This helps the clinician diagnose and locate lesions that may otherwise go undetected, such as retinal holes, tears or vitreoretinal adhesions.

BIO in children is significantly more challenging as they often must be cajoled into allowing the exam or restrained for adequate examination. Use of parents to hold children during the exam and use of toys to get the attention of the child during the exam are often needed to successfully perform the fundus exam. Complete examination of the fundus of a child is no less important than of any other patient who seeks eye care but often requires efficiency and precision (as well as many human arms). Since time is a rate limiting aspect when examining children, preparation and experience will lead to success. Scleral depression is a necessary element in the examination of the premature infant for retinopathy of prematurity and the critical elements of this disease and the examination to diagnose this disease is discussed at length in this chapter.

BINOCULAR INDIRECT OPHTHALMOSCOPY (BIO)

Background

Binocular indirect ophthalmoscopy (BIO) consists of a headband apparatus, optical viewing system, and rheostatically controlled illumination source (Figure 1). The light beam from the BIO is directed into the child's eye which produces reflected observation beams from the retina. With a high plus powered condensing lens, these beams create an aerial image at its focal distance in front of the patient's eye (Figure 2). The resultant image is real, magnified 1.5x to 3.5x, reversed left to right, inverted top to bottom, and located between the examiner and the condensing lens (Figure 3).

Figure 1. Binocular indirect ophthalmoscopy (BIO) components: headband, optical viewing system and illumination source
(Courtesy of Welch Allyn)

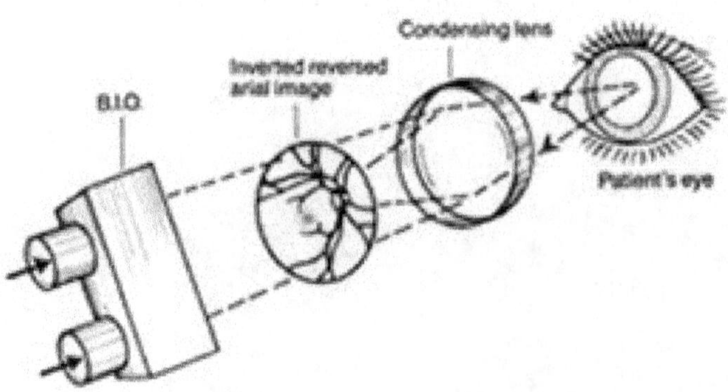

Figure 2. BIO optics: light beams directed into patient's eye, create reflected beams from the retina focused to an aerial image with a condensing len
(Courtesy of Welch Allyn)

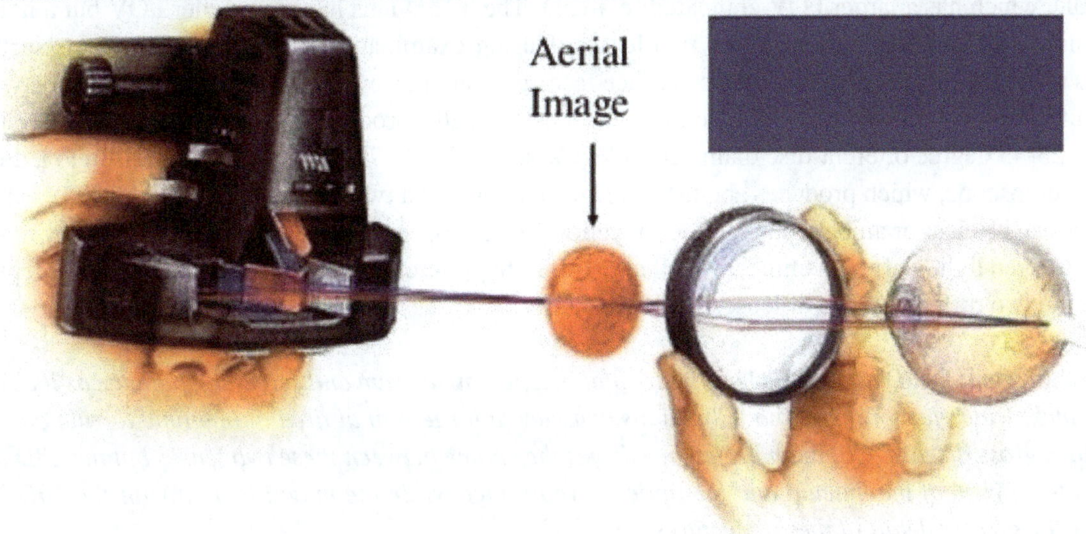

Figure 3. The BIO plus condensing lens creates a real, magnified, reversed, inverted aerial fundus image
(Courtesy of Welch Allyn)

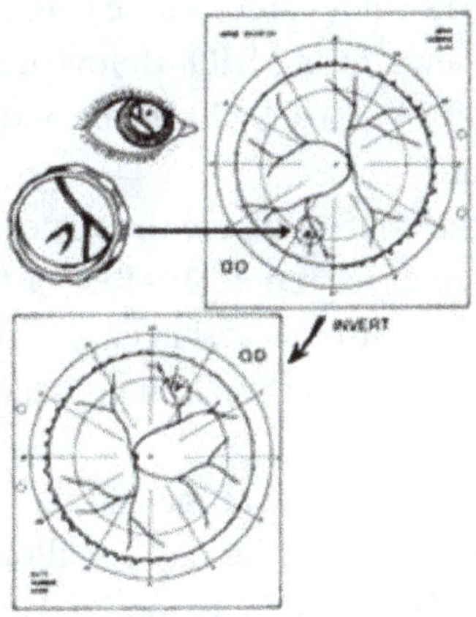

The headband provides proper support with adjustable controls. There are various styles based on manufacturing company. The ocular lens system has knobs that are adjustable to line up with the examiner's pupil distance (PD). Prisms are incorporated into the instrument to create a stereoscopic view. The two images of the examiner's pupils and of the light source are located inside the patient's dilated pupil for 3D viewing. The small pupil BIO allows passage of these points through an undilated pupil and is better for undilated pupil retinal exam or those who do not dilate fully.

The BIO condensing lens is double aspheric lens with antireflective coating. It is available in various powers, including +15D, +20D, and +28D. When the lens provides a larger field of view (FOV), the magnification is decreased and vice versa. For example, the +28D provides a larger FOV compared to 20D, which has a larger FOV compared to +15D. The +15D lens has the smaller FOV but a higher magnification compared to the other two lenses. During examination, the more convex lens surface faces toward the examiner, less convex surface faces the patient's eye. While differences exist between manufacturers, the standard +20D condensing lens typically produces about 2.5x-3x magnification and a 35-45 degree or eight-disc diameter FOV (Casser et al., 1997a). This is in comparison to a direct ophthalmoscope, which produces about 15x magnification and a two-disc diameter fundus FOV. These lenses can be clear or amber color. Amber or yellow lenses appear to increase patient comfort by reducing scattered light. Different clinicians will have different preferences relative to fundus color perception with the two different types of lenses.

Clinical Pearl: *+28D and +20D lens are helpful in a pediatric exam and screening patients as it allows for quick, wide view of the retina. Clinicians can view a large retinal area at one time to rule out any obvious gross disease. Clinician preference drives the choice between these two lenses but the 28D lens provides a view of the macula and the optic nerve at once while the magnification with the 20D lens allow for greater detail of these structures.*

Landmarks of the Retina

Fundus landmarks that are easily seen and recognized include the posterior pole, equatorial retina, peripheral retina, ora serrata, pars plana, ora bays, and vitreous base (Figure 4). Knowing the retinal landmarks assists the clinician in navigating the views during BIO. Below are the definitions of the landmarks:

Posterior Pole: comprised of 60-70% of retina, includes the optic disc, central retinal artery and vein, fovea, macula and vessel arcades (Figure 5).

Equatorial Retina: retina around the equator where the vortex veins exit.

Peripheral Retina: also known as anterior retina, 30-40% of the retina. Divided into superior and inferior retina by the long posterior ciliary arteries and nerves at the temporal and nasal quadrant, at 3 o'clock and 9 o'clock. Short ciliary arteries and nerves run perpendicular to the ora serrata, at the vertical meridians, 6 o'clock and 12 o'clock.

Ora Serrata: far periphery, border between the retina and the pars plana. Gray or "salt and pepper" appearance of the circumferential band. Nasal border has a scalloped appearance (2mm wide nasally). Temporal ora serrata border is smooth (1mm wide temporally. Begins approximately 7mm behind the limbus nasally and 8mm temporally.

Clinical Pearl: *To see the ora serrata most of the time, BIO must be used in conjunction with scleral indentation as described in the premature infant section.*

Pars Plana: have dentate processes (periodic jetties of retinal tissue), more prominent in the nasal quadrant.

Ora Bays: extensions of the pars plana onto the retinal side

Vitreous Base: posterior to the ora serrata, circumferentially oriented, wide band of mottled pigments, however the area just posterior to vitreous base can appear lighter in color than the adjacent retina

Figure 4. Fundus showing landmarks
(Courtesy of Welch Allyn)

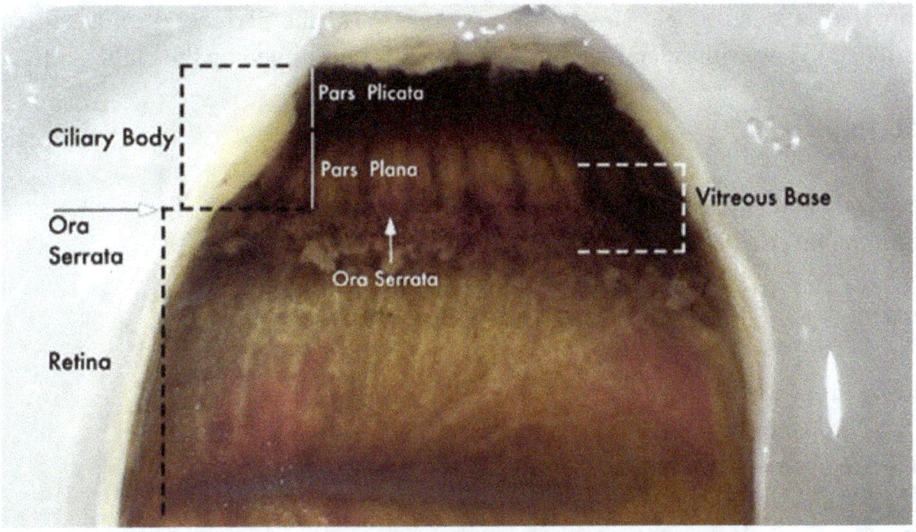

Figure 5. Posterior pole
(Courtesy of Stanford Medicine)

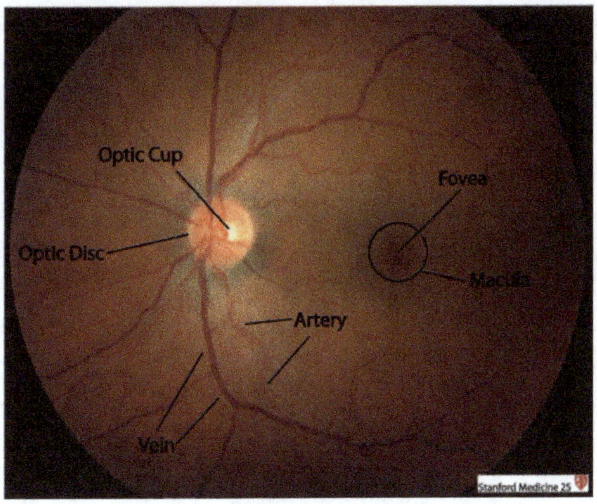

Indications

BIO is a technique used to evaluate the health of the retina. BIO is performed in virtually every eye exam to get adequate visualization of the retina and is particularly important on children with symptoms of floaters, flashes of light, vascular disease, vitreous disease, and blunt ocular trauma. Certain diseases of the retina, such as diabetic retinopathy, should virtually always include BIO for peripheral disease that could alter the course of that patient's treatment. Likewise, many patients will have peripheral findings that may be asymptomatic but require examination to be detected, such as choroidal nevi.

Advantages

BIO exam provides a stereoscopic view with a large FOV of the peripheral retina. It can provide a complete peripheral view with scleral indentation, and it is not limited by the child's refractive error.

Disadvantages

BIO exam needs dilated pupils, child may experience glare and discomfort. There is low magnification, and the images are inverted and reversed.

Equipment

1. Diagnostic drops to dilate eye
   a. 0.5% Proparacaine ophthalmic solution
   b. 1% Tropicamide ophthalmic solution
   c. 2.5% Phenylephrine ophthalmic solution
   d. Cyclopentolate 1% or 2% can be used in addition to the above drops in the pediatric population to achieve better cycloplegia for cycloplegic refraction if needed in addition to the dilated fundus exam.

Clinical Pearl: *While hypersensitivity reactions are rare, it should be noted that the youngest patients, those with cardiac disease, and some patients with Trisomy 21 may experience a reaction so the clinician should educate the family and be vigilant.*

2. Binocular Indirect Ophthalmoscope (BIO)
3. Reclinable / adjustable chair
4. Condensing lens: +20D or +28D

Clinical Pearl: *+15D: higher magnification and smaller field of view, rarely used in clinic.*

Clinical Pearl: *+20D: most commonly used, offers the ideal combination of magnification and field of view.*

Clinical Pearl: *+28D: lower magnification, larger field of view, good for small pupils and the preferred lens by most pediatric clinicians.*

5. Small toy for fixation

Clinical Pearl: *Examples of good toys for fixation during BIO include glow in the dark finger puppets, lighted hand-held toys, spinning toys, and noise makers.*

Procedure

Step 1: Dilate the pupils with 1 drop of Proparacaine Hydrochloride ophthalmic solution 0.5%, 1 drop of Phenylephrine Hydrochloride ophthalmic solution 2.5% and 1 drop of Tropicamide ophthalmic solution 1% (or cyclopentolate as discussed above)
Step 2: BIO can be done in several ways.

1. The supine position or upright position in a reclinable chair is best for older children.
2. For infants and toddlers, it is best to have them sitting on their parent's lap. The parent can help restrain the child by holding on to their lower body, feet and hands but restraint is recommended only if needed.
3. For premature infants, the technique will be different and discussed in the section on ROP

Step 3: With one hand, hold a toy as your target while viewing the different quadrants or have child count your fingers while viewing the different quadrants

Clinical Pearl: *Cajoling a good look at the retina is the balancing act of the talented pediatric clinician, using a toy distraction at the same time as employing the use of the equipment to view the back of the child's eye.*

Clinical Pearl: *The parent can support the young child's head while the examiner performs BIO and views the various quadrants.*

Step 4: With another hand, hold the condensing lens such that the less convex lens surface faces the right eye. This side has the white or silver line encircling the lens

Clinical Pearl: *Hold the lens in your dominant hand and the toy in your non-dominant hand. As you improve in your skills, it is best to be ambidextrous.*

Step 5: Create an optical viewing system consisting of your fixation line through the BIO oculars to the aerial image through the condensing lens' optical center through the center of the pupil to the fundus area of the patient. Pretend there is an imaginary rod through these points
Step 6: Trombone the lens towards and away from the eye continuously as you make fine adjustments in the lens tilt and vertex distance to create a distortion free, full lens view with your condensing lens. Remember to bend the torso in unison with the lens to maintain alignment as the condensing lens is titled to view various fundus areas
Step 7: Using the pupil as your rotation point, adjust illumination as needed and view any specific retinal area by rotating yourself and the light source in the opposite direction of the retinal area being view. The light source is directed onto the retina from 180 degrees away
Step 8: Tilt your head and reposition the light beam and ocular alignment through the pupil along with your torso movements all at the same time as you view each quadrant from posterior to anterior retina, from posterior pole to equator to ora serrata
Step 9: Repeat this procedure for each quadrant. The patient should be directed to look in the direction of the quadrant to be examined.

Clinical Pearl: *In a young child, examine the quadrant the child is fixating at, and view overlapping areas as quickly as you can.*

Clinical Pearl: *Try to point the illuminating light source slightly above the pupil instead of the center of the pupil to allow for better visualization in a small pupil or poorly dilated pupil. This will reduce pupil constriction from the illumination light.*

Clinical Pearl: *When performing BIO, you must have sufficient light to visualize small retinal lesions and color differences. If unable to obtain a view due to a child's light sensitivity, try a yellow filter or attempt to examine the posterior pole first with lower intensity light so the peripheral exam will not be as obtrusive.*

Step 10: Repeat steps 4-9 to examine the left eye by leaning over the child and rotating the lens.

Clinical Pearl: *Flexibility is key when performing BIO on a toddler. You must view the quadrant in the order the child permits while still being thorough. Not seeing the fundus isn't an option just because they are a child; often it is easiest to look into the periphery first since this is less bright for the child. However, in the difficult child/exam, the posterior pole must be viewed at the expense of the peripheral retina if there is no history of trauma or cause for concern regarding the periphery.*

Clinical Pearl: *Remember to prioritize and view the most important elements of the exam first. For example, if you suspect a retinal detachment, look at the posterior pole first to be certain you can appreciate if the macula is involved, then turn your attention to the region of the retina you believe is detached to look for the extent of it and a possible tear or source.*

Clinical Pearl: *Remember that only the condensing lens view is inverted and reversed. If your light beam is directed into the superior fundus, you are looking at the superior retina. As you move more anterior, the new retinal tissue image appears in the condensing lens at its opposite edge closest to the clinician.*

Clinical Pearl: *If the clinician suspects the child is experiencing a reaction to the dilating medications given (rare but more common in infants, particularly those with Trisomy 21 and/or cardiac issues), it is imperative to complete the fundus examination despite the reaction, if possible. Noting in the patient's chart that there was a prior reaction can help the clinician and the patient weigh the risks and benefits of administering this medication again on future examinations. However, the fundus examination may be the clearest opportunity to evaluate for or rule out peripheral retinal pathology.*

SCLERAL INDENTATION

Background

Scleral indentation is a technique that aids in viewing peripheral retina in conjunction with the BIO (Casser et al., 1997b). Scleral indentation increases contrast in the retinal defect from the BIO light beam that is reflected obliquely away from the examiner's view creating a darker choroidal retinal pigment background against the inner translucent retina. When viewing a translucent tissue obliquely, the apparent tissue density is increased, enhancing tissue contrast.

The examiner uses a scleral depressor to elevate and roll the retinal tissue while viewing stereoscopically from multiple angles through the BIO (Figure 6). Scleral indentation between the globe and the orbit displaces the retina inward and creates an elevation, displacing optically inaccessible or poorly defined areas of the retina. This technique enhances the retinal lesion from the surrounding retinal tissue, allowing views of the anterior fundus frequently obscured by the iris, crystalline lens and globe configuration. Scleral indentation requires dexterity and a high level of competency with BIO. The clinician must master the BIO technique before learning the scleral indentation technique.

Figure 6. BIO and scleral indentation
(Courtesy of oculist.net)

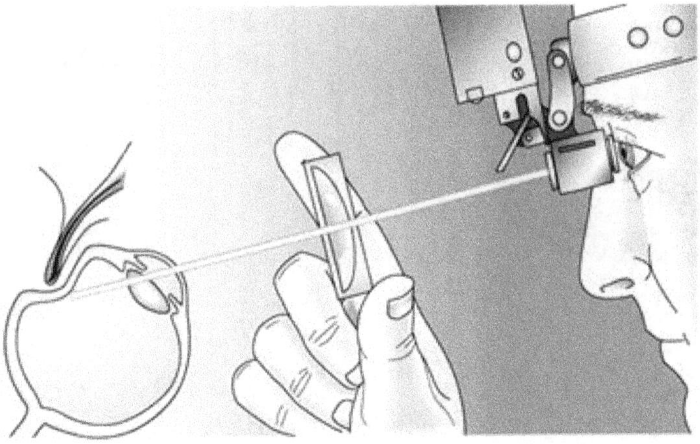

Indication

Scleral indentation allows for greater ease in viewing tissue layer separation and surface irregularities. This helps the clinician diagnose and locate lesions that may otherwise go undetected. It can also help detect lesions that are not well defined such as retinal holes, tears, or vitreoretinal adhesions. Scleral indentation is useful in patients with symptoms of flashes and floaters to rule out peripheral retinal breaks. Also helpful to examine children with risk of peripheral retinal anomalies such as high myopia or those with history of blunt trauma. Remember that a healthy retina does not have round, linear, arc or geometrically shaped lesions in the peripheral retina.

Contraindication

Patients with open globe injury, hyphema, scleral buckle, filtering bleb and those who just underwent ocular surgery should not be scleral depressed.

Clinical Pearl: *Scleral indentation can temporarily increase IOP and should be used with caution in patients with ocular hypertension or glaucoma.*

Equipment (Figure 7, 8, 9)

1. Diagnostic drops to dilate eye
2. Binocular Indirect Ophthalmoscope (BIO)
3. Reclinable / adjustable chair
4. Condensing lens: +20D or +28D
5. Scleral depressor

Figure 7. Equipment used to perform scleral indentation: 20D lens

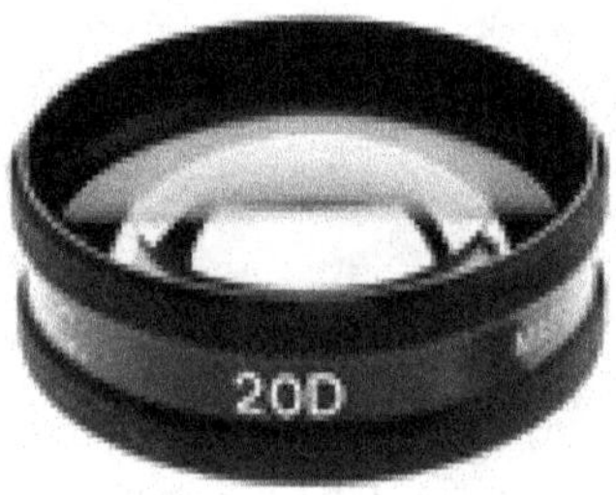

Figure 8. Equipment used to perform scleral indentation: scleral depressor

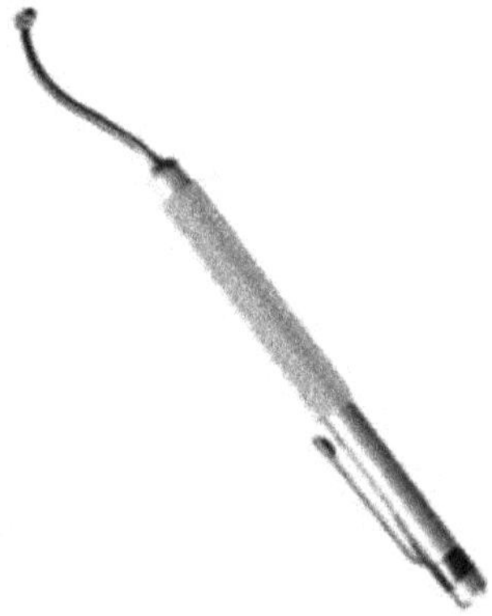

Figure 9. Equipment used to perform scleral indentation: BIO

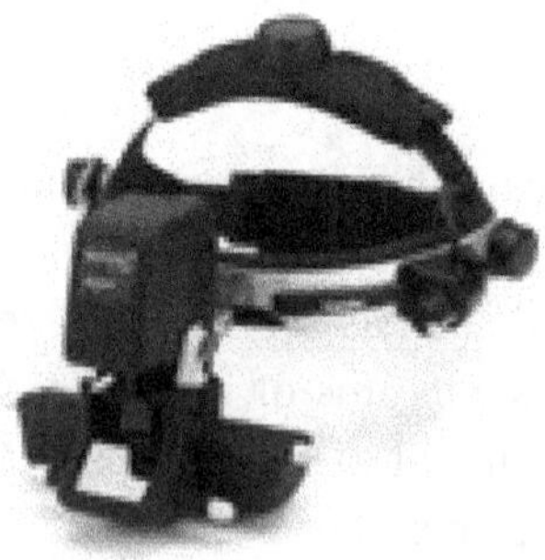

Procedure

Step 1: Eyes are be dilated, and child is seated as described in steps 1 and 2 above for Binocular Indirect Ophthalmoscopy

Clinical Pearl: *When performing BIO you must have a full dilation in order for scleral depression to be performed successfully.*

Step 2: To get a successful view, the clinician's view must be perfectly aligned with the BIO condensing lens, the retinal quadrant being view and the direction of the child's gaze. The clinician must approach on a tangential plane to the pupil

Clinical Pearl: *In scleral indentation, there must be perfect alignment between the clinician, the BIO lens, pupillary center of rotation, the depressor and the retinal quadrant being view.*

Step 3: Direct the patient to look in the opposite direction of the desired quadrant to be view, and then apply the scleral depressor to the lid at a location 5-8mm behind the limbus. Ask the child to slowly change fixation and now look at the direction of the area to be examined

Clinical Pearl: *To view the inferior ora serrata, instruct the child to look as far back as possible towards his/her forehead and the clinician's depressor. After the depressor is on the inferior retina, have the child look towards the depressor and the area of retina to be examined.*

Step 4: As the fixation changes, the scleral depressor should follow along the eye perpendicularly, next, apply gentle pressure tangentially. Look for the red reflex, and watch it darken slightly or appear as a shadow; this signifies that scleral depression is now in the proper location. Practice finding the reflex and the darkened alteration to the reflex corresponding to the depressor position

Clinical Pearl: *The depressor is positioned perpendicular to the eye with its tip tangential to the globe.*

Step 5: Finally, move the condensing lens into the eye's darkened reflex area and look for an elevation of the retina at the opposite side of the lens

Step 6: Scan the retina by adding a little movement to the depressor as you look for the "mouse under the rug" phenomenon

Clinical Pearl: *Move ("rock") the depressor horizontally, vertically, and obliquely to visualize the elevated area.*

Step 7: When examining the 3 or 9 o'clock position, the clinician can drag the lid around or depress on the sclera and globe directly. "When the depressor is pushed perpendicular to the eye or is pressing on a muscle insertion, the patient will feel uncomfortable. Little pressure is required during this procedure" (Dinardo and Walling, 2013). If the child shows signs of pain or discomfort, you are likely depressing too hard, the depressor is not tangential or indentation is too far anterior

Clinical Pearl: *Gentle pressure is applied tangentially, not perpendicularly to the globe with the depressor.*

Clinical Pearl: *If the retinal elevation is seen but not in the proper position, move the depressor in the direction opposite to the area you want visualize, or ask the child to look in that position of gaze.*

Clinical Pearl: *For a child with prominent frontal bone, elevate the chin to get a better view of the inferior quadrant.*

Clinical Pearl: *Younger patients has firmer orbital texture compared to older patients with flaccid lids, thus the clinician needs to reposition the depressor for each clock hour position.*

BIO AND SCLERAL DEPRESSION IN PREMATURE INFANTS

Background

Development of the Normal Retina

The development of the normal retinal vasculature occurs while the fetus is in utero in a relatively hypoxic environment that is supported by the infant's fetal hemoglobin and lower metabolic demands. The retina has dual vasculature supply: the choroidal vessels and the retinal vessels (inner retina). The choroidal vasculature is fully developed by 22 weeks of gestation. The choroid lacks autoregulation in response to hypoxia; therefore, the retina has its own vascular supply to meet the demands of the maturing retina. Retinal vasculature development begins at the optic disk at about 16 weeks gestation through a process called vasculogenesis. Continued development extends the retinal vasculature to the periphery (the ora serrata) by 36-40 weeks of gestation. The retinal vessels reach about 70% of the distance from the optic disk to the periphery by 27 weeks of gestation.

Clinical Pearl: *The formation of the normal retinal vessels depends on a period of physiological hypoxia. Relative hyperoxia that occurs when a baby is born prematurely and exposed to our high oxygen environment inhibits new blood vessel formation by down regulating VEGF.*

Clinical Pearl: *Normal retinal vascularization proceeds from the optic disc to the periphery and is complete in the nasal quadrants at about 36 weeks of gestation and on the temporal side by 40 weeks.*

Clinical Pearl: *The vascularized retina in the premature infant without retinopathy of prematurity normally blends into nonvascularized retina. During the development of disease, the junction between the vascular and avascular retina becomes distinct.*

Retinopathy of Prematurity (ROP)

ROP is a disorder of retinal–blood vessel development. It is a hypoxic retinopathy in a premature baby. In a premature baby, the retinal development occurs in an altered oxygen environment. ROP is a biphasic disease process; the initial phase of vessel growth retardation is followed by a second phase of vessel proliferation.

Very low birth weight premature infant has immature lungs and when a higher level of oxygen is needed both in the natural environment after birth as well as the use of supplemental oxygen given to the infant, the production of VEGF is inhibited, thus there is cessation of normal retinal growth. In utero, the fetus receives IGF-1 (insulin like growth factor) via the placenta. This process is ceased at the time of birth. After birth, IGF-1 is suppressed by a multitude of factors therefore premature infants with prolonged low levels of IGF-1 and slow weight gain are at increased risk of ROP.

During this time, there is progressive increase in metabolic activity in the non-vascularized retina resulting in a hypoxia induced production of VEGF leading to retinal vascularization being re-initiated, and this can sometimes cause pathologically which is when the disease of retinopathy of prematurity can be detected on examination.

NICU Premature Infants

Pre-term babies requiring extensive medical care are often admitted to the Neonatal Intensive Care Unit (NICU). There is a pulse oximeter probe on the premature infant's foot to monitor blood oxygen level. There is a red light and a sensor. As the light travels through the skin to the sensor, it measures the amount of hemoglobin that is carrying oxygen in the blood. This allows the medical staff to determine whether the baby needs more or less oxygen, while reducing the need for painful blood tests. In premature babies, the location of the probe is often rotated several times a day to prevent the light from damaging the premature babies' delicate skin.

The blood oxygen level is titrated, so supplement oxygen is kept at the lowest amount necessary to maintain appropriate oxygen saturation (Cole et al., 2016). The desired level of oxygen saturation is an area of active clinical and basic science investigation, balancing sufficient oxygen for growth and health of the infant's developing organs without the toxic effects of higher oxygen levels (Wright et al., 2006). The role of oxygen in the development of retinopathy of prematurity has been extensively described and the key to the development of retinopathy of prematurity is vascular endothelial growth factor (VEGF).

Classifications of ROP

ROP is classified by the location (zone), severity (stage) and the presence or absence of plus or pre-plus disease (Committee for the Classification of Retinopathy of Prematurity, 1984). Figure 10 illustrates the location of ROP Zones I, II, and III. Figures 11, 12, 13, 14, 15, and 16 are photos representing different severities of ROP. Figures 17 and 18 are photos illustrating plus disease, which is the presence of retinal vascular dilation and tortuosity.

Location of ROP

- Zone I: posterior retina within a 60-degree circle centered on the optic nerve. For ROP exams, the industry standard is to use the 28D lens with the optic nerve at the edge of the lens and observing the retinal vasculature terminates within the lens' view temporally.
- Zone II: as observed with the 28D lens, the retinal vasculature extends beyond Zone I but the retinal vasculature has not fully matured to the nasal ora serrata including in the superonasal and inferonasal quadrants.
- Zone III: retinal vasculature has extended to the nasal ora serrata but the remaining temporal peripheral retina is still not vascularized up to the ora serrata.

Figure 10. Diagram showing locations of ROP zones in a right eye
(Committee for the Classification of Retinopathy of Prematurity, 1984)

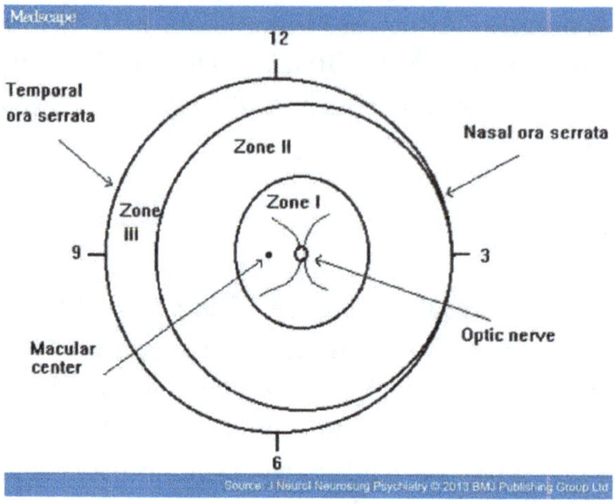

Severity of ROP

ROP is classified in five stages, ranging from mild (stage 1) to severe (stage 5)

- Stage 1: Flat demarcation line between vascularized and nonvascularized retina
- Stage 2: Elevated / ridged demarcation line
- Stage 3: A ridge with extraretinal fibrovascular proliferation
- Stage 4: Partial retinal detachment
- Stage 5: Total retinal detachment

Figure 11. Photo of ROP stage 0. Arrows pointing to vessels that simply end, also known as immature retina
(Courtesy of Brandon Johnson, MD)

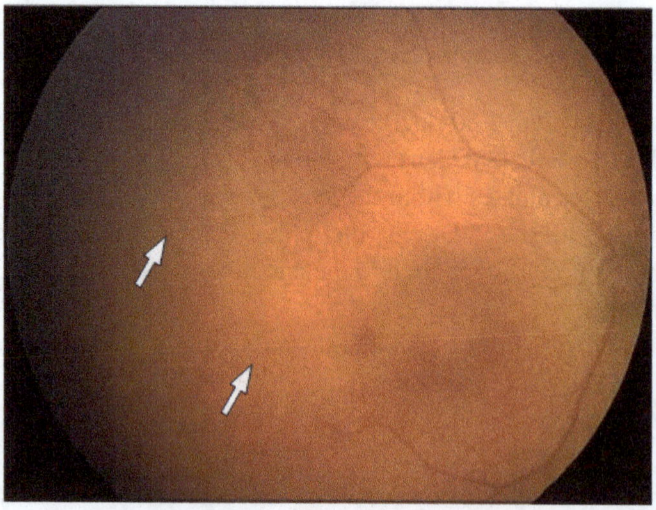

Figure 12. Photo of ROP in zone II, stage 1. Arrow points to demarcation line between the vascular and avascular retina. There is no plus disease
(Courtesy of Brandon Johnson, MD)

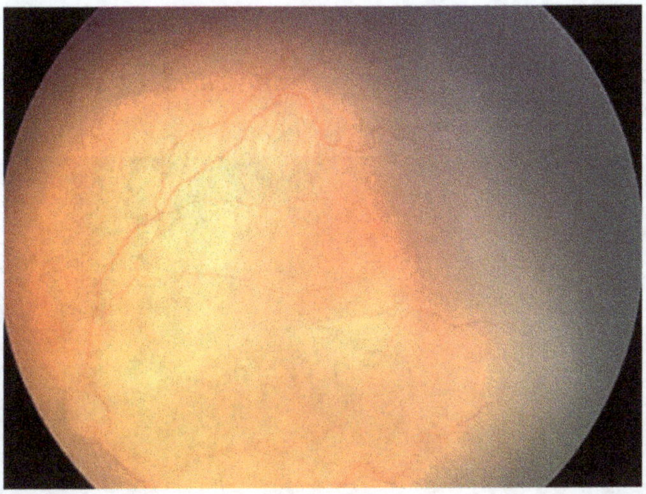

Figure 13. Photo of ROP in zone II, stage 2. Arrows point to a ridge that has volume. There is no plus disease
(Courtesy of Brandon Johnson, MD)

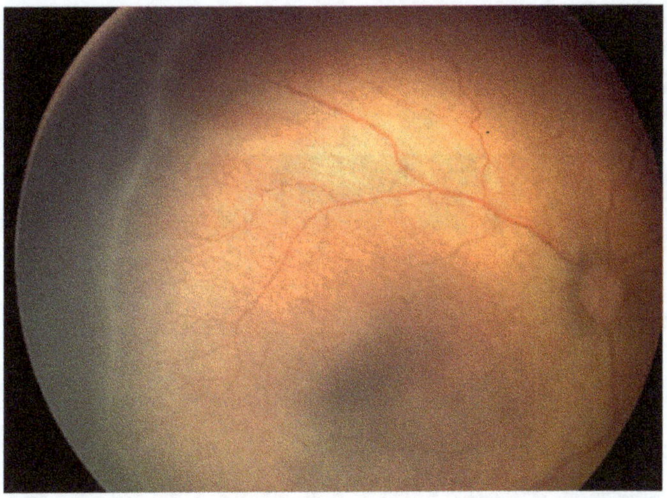

Retinopathy of Prematurity Screening

Retinopathy of prematurity (ROP) screening in premature infants is critical to the prevention of blindness in a small subset of at-risk infants. The screening occurs in the neonatal intensive care unit (NICU) and continues in office after discharge from the hospital. The American Academy of Pediatrics, the American Association for Pediatric Ophthalmology and Strabismus and the American Academy of Ophthalmology periodically update their recommendations, the last publication in 2018 (Fierson et al.)

recommends infants less than 1500g, infants of gestational age less than or equal to 30 weeks or select infants between 1500g and 2000g or older than 30 weeks who are believed by their neonatologist or pediatrician to be at risk for ROP should be screened.

Figure 14. Photo of ROP in zone II, stage 3 showing extra-retinal neovascularization and plus disease
(Courtesy of Brandon Johnson, MD)

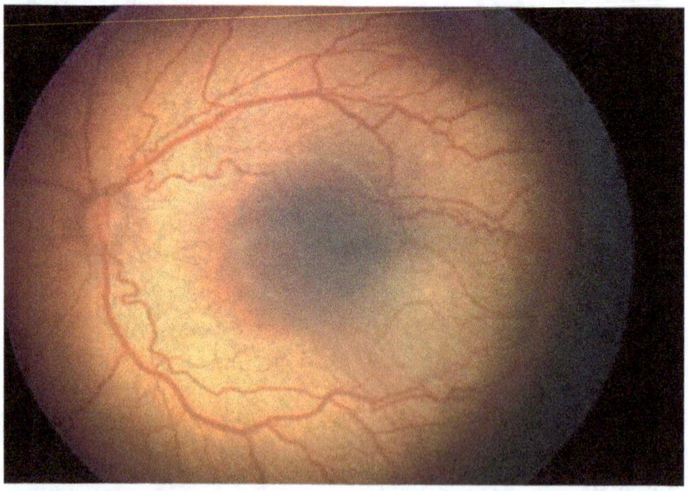

Figure 15. Photo of ROP in zone II, stage 4 showing shallow partial retinal detachment with macula sparing
(Courtesy of Brandon Johnson, MD)

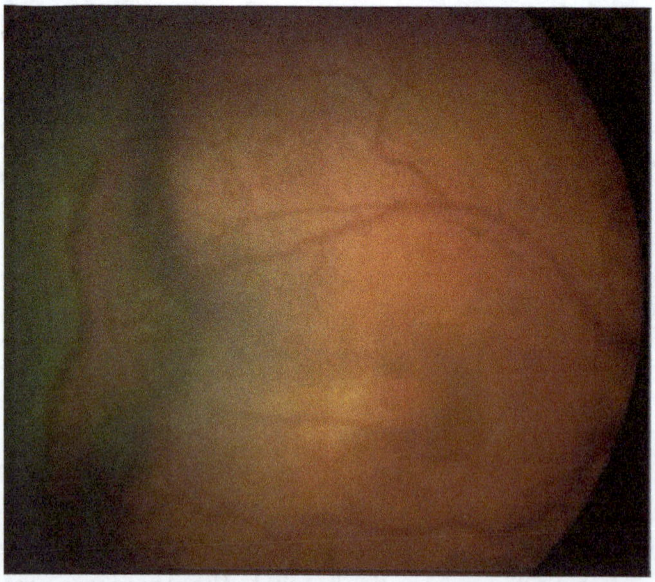

Figure 16. Photo of ROP stage 5 showing total retinal detachment
(Courtesy of Brandon Johnson, MD)

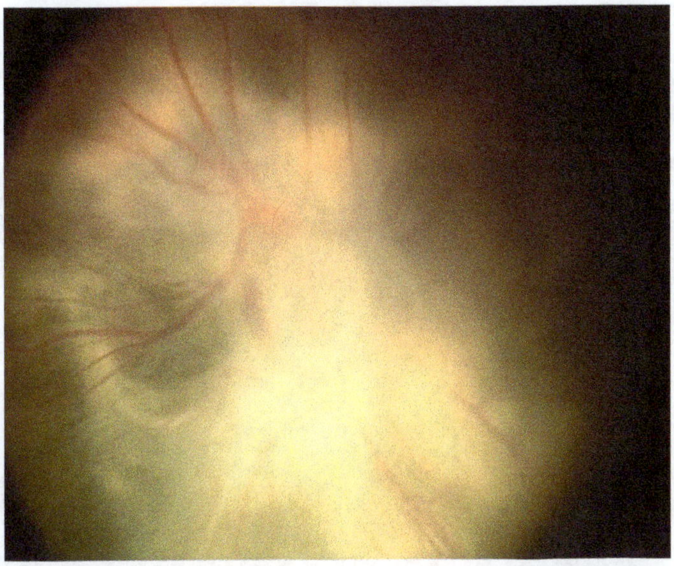

Figure 17. Photo of plus disease. Note presence of retinal vascular dilation and tortuosity in the posterior pole
(Courtesy of Brandon Johnson, MD)

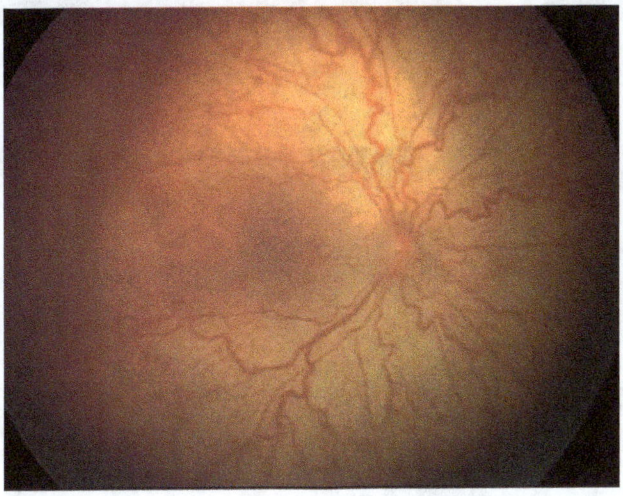

Retinal screening should occur after retinal dilation with the use of binocular indirect ophthalmoscopy, a lid speculum and scleral depression (Figure 19). Separate sterile instruments or instruments cleaned according to the NICU protocol for metal instruments should be used, including attention to clean instruments after the transition to the in-office environment. The difficulty of these examinations and the attention to the vulnerabilities of these infants is critical to successful screening for retinopathy of prematurity. Caring for these at-risk infants is one of the most challenging aspects of pediatric eye care, and the changing guidelines and careful follow up of these infants is key to the avoidance of poor outcomes for this population.

Figure 18. Photo of ROP in zone I, stage 3 with plus disease
(Courtesy of Brandon Johnson, MD)

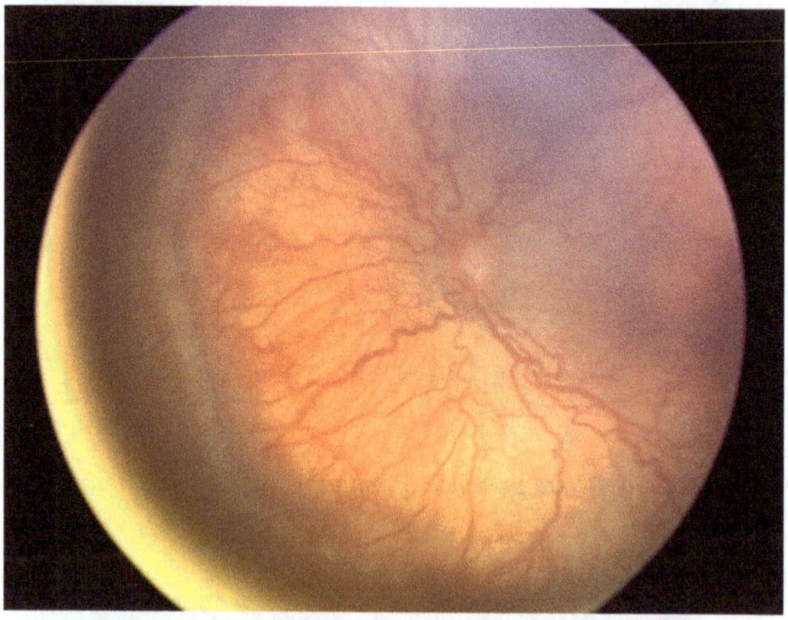

Figure 19. ROP screening procedure

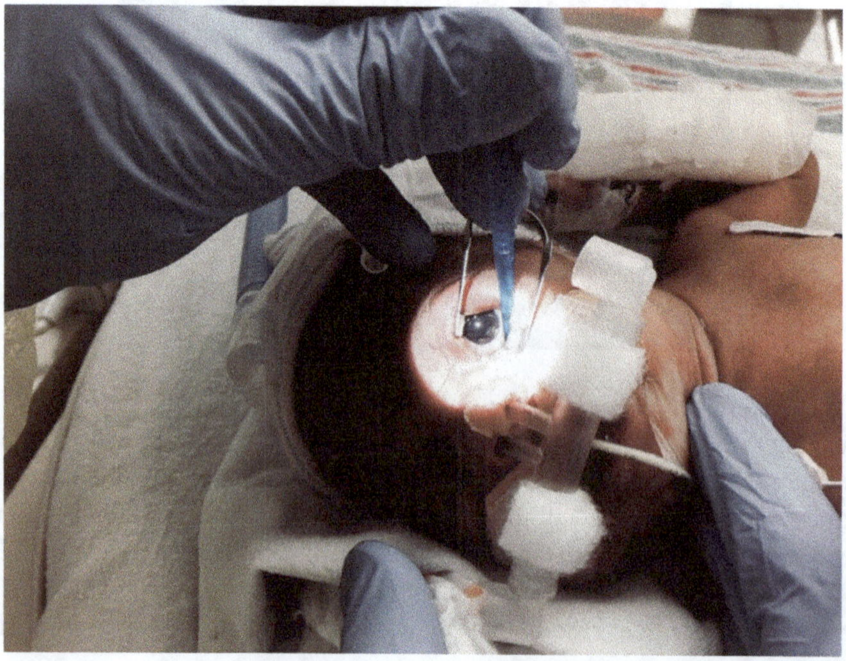

Indication

The clinician must keep in mind the risk factors of developing ROP when examining these infants. Risk factors include birth weight, gestational age, race, oxygen concentration and overall health of the baby. There is higher risk with lower birth weight and extremely premature infants. Many of the co-morbid conditions of prematurity will be seen in the most at-risk infants, such as necrotizing enterocolitis, intraventricular hemorrhage, and pulmonary disease. Retinopathy of prematurity can change very rapidly, and it is the obligation of the examiner to identify the extent of disease or of immature retinal vasculature, document their findings utilizing the nomenclature laid out by Committee for the Classification of Retinopathy of Prematurity (1984) also known as ICROP, and determine next appropriate follow up for that particular infant.

The first eye exam for the premature infant should be based on the infant's postmenstrual age, rather than the chronological age as this is a better correlate with disease (Figure 20). Table 1 is modeled from the American Academy of Pediatrics' 2018 guidelines and shows the timing of eye examinations for premature infants based on postmenstrual and gestational age. Follow up examination depends on the severity of the disease, or the extent of immature retinal vasculature, as determined by screening and continues until the retina is vascularized sufficiently (Table 2). These premature infants are at risk for a lifetime of visual issues so the child will need to be followed for eye care even after the retinopathy of prematurity examinations can be discontinued.

Clinical Pearl: *Determining a baby's gestational age is necessary. It gives the clinician information to set the baby's examination schedule.*

Figure 20. Age terminology during the perinatal period (American Academy of Pediatrics, Committee on Fetus and Newborn, 2004)

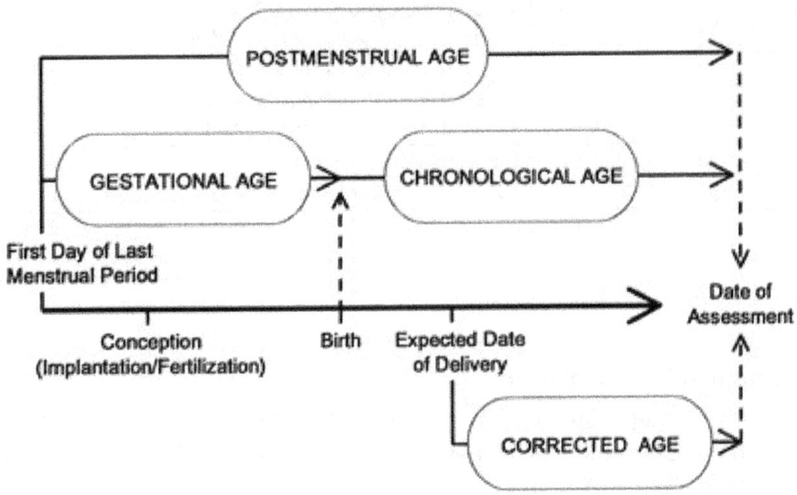

Table 1. Timing of first eye examination based on gestational age (GA) at birth (Adapted from Fierson et al., 2018)

Age	Eye Exam	Eye Exam
22 weeks GA at birth	31 weeks Postmenstrual Age	9 weeks Chronological Age
23 weeks GA at birth	31 weeks Postmenstrual Age	8 weeks Chronological Age
24 weeks GA at birth	31 weeks Postmenstrual Age	7 weeks Chronological Age
25 weeks GA at birth	31 weeks Postmenstrual Age	6 weeks Chronological Age
26 weeks GA at birth	31 weeks Postmenstrual Age	5 weeks Chronological Age
27 weeks GA at birth	31 weeks Postmenstrual Age	4 weeks Chronological Age
28 weeks GA at birth	32 weeks Postmenstrual Age	4 weeks Chronological Age
29 weeks GA at birth	33 weeks Postmenstrual Age	4 weeks Chronological Age
30 weeks GA at birth	34 weeks Postmenstrual Age	4 weeks Chronological Age
31 weeks GA at birth	35 weeks Postmenstrual Age	4 weeks Chronological Age
32 weeks GA at birth	36 weeks Postmenstrual Age	4 weeks Chronological Age

Table 2. Proposed ROP examination follow up schedule. (Fierson et al., 2018) Note that some infants will require an altered frequency of examinations with the goal of examinations to offer treatment at the time when it is most likely to succeed

ROP Follow Up Exam Schedule	ROP Disease Classification
One Week or Less Follow-Up	• Zone I Immature, no ROP • Zone I, Stage 1 or Stage 2 • Immature retina extending into posterior Zone II near the Zone I-II boundary • Suspected presence of AP-ROP • Zone I, Stage 3 ROP requires treatment not observation
One to 2 Week Follow-Up	• Posterior Zone II: immature vascularization • Zone II: stage 2 ROP • Zone I: unequivocally regressing ROP
Two Week Follow-Up	• Zone II: stage 1 ROP • Zone II: no ROP, immature vascularization • Zone II: unequivocally regressing ROP
Two to 3 Week Follow-Up	• Zone III: stage 1 or 2 ROP • Zone III: regressing ROP

Equipment

1. Diagnostic drops to dilate the patient:
   a. 1 drop each eye with Proparacaine Hydrochloride ophthalmic solution 0.5%
   b. 1 drop each eye 2-3 times, 5 minutes apart with Cyclomydril (cyclopentolate 0.2% + phenylephrine 1%)
2. Binocular Indirect Ophthalmoscope (BIO)
3. +28D lens

4. Disposable infant lid speculum (Figure 20) (size may vary based on manufactures) or metal lid speculum
5. Disposable infant scleral depressor (Figure 21) or metal scleral depressor
6. Nurse to assist if in the NICU, trained assistant in the office

Figure 21. Scleral depressor and lid speculum (disposable version shown)

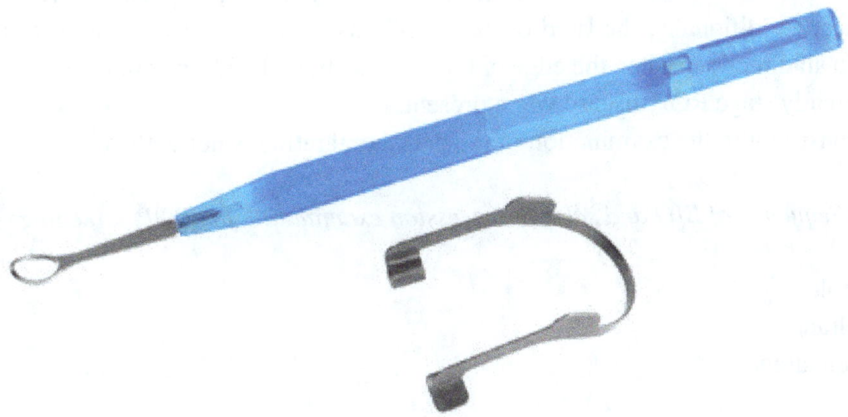

Procedure

Step 1: During the examination while in the NICU, it is highly recommended to have trained assistance with holding the infant, careful observations of the infant's heart rate (HR) and oxygen saturation level throughout the examination as well as general observations of the infant's tolerance of the exam. During bradycardic and apneic episodes, the clinician must pause the eye examination to allow the infant to recover before resuming the exam.

Clinical Pearl: *The use of binocular indirect ophthalmoscopy and scleral depression in an infant especially in a premature baby in the NICU is a little different from older outpatient infants. These patients are more unstable and prone to bradycardia, apnea and oxygen desaturation during the exam. While performing BIO with scleral depression, the clinician must be aware of how the infant is tolerating the exam, best accomplished by having a NICU nurse assisting in the holding and monitoring of the patient during the examination.*

Step 2: The scleral depression technique in infants is the same as when being performed in adults, however, the clinician may notice that the globe is much softer, and the scleral depressor helps to manually move the eye into the position of gaze to view the desired quadrant.

Step 3: Correct positioning of the examiner in relation to the area of retina being examined is important and swaddling the infant to help keep their arms away from their eyes during the exam helps to make the exam efficient and lessen the amount of time that the infant is exposed to this stressful exam technique.

Clinical Pearl: *It is critical to be efficient in the examination. The first look at the fundus is best used to assess the posterior pole vessels for dilation and tortuosity. Try getting the most pertinent information first.*

Step 4: Many examiners prefer the use of a +28D condensing lens instead of a +20D lens. This lens provides a larger field of view despite less magnification and is ideal for quick exams of the posterior pole and periphery. Additionally, the field of view while using a +28D lens extends to the border of Zone I/Zone II in all directions when the edge of the view is aligned with the optic nerve. This helps the examiner consistently stage ROP disease when present.
Step 5: Being consistent in the examination of the peripheral retina benefits the clinician.

Clinical Pearl: *Sequence of BIO and scleral depression examination for ROP screening*

1. Posterior pole
2. Nasal quadrant
3. Temporal quadrant

Step 6: Examine the right eye first, looking at the posterior pole first for plus disease as well as to be certain that the retinal vessels have matured beyond Zone I.
Step 7: Once it is recognized that it is not a Zone I eye, turn your attention to the nasal periphery to look for retinal maturation up to the ora serrata including the superonasal and superotemporal quadrants.

Clinical Pearl: *If the vessels have not matured nasally in the superior and inferior quadrants, then the eye is determined to be Zone II. The region at the termination of the retinal vessels is observed for changes to determine if the vasculature is only immature (stage 0) or if retinopathy of prematurity is developing. If ROP is developing, careful observations as to whether there is only a demarcation line, or a ridge is present, and if there is neovascularization developing in the region of disease. Careful attention needs to be given to the status of the retina to be certain it is still flat and that a retinal detachment isn't starting.*

Step 8: Next, the temporal quadrant is examined in the same manner. If the temporal quadrant is vascularized in the superior and inferior quadrants, then the retinal vasculature is mature (see Figure 10).
Step 9: After completing the right eye, the left eye is examined in the exact same manner. Repeat steps 6-8.
Step 10: Critically, the information gathered is then fully documented in the medical chart of the patient, ideally with drawing of the retinal findings. The information gathered by the clinician is shared with the NICU staff, and if disease is occurring and/or progressing, this information needs to be shared with the family (who may not be present for the exam), including the real risk of blindness from this disease and the importance of close and frequent follow up as determined by the examiner.

When Should Treatment be Performed?

Cryotherapy for retinopathy of prematurity study (CRYO-ROP) (1988) is a multicenter controlled trial that revolutionized our treatment of this blinding disease conducted in the 1980s. It proved that better structural and functional outcomes were achieved with peripheral retinal ablative therapy, using the standard treatment at that time, cryotherapy. Eyes that were recommended to be treated were eyes that had reached threshold disease, defined as Zone I or II ROP with Stage 3 for 5 contiguous or 8 total clock hours, when the presence of plus disease was detected. Plus characteristics are defined as dilation and tortuosity of posterior vessels equal to or greater than those in a standard photograph. Even as the results were being published and the treatment rapidly adopted by providers caring for these premature infants, the development of binocular indirect laser ablative therapy was being adapted and quickly was adopted as the preferred treatment for retinopathy of prematurity. Early treatment for retinopathy of prematurity (ETROP) revised the recommendation for treatment of the peripheral retina with ablative therapy; threshold disease in ROP is no longer the least severe ROP for which intervention should be considered (Good, 2004). ETROP defined Type 1 and Type 2 ROP to guide treatment or observation at levels earlier than what was previously described by CRYO-ROP as time to treat. Type 1 high risk pre-threshold disease that was treated had better structural and functional outcomes, compared with the fellow control eye of the same patient with the same level of disease that did not get treated. Early treatment for Type 2 high risk pre-threshold did not show any added benefit. Fifty-two percent of Type 2 high risk pre-threshold disease regressed without treatment, but close follow up of Type 2 eyes are required as they could evolve to Type I high risk pre-threshold or threshold disease requiring treatment. Table 3 summarizes the clinical characteristics of Type 1 ROP and Type 2 ROP.

Clinical Pearl: *The more posterior the zone at the time of ROP exam, the poorer the prognosis.*

Clinical Pearl: *Eyes with ROP in Zone III typically have a good visual prognosis.*

Table 3. Clinical characteristics of Type 1 and Type 2 ROP

ROP Type	Clinical Characteristics
Type 1 ROP	• Zone I: any stage with plus disease • Zone I: stage 3, no plus disease • Zone II: stage 2 or 3 with plus disease
Type 2 ROP	• Zone I: stage 1 or 2 with no plus disease • Zone II: stage 3 with no plus disease

CONCLUSION

BIO is a challenging and extremely important aspect of pediatric eye care. Learning to perform BIO requires patience and attention to detail. Adding clinical expertise to the technique occurs over years, including what type of condensing lens is best and when scleral depression aids in the exam. All of these elements were covered in this chapter to give the new clinicians an opportunity to form their understanding of the technique and more experienced clinicians to hone the technique over time.

REFERENCES

American Academy of Pediatrics, Committee on Fetus and Newborn. (2004). Age Terminology during the Perinatal Period. *Pediatrics*, *114*(5), 1362–1364. doi:10.1542/peds.2004-1915 PMID:15520122

Casser, L., Fingeret, M., & Woodcome, H. T. (1997a). Binocular Indirect Ophthalmoscopy. In *Atlas of Primary Eyecare Procedures* (2nd ed., pp. 226–229). Appleton & Lange.

Casser, L., Fingeret, M., & Woodcome, H. T. (1997b). Scleral Indentation. In *Atlas of Primary Eyecare Procedures* (2nd ed., pp. 234–237). Appleton & Lange.

Cole, C. H., Wright, K. W., Tarnow-Mordi, W., & Phelps, D. L. (2016). Resolving our uncertainty about oxygen therapy. *Pediatrics*, *112*(6), 1415–1419. doi:10.1542/peds.112.6.1415 PMID:14654618

Committee for the Classification of Retinopathy of Prematurity. (1984). An International Classification of Retinopathy of Prematurity. *Archives of Ophthalmology*, *102*(8), 1130–1134. doi:10.1001/archopht.1984.01040030908011 PMID:6547831

Cryotherapy for Retinopathy of Prematurity Cooperative Group. (1988). Multicenter trial of cryotherapy for retinopathy of prematurity: Preliminary results. *Archives of Ophthalmology*, *106*(4), 471–479. doi:10.1001/archopht.1988.01060130517027 PMID:2895630

Dinardo, A., & Walling, P. (2013). The Lost Arts of Optometry, Part One: A Refresher on Scleral Depression. *Review of Optometry*. Retrieved October 2, 2021, from https://www.reviewofoptometry.com/content/c/42459

Fierson, W. M. (2018). Screening Examination of Premature Infants for Retinopathy of Prematurity. *Pediatrics*, *142*(6), 1–11. doi:10.1542/peds.2018-3061 PMID:30478242

Good, W. (2004). Final results of the early treatment for retinopathy of prematurity (ETROP) randomized trial. *Transactions of the American Ophthalmological Society*, *102*, 233–250. PMID:15747762

Wright, K. W., Sami, D., Thompson, L., Ramanathan, R., Joseph, R., & Farzavandi, S. (2006). A Physiologic reduced oxygen protocol decreases the incidence of threshold retinopathy of prematurity. *Transactions of the American Ophthalmological Society*, *104*, 78–84. PMID:17471328

ADDITIONAL READING

Anand-Apte, B., & Hollyfield, J. G. (2010). *Developmental Anatomy of the retinal and choroidal vasculature*. Elsevier Ltd. Retrieved October 2, 2021, from https://booksite.elsevier.com/brochures/eye/PDFs/Developmental-Anatomy-Retinoid-Choroidal-Vasculature.pdf

Emory University School of Medicine. (2021). *Information for Parents with Infants Still in NICU*. Retrieved October 2, 2021, from http://www.pediatrics.emory.edu/divisions/neonatology/parent_info3.html

Kolb, H. (2011). *Simple Anatomy of the Retina*. Retrieved October 2, 2021, from https://webvision.med.utah.edu/book/part-i-foundations/simple-anatomy-of-the-retina/

The Early Treatment for Retinopathy of Prematurity Cooperative Group. (2010). Final Visual Acuity Results in the Early Treatment for Retinopathy of Prematurity Study. *Archives of Ophthalmology*, *128*(6), 663–671. doi:10.1001/archophthalmol.2010.72 PMID:20385926

U.S. National Library of Medicine. (2021). *Gestational age*. MedlinePlus Medical Encyclopedia. Retrieved October 2, 2021, from https://www.nlm.nih.gov/medlineplus/ency/article/002367.htm

KEY TERMS AND DEFINITIONS

Chronological Age (Postnatal Age): Is the time elapsed after birth.

Gestational Age (Menstrual Age): Is the time between conception and birth. It is measured in weeks, from the first day of the woman's last menstrual cycle to the current date. A normal pregnancy can range from 37 to 42 weeks. Gestational age can be determined before (with ultrasound) or after birth (look at baby's weight, length, head circumference, vital signs, reflexes, muscle tone, posture and condition of the skin and hair).

Oxygen Therapy: Is used to assist in raising blood oxygen levels for the development of organs but need to be titrated carefully to prevent end organ damage, such as retinopathy of prematurity.

Postmenstrual Age: Is the time elapsed between the first day of the last menstrual period and the birth (gestational age) plus the time elapsed after birth (chronological age).

Retinopathy of Prematurity (ROP): A retinal disorder caused by abnormal blood vessel growth in premature infants.

Vasculogenesis: Process involves the proliferation, differentiation, and organization of blood vessels from endothelial progenitors and angioblasts (angiogenesis).

Vascular Endothelial Growth Factors (VEGF): Are substances made by cells that are important in new blood vessel development. They are also associated with pathologic angiogenesis.

Chapter 15
Ocular Emergencies in Children:
Techniques and Procedures to Assist in Diagnosis and Treatment

Joy Harewood
SUNY College of Optometry, USA

Alanna Khattar
BronxCare Heath System, USA

Olivia Bass
Fromer Eye Centers, USA

ABSTRACT

This chapter covers general bedside and chairside examination procedures and instruments used to examine a pediatric patient in an acute care setting. Pediatric patients may present to an emergency room or present emergently in any clinical setting with a wide variety of acute ocular conditions. When working in an emergency room or hospital-based setting, it is unlikely that a clinician will have all of the exam equipment typically used for routine care. The authors review the various ocular imaging techniques used to obtain a view of the internal structures of the eye, orbit, head, and brain when external examination is not sufficient. The procedures described aid the clinician in appropriately and thoroughly evaluating pediatric patients presenting with ocular emergencies.

INTRODUCTION

Pediatric patients may present to an emergency room or present emergently in any clinical setting with a wide variety of acute ocular conditions. When working in an emergency room or hospital-based setting, it is unlikely that a clinician will have all of the exam equipment typically used for routine care. This chapter serves as a guide to aid in managing a wide variety of ocular conditions in a non-traditional setting. The chapter starts by covering general bedside and chairside examination techniques that can

DOI: 10.4018/978-1-7998-8044-8.ch015

be used in an emergency room, followed by discussion of various tests and techniques that aid the clinician in appropriately and thoroughly evaluating pediatric patients presenting with ocular emergencies.

BEDSIDE AND CHAIRSIDE EXAMINATION TECHNIQUES

Indication

Bedside and chairside examinations are useful for infants and toddlers who are usually in the lap of the guardian. Additionally, bedside/chairside exam techniques are indicated when young patients are unable to fit into commonly used equipment due to body habitus or if a patient uses a wheelchair or other assistive devices. These techniques are also useful when certain equipment is unavailable or if a child is unable to be transported from the emergency department for an eye examination.

Background

There are situations where patients are unable to be examined with traditional examination equipment, particularly in the pediatric population. This may be because the patient is an infant, the patient is a toddler who cannot sit in a slit lamp or other eye apparatus, or if it is unsafe for the child to be transferred into a traditional eye examination apparatus due to different abilities. This is even more magnified in an acute-care setting, where an eye examination lane may not be available. In these cases, it is best to adapt the examination to evaluate the child where they can most comfortably sit or rest.

Chairside and bedside techniques discussed largely deal with examination of the front surface of the eye. The posterior segment of the eye can be well viewed with a binocular indirect ophthalmoscope and a condensing lens with the child in almost any position.

Advantages

- Patients can be examined in almost any setting
- Promotes inclusive examinations

Disadvantages

- The view of the eye is less stable
- Examination is more ergonomically taxing for the clinician
- Less detailed view of the eye

Equipment List for Performing a Basic Eye Exam in an Emergency Department Setting

1. Near visual acuity card
2. Adjustable visual acuity chart (ETDRS, Feinbloom number chart)
3. Occluder with pinhole
4. Transilluminator or penlight

5. 20D condensing lens
6. Portable IOP measuring device (i.e. Tonopen, iCare)
7. Eyedrops
    a. Sodium Fluorescein containing ophthalmic solution (or sodium fluorescein strips)
    b. Proparacaine ophthalmic solution 0.5%
    c. Tropicamide 1% ophthalmic solution
    d. Phenylephrine 2.5% ophthalmic solution
8. Binocular indirect ophthamoscope
9. Direct ophthalmoscope

Visual Acuity

All visual acuity should be checked with the child's habitual correction. Checking near visual acuity at an appropriate 40 cm (about 16 inches) for standard measurement can predict a child's distance visual acuity. This can be done with a near visual acuity card or smartphone-based visual acuity card. There are a variety of smartphone apps that can be used to measure accurate visual acuity. Be sure to follow the directions from the manufacturer to get accurate measurements.

There are a variety of charts with a rolling apparatus that can be adjusted easily for use at chairside or besides, namely the ETDRS chart.

The Feinbloom number chart is used extensively in low vision examinations and can be used at various distances to get accurate visual acuity measurements.

Notably, if a child is aphakic (has no natural lens) or has known issues with focusing at near, use a +2.50 loose lens over their habitual distance correction when checking visual acuity at close range. The child may present with bifocals in which case their vision should be checked through the near (bottom) segment.

Anterior Segment Examination

Equipment used to assess the structures and function of the anterior segment include: handheld slit lamp, Tonopen, direct ophthalmoscope, 20D condensing lens and a transilluminator, and transilluminator or penlight for gross examination of large foreign bodies or other more obvious pathology.

A retinoscope or direct ophthalmoscope can be used to examine the cornea and lens for opacities. This is done by standing or sitting roughly an arm's length away from the child and shining the retinoscope or direct ophthalmoscope directly through the center of the eye. You should get a clear red reflex off the retina. Make a note if you see the reflex is absent, or if it appears blocked (a media opacity).

A transilluminator or penlight can be used to check angles by positioning the child sitting upright in a chair or on the edge of a bed. The transilluminator or penlight should then be positioned beside the side of the face, shining the light perpendicular to the eye. Examine the shadow cast by the light to get a rough estimate of the anterior chamber angle.

EYELID SPECULUM

Indication

The use of an eyelid speculum is warranted when the ocular surface must be exposed in a child who is resistant to keeping their eyelids open. The eyelid speculum is useful for the evaluation of either the anterior or posterior segment of the globe. Procedures which may require in-office use of an eyelid speculum include the removal of an anterior segment foreign body, irrigation procedures, intraocular pressure measurements, evaluation of medically necessary contact lenses, forced duction testing and retina examinations for pathology such as retinopathy of prematurity (ROP), retinoblastoma, Coats' disease, persistent fetal vasculature and TORCH Syndromes. An eyelid speculum is commonly used during ophthalmic operative procedures and exams under anesthesia requiring access to the ocular surface.

Importantly, the use of an eyelid speculum should be reserved for necessary scenarios that consist of poor patient cooperation and critical examination of the globe. Procedures such as IOP measurements and contact lens evaluations on infants and school-aged children should typically be successfully obtained without the use of a speculum.

Background

Eyelid speculums are usually metallic and made of surgical steel; however, plastic disposable speculae are available and commonly utilized for ROP screenings. Eyelid speculae consist of two parallel arms, each with a ring, as seen in Figure 1A, or a blade, as seen in Figure 1B, that is contoured to rest against the globe. The blade or ring acts to refrain the eyelids from blinking. The other end of the arms is eventually angled toward the base and are joined by either a hinge or locking mechanism, seen in Figure 1C, which is used to adjust the blade spread, or opening width. The blades are slipped underneath the upper and lower eyelids and effectively resist the force of the activated orbicularis oculi during forced eyelid closure. The blade spread allows for effectual access to the globe.

Advantages

- Improved access to the ocular surface
- During instances such as retina exams, eyelid speculums allow the examiner to manually manipulate additional instruments (condensing lens and spatula or scleral depressor)
- Available in many sizes to accommodate various eyelid sizes

Disadvantages

- Patient discomfort
- The patient must still cooperate with proper fixation (unless also using depressor or spatula to alter fixation)
- Possibly associated with inducing iatrogenic, post-procedure ptosis, especially in patients with smaller palpebral apertures (Crosby et al., 2013)

Figure 1. A: Hinged eyelid speculum. B: Eyelid speculum with blades. C: Eyelid speculum with locking mechanism

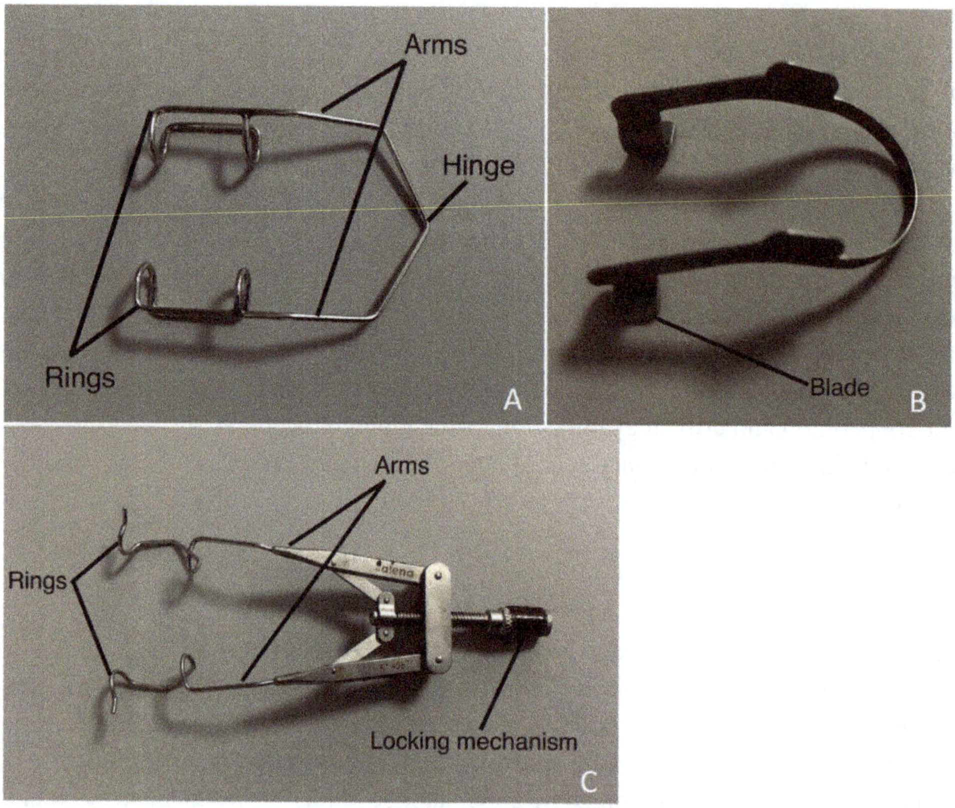

Equipment

1. Eyelid speculum
2. Proparacaine 0.5% ophthalmic solution
3. Balanced salt solution (BSS) or artificial tears (as needed)
4. Depressor or spatula (as needed)

Procedure

Step 1: Instill 1 drop of proparacaine 0.5% ophthalmic solution to the eye
Step 2: Insertion of the speculum

1. Select an appropriately sized eyelid speculum based on the child's eyelid length
    a. Pediatric eyelid speculums are available in smaller blade sizes (about 7 mm to 13 mm) and are useful for neonate and infant exams
    b. Adult eyelid speculums are available in larger blade sizes (14 mm and larger) and are useful for school-aged children and older

2. Reduce the distance between the blades or rings with the concave aspect of the blade/ring facing the globe.
   a. Hinged mechanism (Figure 2A): Pressure should be applied simultaneously to each arm of the speculum so that the proximity is minimized between the two blades or rings
   b. Lock mechanism (Figure 2B): The distance between the two parallel arms of the speculum should be minimized by rotating the thumbscrew at the base
3. Pull the upper eyelid up and insert the upper blade/ring into the conjunctival sac of the upper eyelid
4. Pull the lower eyelid down and insert the lower blade/ring into the conjunctival sac of the lower eyelid
5. Increase the distance between the arms to maintain maximum distance between the eyelids
   a. Hinged mechanism: Release pressure applied between the two parallel arms
   b. Lock mechanism: Rotate the thumbscrew in the opposite direction until the palpebral aperture is widened to an appropriate distance.
6. If the child's fixation needs manipulation, ensure the eye is still anesthetized and utilize the depressor (or spatula)
7. The depressor (or spatula) should be applied to the conjunctiva (never the cornea) in the direction of the location you wish the child to look in (e.g., if you want the child to look temporally, apply pressure down and temporally with the depressor to the temporal conjunctiva)

Figure 2. A: Hinged speculum ready for insertion. B: Eyelid speculum with locking mechanism ready for insertion

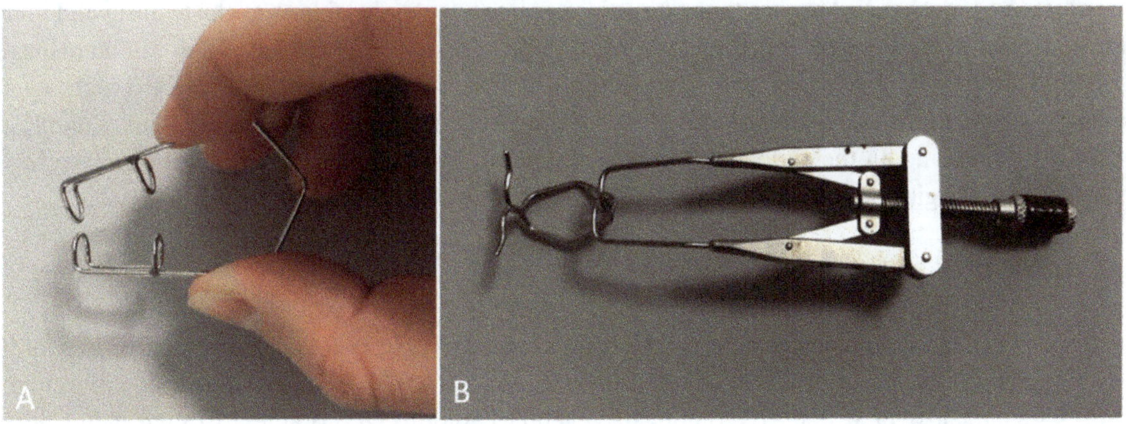

Clinical Pearl: *For prolonged procedures, it is recommended to intermittently apply balanced salt solution or artificial tears to the cornea to improve patient comfort and corneal clarity as needed.*

Clinical Pearl: *When interpreting intraocular pressure (IOP) measurements made while an eyelid speculum is in place, it is important to consider that the presence of an eyelid speculum raises IOP an average of 4 mmHg (Epley et al., 2002).*

Step 3: Removal of the speculum

1. Reduce the distance between the blades or rings
    a. Hinged mechanism: Pressure should be applied simultaneously to each arm of the speculum so that the proximity is minimized between the two blades or rings
    b. Lock mechanism: The distance between two parallel arms of the speculum should be minimized by rotating the thumbscrew at the base in the original direction
2. Have the child look up. Pull the lower eyelid down and remove the lower blade/ring from the conjunctival sac of the lower eyelid
3. Have the child look down. Pull the upper eyelid up and remove the upper blade/ring from the conjunctival sac of the upper eyelid

Clinical Pearl: *Some clinicians recommend considering an exam under anesthesia if a non-emergent procedure warrants the use of an eyelid speculum and the child is older than 12 months. This is due to inadequate cooperation and psychological stressors that may occur during the procedure.*

Clinical Pearl: *Care must be taken to prevent corneal abrasions on insertion and removal of the eyelid speculum, especially as the child may not be aware of discomfort at the time due to anesthesia.*

SIMPLE EYELID LACERATION

Indication

If a pediatric patient has had trauma to their eyelid, it is important to be able to evaluate the eyelid injury and determine the best course of action. In some instances, a simple eyelid laceration can be managed in office. However, if the eyelid margin, canalicular system or canthal tendons are involved or the eyelid laceration is full thickness, the child should be referred for eyelid laceration repair by an oculoplastic specialist. Depending on the child's age, even a simple eyelid laceration may be best managed by an oculoplastic or surgical specialist to ensure the best outcomes for the patient.

Background

On initial presentation, it is important to first obtain a thorough history to determine the etiology of the eyelid laceration. An open globe must be ruled out by exam, and then it must be determined if the clinical features are indicative of a simple or complicated eyelid laceration. The complexity of the eyelid laceration will determine whether it can be managed in-office by a clinician who is not a specialist in surgical eye care, or if it should be referred to a hospital/oculoplastic specialist for repair. Another indication for referral is if the child is not cooperative and sedation is necessary for the eyelid laceration repair.

Equipment

1. Balanced salt solution (BSS) or Sterile irrigating solution
2. Povidone-iodine solution
3. Adhesive surgical tape or Cyanoacrylate tissue adhesive

Figure 3. Eyelid laceration involving the upper eyelid of a pediatric patient

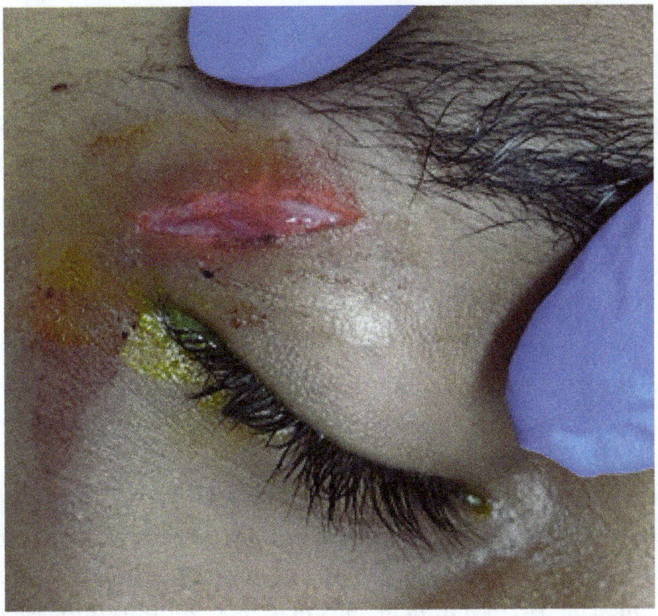

Procedure

Step 1: After it has been established that the child does not have a ruptured globe, the wound should be thoroughly irrigated with saline and any visible foreign body particles should be removed
Step 2: Eyelid lacerations that are superficial and horizontal, follow skin lines, and take up less than 25% of the eyelid margin can be managed without surgery. In some mild cases, only an antibiotic ointment is used for coverage
Step 3: If the eye does not require a sutural repair, but needs more than antibiotic coverage, an adhesive can be used along the laceration to repair the tissue (Brown et al., 2007)
Step 4: Prior to repairing a simple eyelid laceration, the child should be placed in a supine position and the wound cleaned using a full-strength povidone-iodine solution (Cochran & Czyz, 2020)
Step 5: When placing the adhesive, bring the edges of the laceration in apposition without overlapping and then apply the adhesive along the lid laceration and allow it to dry. Care must be taken to not place glue onto other ocular structures or to glue the eyelids together

Clinical Pearl: *Depending on the etiology of the eyelid laceration, systemic antibiotic prophylaxis may be warranted. If the eyelid lesion was from a dog bite, rabies prophylaxis may be considered if the dog was suspected to have rabies or the attacking animal is unknown. It is also important to determine the date of the child's last tetanus shot (Gardiner, 2019).*

FOREIGN BODY REMOVAL

Indication

Corneal and conjunctival foreign bodies can cause significant discomfort for the pediatric patient and must be removed accordingly. There are several different techniques/tools that can be used to remove corneal or conjunctival foreign bodies. These will each be discussed below, from least to most invasive.

Background

Prior to beginning the removal process, obtaining a thorough history from both the child and parent/guardian is critical to determine if there is concern for an intraocular foreign body. If there is concern for an intraocular foreign body, it is prudent that the child be referred for further imaging (see neuroimaging section) and consideration for surgical intervention if warranted.

Once it has been determined that there is no risk of an intraocular foreign body, the process of removal of the corneal or conjunctival foreign body can begin. Prior to removal it is important to thoroughly examine both eyes (even if child is only symptomatic in one eye) with lid eversion, evaluating for any debris that may be present. The use of a topical anesthetic is helpful to improve comfort during examination, and throughout the foreign body removal procedure.

Prior to foreign body removal, it is necessary to discuss with the guardian the risks, benefits and alternative options relating to removal and obtain their consent on behalf of the pediatric patient. Older pediatric patients should be included in the discussion as well, but consent must still be given by their guardian.

With pediatric patients, especially of younger age, the less invasive the procedure is for foreign body removal the more tolerated it will be. With foreign body removal, the initial approach should be the least invasive.

Advantages

- The source of child's initial discomfort is removed
- Allows the healing process to begin

Disadvantages

- Discomfort from residual corneal/conjunctival abrasion post-removal
- Increase in pain after foreign body removal until healing takes place

Equipment

Note that not all of the following pieces of equipment will be needed each time a foreign body removal is performed. This list includes different equipment options that can be used for foreign body removal.

1. Anesthetic eye drop such as proparacaine 0.5% ophthalmic solution
2. Balanced salt solution (BSS) or Sterile irrigating solution

3. Cotton swab applicator
4. Spud
5. Needle gauge
6. Alger brush
7. Speculum

Figure 4. Top: A needle gauge attached to a cotton swab applicator for ocular foreign body removal. Middle: An Alger brush with an attached burr that can be used to remove a rust ring from the cornea. Bottom: A spud used for ocular foreign body removal

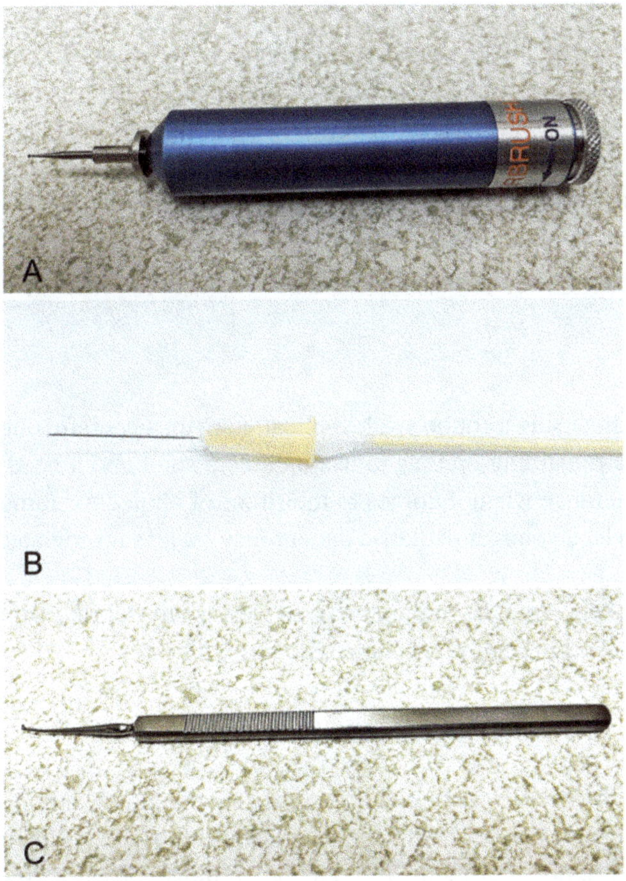

Procedure

Prior to foreign body removal using any of the following techniques, a drop of a topical anesthetic should be instilled in the affected eye. Sodium fluorescein dye can be instilled to check for a Seidel sign (details provided later in this chapter) as well as to highlight the location of foreign bodies and mucus clumps which may contain foreign bodies as well.

Using BSS Sterile Irrigating Solution

Balanced salt solution (BSS) or Sterile irrigating solution can be used if the foreign body is superficial to dislodge it while rinsing the eye. When irrigating, the solution should not be pointed directly at the foreign body, but applied at an angle.

Clinical Pearl: *Folding 2-3 paper towels in half on the diagonal twice, into a triangular shape, with the long end placed under the eye can be effective at capturing solution that spills out of the patient's eye.*

Cotton Swab Applicator

The next least invasive approach is using a cotton swab applicator to remove very superficial conjunctival foreign bodies and corneal foreign bodies in limited situations. If using a cotton tipped applicator on the cornea, be mindful as it can cause significant disruption. There is also the risk that the cotton swab can embed the foreign body deeper in the cornea as well, so the clinician must be very careful when employing this technique. After the eye is anesthetized, a cotton swab can be soaked in proparacaine ophthalmic solution or BSS/Sterile Irrigating Solution and then can be used to attempt to lift more superficial foreign bodies off the ocular surface.

Spud

If rinsing the child's eye and using a cotton swab applicator are unsuccessful due to the extent the foreign body is embedded, some remaining options to use include a spud and a needle gauge. Most clinician will have a personal preference when it comes to their tool of choice for removing a foreign body. Of the more invasive methods, a younger pediatric patient may be less intimidated by a spud compared to a needle gauge.

A spud can be used to scoop out the foreign body, as well as any debris surrounding the foreign body. A magnetic spud can also aid in removal of a metallic foreign body.

Needle Gauge

If using a needle gauge, the needle gauge can be gripped by the plastic end opposite of the bevel, or a syringe or cotton tip applicator can be attached to the plastic end of the needle gauge. This can allow for increased stability of the provider during the foreign body removal process. Needle gauges are available in different sizes, with an 18-gauge needle being larger and a needle gauge of 25 being smaller and better for smaller foreign bodies (Augeri, 1991).

The tip of the instrument being used lifts under the edge of the foreign body to then remove it off the cornea. In general, a needle gauge will result in a smaller residual corneal abrasion than a spud due to the smaller size.

The cornea must be approached tangentially (never perpendicularly) when performing a foreign body removal to prevent penetration through Bowman's membrane or the stroma (Augeri, 1991). When possible, provide the child with a target to focus on or a direction to look in while the examiner approaches the eye to remove the foreign body. For example, it is useful to place a sticker on the slit lamp or to ask the guardian to stand behind you and encourage the child to fixate on the guardian to assist in achieving desired fixation. When using a needle gauge, approach the cornea with the bevel facing outwards.

Alger Brush

Metallic foreign bodies that have been present for as little as four hours can lead to a rust ring formation (Guier & Thomas, 2021). An Alger brush can be used to remove the rust ring if tolerated by the child. Prior to using the Alger brush, it is recommended to turn it on so that the child and guardian hear the sound and know what to expect. The approach of the Alger brush should be tangential and gentle pressure should be applied. The use of an Alger brush will increase the area of a residual corneal abrasion.

Use of a Speculum/ Exam Under Anesthesia

If the child is unable to keep their eyes open for foreign body removal, a speculum may be employed. It must also be considered that a child is not able to be positioned in the slit lamp, or if child is unable to tolerate foreign body removal at the slit lamp, as well as in cases where the foreign body is deeply embedded and a risk of scarring leading to visual loss may take place with removal attempt, an exam under anesthesia may be necessary to allow for successful removal of the foreign body.

Corneal Management Post-Foreign Body Removal

A residual corneal epithelial defect is often inevitable when performing a foreign body removal of the cornea. This defect should be measured with use of fluorescein staining of the cornea and documented. A broad-spectrum antibiotic should be prescribed four times a day for one week after removal. Follow up in 24 hours is recommended to evaluate the healing process and assess for any signs of infection.

PRESSURE PATCHING

Indication

Situations that may benefit from the use of a pressure patch are when a patient may be in pain due to a large corneal abrasion or foreign body removal and residual corneal abrasion. The goal is to facilitate wound healing by reducing the likelihood of mechanical disruption.

Background

Pressure patching can be beneficial in an emergency room setting, especially with pediatric patients. While bandage contact lenses are now used more often therapeutically than a pressure patch, a bandage contact lens is not feasible to use in all situations. A bandage contact lens is not always ideal when there is concern for the pediatric patient being lost to follow up. Additionally, the risk of microbial keratitis developing if a bandage contact lens is not removed in an appropriate time frame is cause for concern. In these instances, a pressure patch is a feasible alternative to the use of a bandage contact lens. With a pressure patch, if the child does not return for follow up, the guardian is able to remove the patch. This may not be the case for a bandage contact lens. If the child and the guardian are not habitual contact lens wearers, removal of a bandage contact lens may be problematic.

Advantages

- Keeps eye closed to facilitate healing
- Prevents excessive eye rubbing by the child
- Easier than inserting a bandage contact lens in a very young or uncomfortable child
- Not inhibited by tearing or crying as the insertion of a bandage contact lens may be

Disadvantages

- Loss of binocularity
- Loss of visual field
- Potential for increased risk of ocular infection due to increased moisture underneath the pressure patch
- Risk of growth of infectious organisms in contact lens wearers

Equipment

1. Two eye pads or folded pieces of gauze
2. Medical tape

Procedure (American Academy of Ophthalmology, 2020; Allen, 2016)

Step 1: Clean the periocular area, extending to the mid to lower cheek with a wipe or lightly with an alcohol pad, being sure to avoid contact with the eye

Step 2: Instill ¼" ribbon of a topical ophthalmic antibiotic ointment (e.g., erythromycin) into the lower fornix of the eye. A drop of a broad-spectrum antibiotic eye drop can also be used in lieu of an antibiotic ointment, although the ointment may provide more comfort

Step 3: Instruct the child to close both eyes

Step 4: Two eye pads or folded pieces of gauze are placed gently against the affected eye. The two eye pads can be placed directly on top of one another, or the bottom eye pad can be folded in half to apply additional pressure to keep the eye closed, with the other eye pad placed over top

Step 5: Place medical tape to secure the patch. Ensure the child continues to keep their eye closed while the tape is applied. If needed, the guardian can be asked to hold the patches in place while the clinician applies the tape

Step 6: The lower cheek should be pulled up firmly while the tape is being applied to the closed eye. Multiple strips of tape can be applied to secure the patch

Step 7: The pressure patch should be left in place for 24 hours, with a follow up scheduled the next day to evaluate the eye and the healing process

Clinical Pearl: *With a small corneal abrasion, if the clinician determines the child is not likely to rub the eye, neither a pressure patch nor a bandage contact lens may be necessary. The clinician should prescribe an age-appropriate broad-spectrum antibiotic to be applied four times a day in the affected eye, with an appropriate follow up scheduled to ensure healing is taking place.*

Figure 5. A properly placed pressure patch secured with medical tape covering the right eye

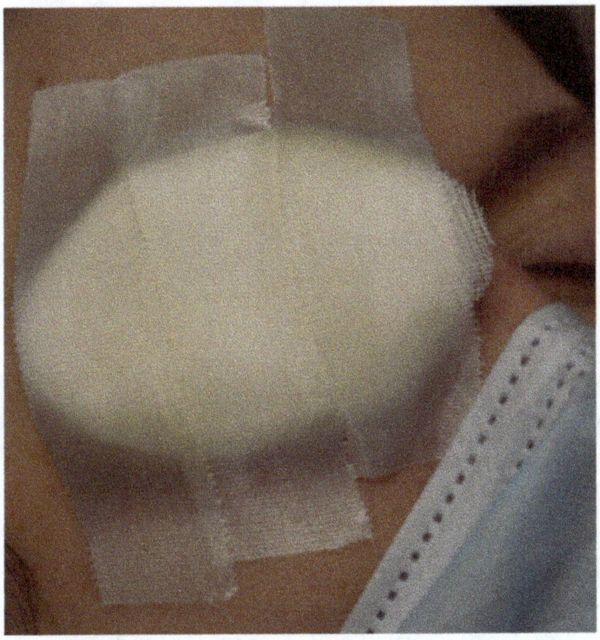

BANDAGE CONTACT LENS

Indication

Bandage contact lenses in the pediatric emergency room setting are most often used to aid in the healing of corneal abrasions whether from trauma or secondary to foreign body removal. They also help with pain management during the corneal healing process.

Background

Bandage contact lenses can be used on pediatric patients of all ages. Success with insertion of a contact lens depends less on age and more on the child's tolerance with having their eyelids manipulated during contact lens insertion, all while experiencing eye pain.

Examples of contact lenses that have been FDA approved for therapeutic use are Acuvue Oasys with Hydraclear Plus (Johnson & Johnson Vision), Air Optix Night & Day Aqua (Alcon) and PureVision (Bausch & Lomb). Bandage contact lenses come in plano power, or if the patient's refractive error is known, an appropriate power of bandage contact lens can be used.

Advantages

- Allows the affected eye to see during the healing process
- Allows the child to return to school and participate in their regular daily activities
- Does not draw unwanted attention to the affected eye (compared to an eye patch)
- Topical ophthalmic medications can be instilled over the bandage contact lens

Disadvantages

- Contraindications include (Lim & Lim, 2020):
    - Infectious keratitis
    - Significant exposure keratopathy with inadequate eyelid position/movement
    - Corneal anesthesia
- Risk of visually devastating complications if child is lost to follow up

Equipment

1. Bandage contact lens
2. Speculum (as needed)

Procedure

Step 1: Select the appropriate bandage contact lens
Step 2: Seat the child in the exam chair or comfortably in the guardian's lap. Neonates and infants should be swaddled to keep their arms and legs still. After swaddling, ask the guardian to hold the child's head still while you insert the lens
Step 3: A speculum can be used if needed to keep the eye open for insertion of the contact lens
Step 4: If child is unsettled during a direct approach with the contact lens, ask the child to look up, place the contact lens on the inferior sclera, and then ask the child to look straight ahead. In combination with blinking this will move the lens onto the cornea
Step 5: After insertion, the bandage contact lens should be assessed for a proper fit in the slit lamp if possible. With a bandage contact lens, it is critical to ensure that the lens is not too loose, because this may cause more damage and inhibit the healing process
Step 6: The first follow up visit should be one day after contact lens placement. Monitor the child daily until the corneal wound has healed. When it is time to remove the bandage contact lens, first apply an ocular lubricant to the patient's eye. The examiner can then use their finger to slide the contact lens onto the patient's bulbar conjunctiva prior to removal. It is not recommended that the child or guardian remove the contact lens themselves.

Clinical Pearl: *Another tool available to the eye care provider that can aid in the healing of the ocular surface are amniotic membranes. Amniotic membranes can be used in the pediatric population; however, they are less likely to be used compared to a bandage contact lens. Amniotic membranes are best for treating acute chemical burns and severe ocular surface disease that are poorly healing.*

SEIDEL SIGN

Indication

When a pediatric patient presents with a history of ocular trauma, it is prudent that an open globe injury be ruled out. The open globe may be due to an injury to either the cornea or the sclera.

Background

An open globe is one of the true ocular emergencies an eye care provider will encounter. It is critical to assess for a Seidel sign in any patient that has a history of ocular trauma. There are a number of clinical signs on examination that may indicate an open globe in addition to a full thickness corneal or scleral laceration, including a pupillary defect (peaked or irregular pupil), bullous subconjunctival hemorrhage, a deep or shallow anterior chamber that is asymmetric when compared to the other eye, blood in the anterior chamber, and a laceration through the eyelid. It is also important to take a thorough patient history to determine if they may be at risk of an open globe due to postoperative complications or due to a degenerative condition.

In the absence of a positive Seidel test result, but the clinician has high suspicion for a globe rupture, it is recommended the child undergo a computed tomography (CT) scan of the orbits to assess for signs of a globe rupture.

Advantages

- Quick, non-invasive test
- Requires readily available standard equipment

Disadvantages

- Possible to have a false negative result in certain instances such as
  - self-healing, small full thickness corneal laceration
  - larger laceration that has been plugged
  - posterior globe rupture

Equipment

1. 0.5% proparacaine ophthalmic solution
2. Sterile fluorescein strips
3. Saline solution

Procedure

Step 1: Instill a drop of topical anesthetic such as 0.5% proparacaine ophthalmic solution in the affected eye.
Step 2: Slightly moisten a sterile fluorescein strip with saline

Step 3: Apply the fluorescein strip in and around the area of concern (Cain and Sinskey, 1981). Alternatively, the dye may be placed on the superior bulbar conjunctiva and the dye will then flow inferiorly over the cornea
Step 4: To spread the dye, ask the child to blink
Step 5: Using the cobalt blue light source, evaluate for a fluorescent, green flow of liquid exiting the wound, streaming downwards with gravity (Cain & Sinskey, 1981). This indicates a positive seidel test. The center of the flowing liquid will not be green in color because there will not be fluorescein present in the aqueous humor that has leaked from the eye
Step 6: Upon identification of a positive Seidel sign, the child must be immediately referred to a hospital where they can undergo further evaluation and surgical intervention. Prior to the patient leaving for the hospital, a protective eye shield should be placed over the affected eye, and securely taped in place using medical tape. This allows for protection of the injured eye in the interim. A topical antibiotic eye drop can also be instilled to begin to target potential microbes on the ocular surface

Clinical Pearl: *If the child appears to be in pain, immediate instillation of a topical anesthetic can significantly improve cooperation and participation during the examination*

CORNEAL AND CONJUNCTIVAL CULTURING

Indication

Corneal culturing, which is more casually referred to as swabbing, is indicated when a corneal ulcer is large (>3mm), within 1 mm of the visual axis, presence of multiple ulcers, or if the ulcer is resistant to previously prescribed treatment. Additionally, culturing should be considered if the patient has recently undergone surgery or is immunocompromised (Robinson et al., 2016).

Conjunctival culturing is indicated when a patient presents with ophthalmia neonatorum, or conjunctivitis within the first month of life and when childhood conjunctivitis is resistant to previously prescribed treatment (Prentiss & Dorfman, 2008).

Background

Culturing a corneal ulcer or a conjunctivitis associated with purulent discharge is the most effective way to ensure proper treatment is initiated. Several organisms exist that can penetrate an intact cornea (*Listeria* species, *Shigella, Neisseria gonorrhoea, Neisseria meningitidis, Cornyebacterium diptheriae, Hemophilus influenzae*, and *Acanthamoeba*) leading to severe vision impairment. These organisms are associated with subtle signs that can be challenging to identify in an emergency room setting. Therefore, it may be best to culture any pediatric eye with a suspected ulcer or recalcitrant conjunctivitis that presents to an emergency room setting.

The most common factors that can cause a non-viral keratitis in the pediatric population are ocular trauma (usually causes a bacterial infection but can also be fungal) followed by contact lens wear. Systemic diseases associated with pediatric keratitis include hypoxic encephalopathy, pulmonary stenosis, malnutrition, co-existing congenital abnormalities and severe prematurity. Ocular diseases such as trichiasis, blepharitis, and exposure keratopathy can increase a child's chance of developing bacterial keratitis (Al-Otaibi, 2012).

When a patient presents with ophthalmia neonatorum, or conjunctivitis within the first month of life, a conjunctival culture should be obtained. Neonatal conjunctivitis is usually chemical, bacterial, or viral. Chemical conjunctivitis may occur paradoxically secondary to prophylactic application of silver nitrate to prevent ophthalmia neonatorum; this is seen less frequently as erythromycin ophthalmic ointment has largely replaced silver nitrate. Iatrogenic induced perinatal conjunctivitis usually occurs 24 to 48 hours after birth. These patients will present with edematous eyelids and watery discharge. Gram staining will show white cells without the presence of bacteria. After discontinuation of all ophthalmic medications, symptoms should resolve in 48 hours. If improvement is not appreciated, a culture should be obtained (Prentiss & Dorfman, 2008).

Transmission of bacterial and viral infections can occur during birthing through an infected mother's birth canal. Infections include *Chlamydia trachomatis* (presents between 5 and 14 days of life), *Neisseria gonorrhoeae* (presents between 2 and 5 days of life), and herpes viruses (Prentiss & Dorfman, 2008).

Additionally, gram-negative enteric, staphylococcus and streptococcus species can be acquired in a neonate (Prentiss & Dorfman, 2008). Table 1 summarizes the nutrient agars for detection of various suspected organisms.

Table 1. Nutrient agar plate/tube

Media	Growth Supported
Blood agar (Figure 6A)	Most bacteria and fungi, excluding Neisseria, Haemophilus and Moraxella
Chocolate agar (Figure 6B)	Haemophilus Moraxella Neisseria
Sabouraud dextrose agar (Figure 7D)	Fungi
MacConkey	Gram negative bacteria (helpful in differentiating Pseudomonas)
Inhibitory mold agar (IMA) with gentamicin	Fungi
Thioglycollate broth (Figure 7B)	Wide range of bacteria including anaerobic and fungi
Löwenstein-Jensen medium	Mycobacteria Nocardia
Non-nutrient agar with Escherichiia coli	Acanthamoeba
Brain heart infusion	Streptococci Meningococci Yeast Fungi
Cooked meat broth	Anaerobic bacteria Fastidious bacteria
Viral and chlamydia **(Figure 7A)**	Virus Chlamydiae
ESwab™ (COPAN Diagnostics Inc., 2019) (Figure 7C)	Aerobic bacteria Anaerobic bacteria Fastidious bacteria

(Robinson et al., 2016)

Figure 6. A: Blood agar plate. B: Chocolate agar plate

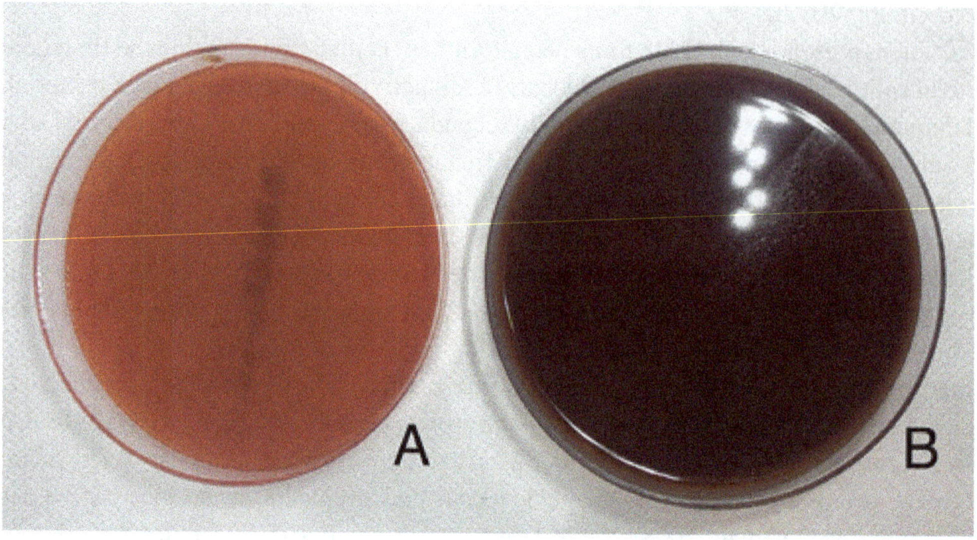

Advantages

- Allows for a pathology-driven treatment plan

Disadvantages of Procedure

- Requires access to a laboratory
- May take weeks to receive results
- Susceptible to laboratory error

Equipment

1. Synthetic (rayon on Dacron) swab (Figure 7E)
    a. Swab cannot have a wooden handle
2. Indicated nutrient agar plate/tube
3. Topical anesthetic (proparacaine 0.5% ophthalmic solution)
4. Eyelid speculum (as needed)
5. Patient identifier labels (as needed)

Clinical Pearl: *While some advocate the use of a spatula or blade to obtain a corneal culture, a swab is likely the most comfortable option for the pediatric patient.*

Figure 7. A: Viral and chlamydial tube. B: Thioglycollate broth tube. C: ESwab tube. D: Sabouraud dextrose agar tube. E: Synthetic rayon swab

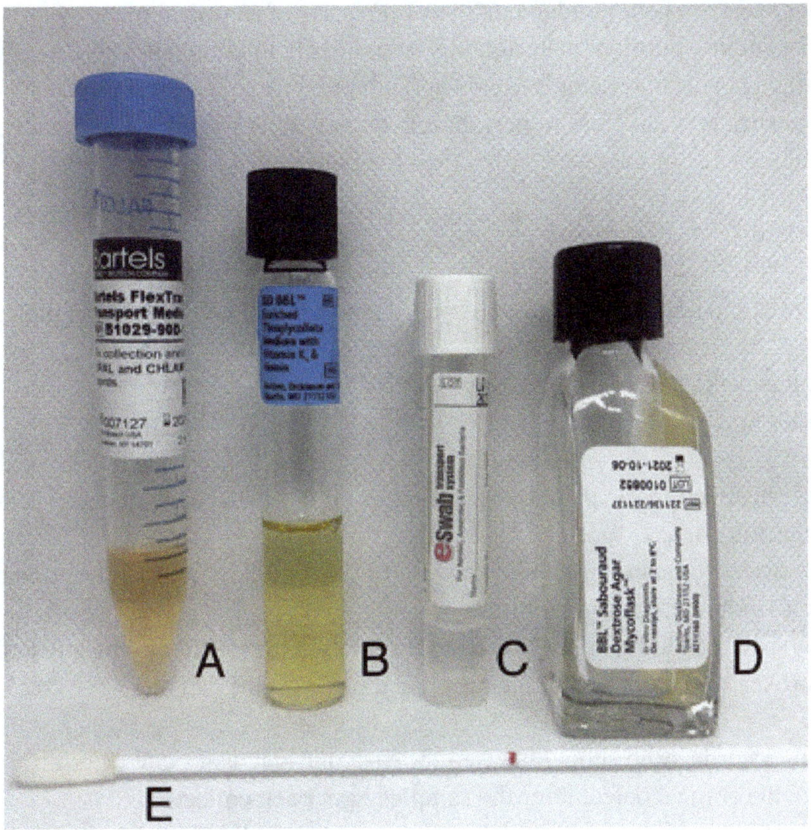

Procedure

Step 1: Educate the guardian and the child regarding the procedure and obtain consent from the guardian
Step 2: Instill the topical ophthalmic anesthetic, preferably proparacaine 0.5% ophthalmic solution as it is less bactericidal
Step 3: Consider the use of an eyelid speculum when culturing a corneal ulcer if it is suspected that the child will not be able to keep their eyelids open
Step 4: Align the child in the slit lamp if possible

Clinical Pearl: *If the patient is unable to be examined in the slit lamp, consider using a binocular indirect ophthalmoscope and 20D lens to direct adequate lighting and magnification to the cornea or conjunctiva as necessary (see chairside/bedside examination techniques).*

Step 5: Direct fixation by giving the child something to look at throughout the entire procedure
Step 6: Corneal ulcer (Robinson et al., 2016)

1. To obtain the greatest microbial yield, scrape the ulcer with the swab at the base (center floor of ulcer) and/or leading edge (peripheral ulcer between the floor and the margin) of the infiltrate. Refer to Figure 8 for a better understanding of the parts of a corneal ulcer.
    a. Avoid sampling purulent material, this is less likely to yield a positive result
    b. To obtain an adequate sample, apply enough pressure to indent the cornea
    c. If the cornea appears close to perforation, do not apply pressure and obtain the sample from the leading edge of the ulcer, rather than the base

Step 7: Conjunctivitis:

1. Swab the lower and upper conjunctiva (if possible) two to three times using the cotton swab

Step 8: Remove the eyelid speculum (if used)
Step 9: Transfer the specimen

1. Transfer the specimen to the plate by spreading it on the surface of the agar. Avoid breaking the surface of the solid agar
2. Using your swab, you can optionally draw a "C" on the plate, this conventionally represents a corneal versus conjunctival or lid culture
3. Transfer the specimen to the tube by mixing the swab in the broth. The plastic handle of the swab should be broken or cut off so that the tube can close with the cap on

Step 10: A separate sterile swab should be used for each nutrient agar plate or broth
Step 11: Measure the corneal defect after the samples have been collected
Step 12: Label each plate and tube with the necessary patient identifiers as required by the lab with which you are working. Label the structure and eye from which the sample was collected
Step 13: Initiate empirical-based treatment after culturing is performed so as not to interfere with accuracy of laboratory results. Empirical treatment should be started prior to receiving laboratory results

Figure 8. Descriptive parts of a corneal ulcer

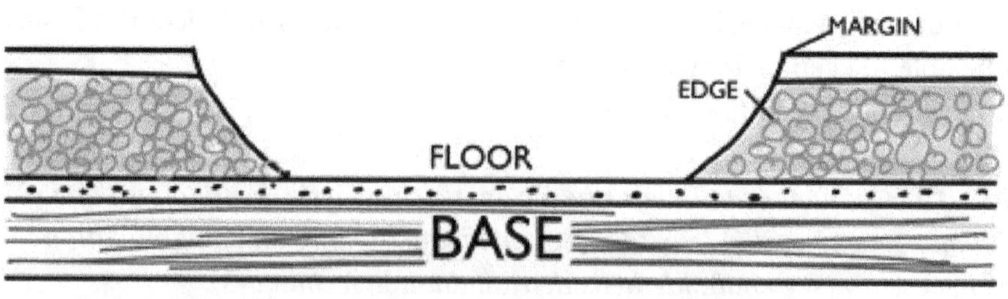

Clinical Pearl: *It is useful to have the pediatric patient look at a sticker placed on the slit lamp or have their guardian stand behind the examiner as a fixation target to maintain attention.*

Clinical Pearl: *Conjunctival culturing can be performed outside of the slit lamp, particularly if that provides better access to the patient and eyelid control.*

CHEMICAL BURNS: pH TESTING AND IRRIGATION

Indication

pH testing and irrigation of ocular structures is indicated when a patient presents with an ocular injury of known or suspected contact with a chemical agent.

Background

Ocular chemical burns result in pain and discomfort to the patient and pose the risk of causing long-term detriments to vision and quality of life. Severity of sequelae is determined by the extent of conjunctival, corneal and limbal involvement. Chemical burns can result in entropion (inward turning of the eyelids) and secondary infection (Haring et al., 2016). Children 1 to 2 years of age have the highest rate of injury per 100,000 cases (Bates & Zanaboni, 2020).

Chemical burns are caused by either acidic or alkaline agents. Alkaline agents result in cellular membrane lysis which can cause rapid penetration of the cornea, consequently having the potential to be more injurious. Acidic agents cause more limited damage to the eye as they produce proteins which act as a barrier to intraocular invasion; hydrofluoric acid is a notable exception that can cause corneal penetration (Bates & Zanaboni, 2020). Common alkaline agents include cement, lime, sodium hydroxide (found in oven and drain cleaners), chlorine bleach and ammonia. Common acidic agents are sulfuric, hydrochloric, hydrofluoric and battery acids (Haring et al., 2016). More recently, laundry detergent pods, which are highly alkaline, have been found to be a frequent cause of pediatric corneal burns. Notably, pediatric chemical injuries almost always occur in the home as a result of access to household cleaners (Breazzano et al., 2018).

When a child presents with an acute ocular chemical injury, the pH should be returned to a normal limit of 7.0 – 7.2 as quickly as possible. Prior to treatment, visual acuity should be quickly assessed and pH should be measured with pH indicator strips or litmus paper, if possible.

Litmus paper changes color with contact of substances of different pH's, allowing the identification of residual acidic or alkaline agents on the ocular surface. Irrigation with a saline solution is performed to remove the offending chemical agent from the ocular surface and return the pH of the ocular surface back to normal as quickly as possible. In an emergency setting irrigation should be performed as quickly as possible. Irrigation should be performed prior to coming into the office or emergency room. If an eye care consult is needed, irrigation should be started prior to calling the eye care provider.

Advantages

- Assessing the pH of the ocular surface assists the clinician in interpreting the effectivity of irrigation in an acute chemical burn

Disadvantages

- Litmus paper can be degraded, especially if light exposed
    - According to the manufacturer, degradation of the paper can be avoided by storing it in a closed bag or vial and in a cool (68 - 86 degrees F), dry place (Precision Laboratories, 2020)
    - Reliability of litmus paper is uncertain (Monaghan et al. (2019) found that 5% of readings are unreliable)
- The effectiveness of litmus paper following irrigation has never been studied or verified

Equipment

1. Litmus or pH paper (Figure 9)

Procedure (Bates & Zanaboni, 2020; Brady, 2020)

If possible, assess the pH of the ocular surface with pH or litmus paper prior to irrigation to elicit the severity of the offending agent.

Step 1: Place a dry strip of the litmus paper into the lower fornix of both eyes (even if history indicates only one eye is affected)

Step 2: The pH paper will change color based on the offending agent

1. Compare the color of the paper to the provided manufacturer's key (typically, red is acidic and blue is basic)
2. The goal is to achieve a pH of roughly 7 as quickly as possible

Figure 9. Unused Hydrion litmus paper (right) with provided color coded key (left)

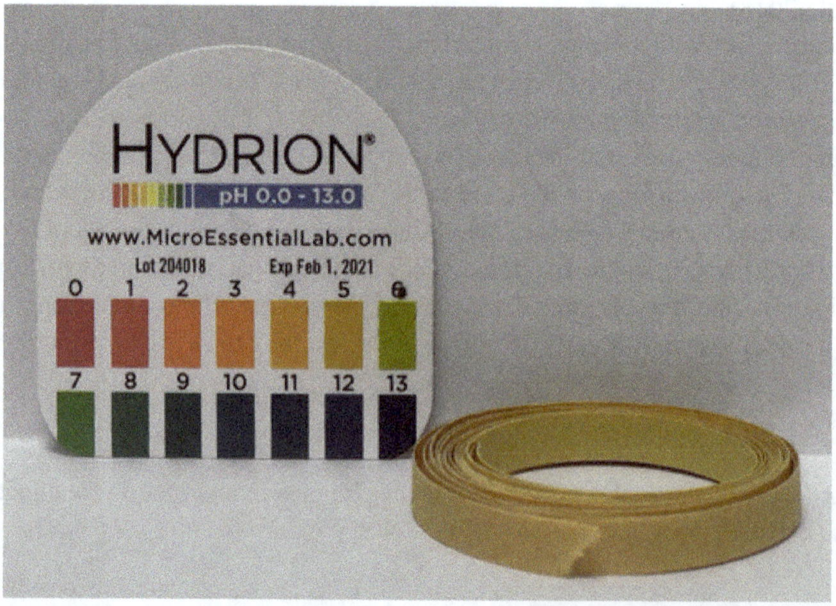

Irrigation

Equipment

1. Topical ophthalmic anesthetic
2. Normal (0.9%) saline, balanced salt solution (BSS), or Ringer's lactate
    a. Contact lens solution can be used if the above solutions are not available
    b. Tap water can be used in emergent situations in the absence of all other solutions
3. Drainage basin and/or towels
4. Eyelid speculum as needed
5. Cotton or rayon tipped swab

Procedure

Step 1: Place the child in a supine position and turn their head slightly toward the eye you are going to irrigate
Step 2: Place a drainage basin or ample towels along the inferior temporal aspect of the cheek where fluid can collect (you can ask the child to do this for you if they are capable)
Step 3: When necessary, place a drop of topical anesthetic in the lower fornix to improve comfort. Of note, topical anesthetics can affect the pH of the ocular surface. If the child shows improved toleration of the procedure with the use of a topical anesthetic, it can be reapplied every 5-10 minutes as needed; however, repeated application of topical anesthetics is controversial as they can cause corneal melts. Therefore, repeat instillation of topical anesthetics should be used only if absolutely necessary.
Step 4: Retract the eyelids using your fingers or an eyelid speculum (*see Eyelid Speculum section*).
Step 5: Begin irrigation using your chosen solution, covering the entire ocular surface, including the superior and inferior fornices. Try to direct the stream away from the punctum. Ask the child to move their eyes in all directions while applying irrigation

1. Severe acidic or alkali burns should be irrigated for **at least 20 minutes,** 30 minutes is preferable.

Step 6: Swab the upper and lower fornices with a cotton or rayon swab to remove any residual chemical agent
Step 7: Periodically pause irrigation for about one minute and then remeasure the pH of the inferior fornix using the litmus paper. Continue to irrigate if the pH is abnormal

Irrigation with a Morgan Lens

Equipment

1. Normal (0.9%) saline, balanced salt solution (BSS), or Ringer's lactate
    a. Tap water can be used if absolutely necessary in the absence of all other solutions
2. Morgan lens (Figure 10)
    a. IV tubing
    b. IV pole

Procedure

Step 1: Severe burns may require prolonged irrigation with the assistance of a scleral Morgan Lens

1. Optional: Instill one drop of a topical anesthetic
2. Hang the bag of saline several feet above the child's head
3. Attach the lens to the saline tubing
4. Open the intravenous tubing to allow fluid to flow
5. Ask the child to look down, retract the upper lid and place the lens inside the superior fornix. Ask the child to look up, retract the lower lid and place the lens inside of the inferior fornix
6. Increase the flow rate by further opening the intravenous tubing

Step 2: Continue to irrigate until the pH has returned to normal
Step 3: Post-irrigation treatment:

1. If pain, photophobia, and/or anterior chamber inflammation is present, a cycloplegic is recommended two to three times a day
2. Epithelial defects require the use of a broad spectrum topical antibiotic four times daily
3. Moderate to severe epithelial defects may benefit from the use of a bandage contact lens or amniotic membrane
4. If there is notable anterior chamber or corneal inflammation, consider a topical steroid at least four times a day (more based on severity), concurrently with a topical antibiotic
5. Patients should be seen daily for improvement, removal of bandage contact lens and tapering of steroid drops as necessary
6. The patient should use preservative free artificial tears frequently to the affected eye(s)

FORCED DUCTION TESTING

Forced duction testing is used to assess if an extraocular muscle limitation is due to paralysis of the muscle or a mechanical restriction of the muscle. If a pediatric patient presents with an eye muscle restriction, depending on cooperation it may be possible to evaluate using forced duction testing.

Equipment

1. Cotton swab applicator or forceps
2. 0.5% proparacaine ophthalmic solution

It is possible to use either a cotton swab or forceps, but a pediatric patient will likely be less resistant to the use of a cotton swab.

Figure 10. Sterile water and Morgan Lens for irrigation

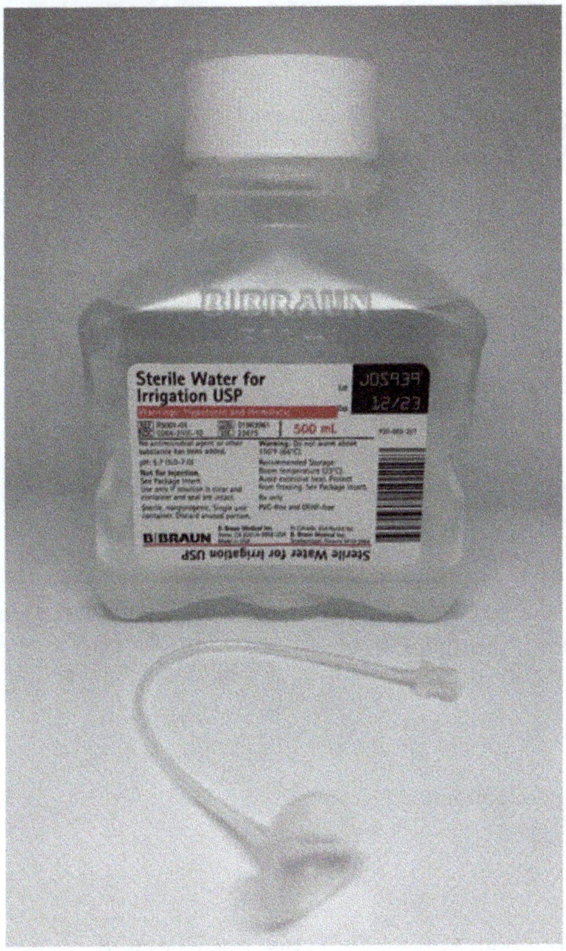

Procedure

Step 1: First place two drops of a topical anesthetic such as 0.5% proparacaine ophthalmic solution in the eye

Step 2: If using a cotton swab, push on the conjunctiva of the deviated globe to see if the eye can be moved. If using forceps, pull on the bulbar conjunctiva to evaluate if it is possible to move the eye. Avoid contact with the cornea since doing so can cause a corneal abrasion

Step 3: If the eye cannot be moved by force, this is suggestive of a restriction. If the eye can be moved by force this is indicative of paralysis of the muscle (Biousse and Newman, 2009).

Clinical Pearl: *If the patient is able to cooperate, forced duction testing can be facilitated by having the child look in the direction of the restriction. The cotton swab can then be used to attempt to further move the eye in the restricted direction.*

Clinical Pearl: *In small children, try to keep the patient from seeing the forceps prior to and during the procedure to improve patient cooperation.*

NEUROLOGICAL TESTING

Indication

Cranial nerves II, III, IV and VI are always tested as part of ocular motility testing. This section covers cranial nerve tests for other cranial nerves, most significantly with a focus on cranial nerve V and VII. Cranial nerves I, VIII, XI and XII are also discussed as part of the holistic evaluation of neurological functioning in an emergency room setting.

CN I

Cranial nerve I, the olfactory nerve, can be tested easily in an emergent setting to assess for anosmia. The olfactory nerve may be damaged with head injuries, so if a patient presents after this type of trauma it may be warranted to perform this quick test.

Equipment

1. Standard 70% isopropyl alcohol pad

Procedure

Step 1: Have the patient close both eyes and hold one nostril closed
Step 2: Hold the 70% isopropyl alcohol pad 30cm from the child's nose
Step 3: Gradually bring the alcohol pad towards the nose until child can identify the odor (Kurtz & Carlson, 2003). Record the distance
Step 4: Repeat again with the other nostril
Step 5: If the patient is unable to detect the odor of the alcohol pad until it is very close to their nose they are anosmic (Davidson & Murphy, 1997)

CN V

CN V, the trigeminal nerve can be assessed in children easily and quickly during examination. CN V has both sensory and motor functions. The three branches of the trigeminal nerve are the ophthalmic (V1), maxillary (V2) and mandibular (V3) branches. Damage to the trigeminal nerve in children can occur secondary to trauma (Rogan & Fang, 2020)

Equipment

1. Tissue

Procedure

Step 1: Have the child sitting comfortably and looking straight ahead
Step 2: Using a tissue, show the child what will be used to touch different parts of their face, then have child close their eyes
Step 3: To assess the sensory function of CN V, with the tissue touch the child's face on either side of the midline of the forehead, cheek, and on the chin. The points of touch should be symmetric to the midline on each side of the face

1. Alternatively, the examiner can touch both sides of the forehead or cheek or chin at the same time and ask the child if the touch feels equal between the two sides
2. For a gross assessment in an emergency room setting this can be performed by lightly tapping the six locations with your fingers instead of using a tissue

Step 4: Ask the child to state where they feel the tissue touch their face, and if there is a difference when comparing one side to the other
Step 5: To assess motor function of CN V, have the child clench their teeth to evaluate for a flexing of the masseter muscle on either side of their face. If there is poor flexure, this may indicate a deficiency along the mandibular branch of the nerve

CN VII

CN VII, the facial nerve, has both sensory and motor divisions. The evaluation of the somatic motor and parasympathetic divisions will be discussed here. There are many potential etiologies for a facial nerve palsy, aka a Bell's palsy. An idiopathic Bell's palsy is a diagnosis of exclusion; therefore, if a patient presents with a facial nerve palsy a work up must be performed to rule out all other etiologies. Potential etiologies of a CN VII palsy in pediatric patients are hemorrhaging, infection, oncological disorders and trauma (Lorch & Teach, 2010). Neuroimaging such as CT/MRI can help evaluate certain etiologies and blood work can rule out infectious causes.

Equipment

None

Procedure

Examine the patient's face, evaluating the left and right sides for any asymmetry, being sure to look separately for any asymmetries in the upper and lower face

Step 1: Evaluate if there is a loss of the nasolabial fold or facial wrinkles on one side
Step 2: Ask the child to blow out both of their cheeks at the same time
Step 3: Ask the child to smile and frown and purse their lips or try to whistle
Step 4: Next, place all four fingers of both of your hands on the child's eyelids and gently pull down. Ask child to try to raise both eyebrows and note if there is a difference between them.

Clinical Pearl: *It may be helpful to show the pediatric patient what you would like them to do by performing the task first.*

Step 5: Additional testing of the eye muscles involves instructing child to close their eyes tightly. The provider attempts to pull the eyes open while the patient tries to keep them shut. This is testing the orbicularis oculi muscles and compares the ability of each side to resist being pulled open (Kurtz & Carlson, 2003) A patient with a facial nerve palsy may be unable to close their eye.

Clinical Pearl: *It may be helpful to show the pediatric patient what you would like them to do by performing the task first.*

Step 6: It is important to document the palpebral fissure size of both eyes, as well as to evaluate the pattern of upper lid creases

CN VIII

CN VIII, the vestibulocochlear nerve is responsible for hearing as well as maintaining balance and equilibrium. Direct trauma, tumors, meningitis, congenital malformations, infections and vascular injury can all cause damage to CN VIII (Hwang et al., 2016; Bordoni et al., 2021). Patients may present with symptoms such as nystagmus, tinnitus and vertigo in addition to sensorineural hearing loss (Bordoni et al., 2021).

Equipment

None

Procedure

Step 1: Have child close their eyes
Step 2: Starting about 50cm away rub your index and thumb together, slowly moving closer to the patient's ear (Kurtz & Carlson, 2003)
Step 3: Have the child close their eyes, and repeat for the other side, and compare the distance at which the child was able to identify the sound

Clinical Pearl: *Alternatively, the child can also be asked to hum, and relay if they hear the humming sound louder in one ear versus the other (Kurtz & Carlson, 2003)*

CN XI

CN XI, the accessory nerve, innervates the sternocleidomastoid and trapezius muscles. It is rare for a lower cranial nerve to have an isolated dysfunction in children; if there is damage to a lower cranial nerve it usually presents as a combined dysfunction with other cranial nerves (Hwang et al., 2016). Posterior fossa tumors can cause lower cranial nerve dysfunction (Hwang et al., 2016).

Equipment

None

Procedure to evaluate trapezius muscle innervation (Kurtz & Carlson, 2003)

Step 1: First observe the child's shoulder heights relative to each other

Step 2: Next, ask the child to shrug both shoulders simultaneously, comparing the height of each shoulder during the shrug

Step 3: An additional test is to place both hands on the child's shoulder and push down gently. Ask the child to shrug both shoulders and compare the force of each shoulder pushing against the resistance of your hands

Procedure to evaluate sternocleidomastoid muscle innervation (Walker et al., 1990)

Step 1: While facing that child, place your right palm on the child's left cheek

Step 2: Ask the child to turn head to the left while the examiner is simultaneously applying resisting force in the opposite direction evaluating the right sternocleidomastoid as this is performed

Step 3: Reverse the procedure to evaluate the left sternocleidomastoid muscle

CN XII

CN XII, the hypoglossal nerve is a motor nerve that innervates most of the muscles of the tongue. Trauma, inflammation of the skull base and brainstem tumors can all cause CN XII dysfunction (Hwang et al., 2016).

Equipment

None

Procedure (Kurtz & Carlson, 2003)

Step 1: Have the child stick out their tongue

Step 2: If the tongue sticks out straight along the midline this cranial nerve is not damaged. If the tongue deviates to one side or the other this is an abnormal response

DOLL'S HEAD MANEUVER

The doll's head maneuver is a technique that can be used in pediatric patients as young as neonates or comatose patients to evaluate the oculocephalic reflex. This technique is used for neurologic examination of CN III, VI and VIII and evaluates the integrity of the brainstem. This maneuver should not be performed in patients with a cervical injury (Biousse & Newman, 2009).

Equipment

None

Procedure (Pullen, 2005)

Step 1: If the child is not comatose, prior to beginning the maneuver, ensure that the pediatric patient is looking at the examiner

Step 2: Turn the child's head briskly but gently from side to side horizontally. If the child is unable to hold their eyes open, hold their upper eyelids open while turning their head

Step 3: The eyes should conjugately deviate in the direction opposite of the head turn, such as the eyes moving to the right as the head is turned to the left. This is a positive result. If the horizontal eye movements are dysconjugate this suggests a potential third or sixth nerve palsy, or internuclear ophthalmoplegia

Step 4: If the patient's eyes stay fixed at midline or move in the same direction as the head turn the oculocephalic reflex is absent indicating a negative result; do not move when their head is rotated this is a negative result

Step 5: A similar test can be performed moving the head vertically, with the eyes again moving in the opposite direction of the head indicating a positive result

Clinical Pearl: *A fixation target such as a video can also be used if the child will not focus on the examiner.*

ADDITIONAL LABORATORY TESTS

Indication

Additional laboratory tests are indicated when a pediatric patient presents with a hyphema or a uveitis that is either one or a combination of the following features: bilateral, chronic, recurrent, and granulomatous.

Background

Pediatric patients can present with urgent and emergent ophthalmologic findings that suggest the presence of an underlying systemic condition. These findings may warrant laboratory testing to identify an underlying cause.

Laboratory testing should be considered in a patient who presents with a hyphema. Testing would include screening for a blood dyscrasia such as sickle cell trait or sickle cell disease. Sickled red blood cells can block the trabecular meshwork of the iridocorneal angle and increase intraocular pressure. Additionally, patients with sickle cell disease are more likely to have spontaneous hyphemas. A hyphema can also indicate the presence of other diseases of the blood such as leukemia, hemophilia, or von Willebrand disease (Syed, 2021; Bagheri, 2017a).

A pediatric patient that presents with bilateral, chronic, recurrent, or granulomatous anterior uveitis requires a panel of lab work to determine the causative agent. Juvenile idiopathic arthritis (JIA) is the most common disease associated with pediatric uveitis. JIA-related uveitis is typically bilateral and seen in females. Additional causes of childhood uveitis include toxocariasis and toxoplasmosis (Bagheri, 2017b). It can be either granulomatous or non-granulomatous. Other causes of uveitis in infants include TORCH infections (**T**oxoplasmosis, **R**ubella, **C**ytomegalovirus, **H**erpes simplex virus) and retinoblastoma; however, the cells seen in cases of retinoblastoma are likely representative of tumor seeding rather than a systemic inflammatory process.

Suggested Systemic Work-Up

1. Hyphema (Syed, 2021; Bagheri, 2017a).
    a. Laboratory studies
        i. Hemoglobin electrophoresis
        ii. High performance liquid chromatography (HPLC) of blood
        iii. Deoxyribonucleic acid (DNA) testing
        iv. Prothrombin time/INR
        v. Partial thromboplastin time
        vi. Complete blood count (CBC) with platelet count
        vii. Protein C
        viii. Protein S
2. Uveitis (Bagheri, 2017b)
    a. Laboratory studies
        i. Rheumatoid factor
        ii. Antinuclear antibodies
        iii. HLA-B27
        iv. Complete blood count (CBC) with differential
        v. Erythrocyte sedimentation rate (ESR)
        vi. C-reactive protein (CRP)
        vii. Anti-neutrophil cytoplasmic antibodies (ANCA)
        viii. Angiotensin-converting enzyme (ACE)
        ix. Urinalysis/renal function tests
    b. Rheumatology consult
    c. Radiographs of affected joints

OCULAR IMAGING

B-Scan Ultrasound

Indications

Indications for B-scan ultrasonography include cases of ocular trauma to rule out globe rupture, lens dislocation, to further investigate posterior vitreous detachments, retinal tears and retinal detachment and finally to rule out a retrobulbar hematomas and intraocular foreign bodies. B-scan can also be useful to view the intermediate and posterior segment when there is a poor view such as in cases of small pupils, dense cataracts, corneal opacification, vitreous inflammation, and vitreous hemorrhage.

B-scan technology is also useful to characterize tumors, eyelid inflammation and extraocular inflammation. Finally, it can also be used to further investigate optic nerve disease such as optic nerve edema and other optic nerve head anomalies.

Background

B-scan, or brightness scan, ultrasonography utilizes measurement of sound wave reflection and attenuation to examine the internal structures of the eye. If there is more attenuation of the signal, the anatomy will appear hyperechoic (white), while less attenuation will appear anechoic (black). Denser tissue will be hyperechoic, while less dense tissue will be anechoic. It is important to approach ocular ultrasonography in a stepwise and organized manner to get the best possible information. This technique has been shown to be highly effective in the determination of ocular integrity in emergency settings (Yoonessi et al., 2010, p. 914).

Advantages

- Quick
- Cost effective
- The unit is small and can serve multiple purposes other than ocular examination
- Ionizing radiation is not required
- Can identify intraocular foreign bodies that are radiopaque
- Can be performed on patients with implanted metallic devices

Disadvantages

- Low resolution image
- Poor penetration of sound waves past the globe and orbit
- The quality of the image is dependent on the ability of the clinician to use the instrument, thus there can be inter-observer variability (Oberfoell et al., 2017, p. 1582)

Equipment

1. B-scan ultrasound unit and probe (Figure 11)
2. Ultrasound coupling gel (Figure 11)

Figure 11. A: Ultrasound unit. B: Ultrasound coupling gel. C: Ultrasound probe (Clockwise)

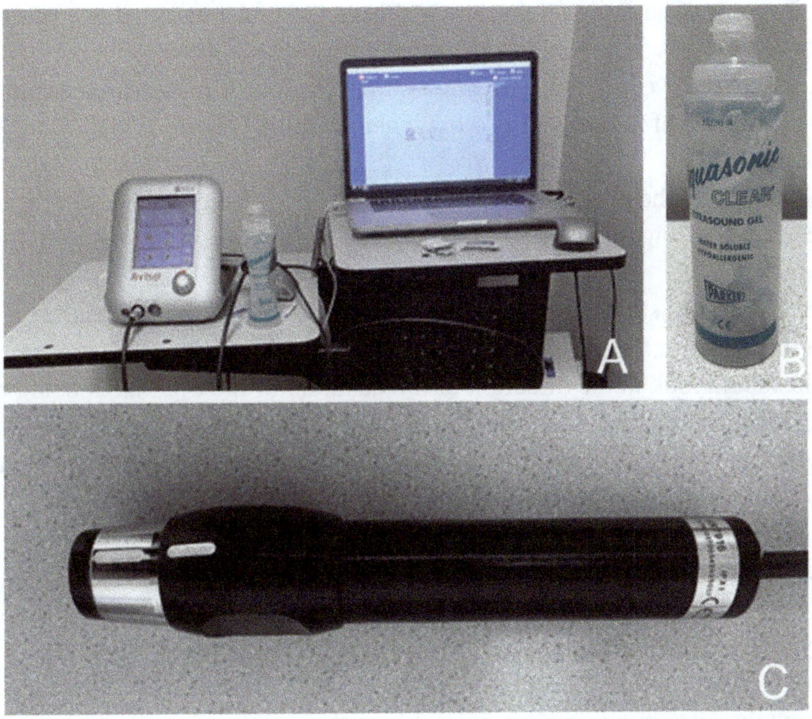

Procedure

Step 1: The child should be seated comfortably with their eyes closed. This technique can be performed supine or with the child slightly reclined for better access to the eye. This scan can also be performed directly on an anesthetized eye (consider using proparacaine hydrochloride ophthalmic solution). However direct application to the eye is not as well tolerated in a child so is less recommended
Step 2: Turn the gain on the machine on high
Step 3: Apply ultrasound gel to the ultrasound probe

Clinical Pearl: *If ultrasound coupling gel is not available, a thick artificial tear ophthalmic ointment or gonioscopy coupling solution like Goniosol can be used.*

Step 4: The ultrasound probe will have a marker, generally a dot or a line. This indicates where the superior part of the scan will be represented on the image (e.g., if the line is oriented directly superiorly, the superior part of the eye will be at the top of the scan)

Step 5: There are three types of scans used to view the eye:

1. Longitudinal scan – Orient the probe with the marker perpendicular to the limbus. This allows you to examine a particular clock hour of the eye. The area scanned will be opposite to where the probe is placed (e.g., if the probe is at 6'o'clock, the area represented will be the 12'o'clock meridian) (Figure 12A)
2. Transverse scan – The probe is placed parallel to the limbus. This will scan the lateral aspect of the globe. By convention horizontal scans will have the probe oriented towards the nose (Figure 12B)
3. Axial scan – With the eye looking straight forward, the probe is placed on the center of the cornea. This allows for a scan of the macula and optic nerve region (Figure 12C)

Step 6: Apply the probe to the eye gently, resting your hand on the child's nose area or on the cheek. Aim to get a clear image using the least amount of pressure possible, so as not to deform the integrity of the eye
Step 7: It is often easiest to start by locating the optic nerve, which will appear as a triangle shaped anechoic area in the posterior aspect of the eye
Step 8: The child should look in the direction of the quadrant of the eye that is being evaluated. Place the probe directly opposite to where the patient is looking (e.g., to view the superior aspect of the eye, have the patient look up and place the probe inferiorly). Scan the area of interest using the probe orientations listed above
Step 9: Examine inferior, superior, nasal and temporal by using the same technique
Step 10: The examination can be repeated at a lower gain to improve resolution of the retina and finer structures. This can also help to identify hyperechoic structures such as optic nerve head drusen, which will be highly hyperechoic at high and low gain
Step 11: Pathology of interest can be captured in a still image and/or saved as a video. The method of capture depends on the ultrasound unit, but it is often either by stepping on a foot pedal or pressing a button on the B-scan unit

COMMUTED TOMOGRAPHY (CT) SCAN

Indications

Commuted tomography (CT) scans can be used when a more detailed image of ocular structures is desired and for views of the internal structures of the eye and the brain. It can be used in cases of ocular trauma to rule out orbital fractures and globe rupture. It can also be used to further investigate proptosis, ptosis and peri-ocular inflammation such as preseptal cellulitis and orbital cellulitis. Other uses include further investigation of extraocular muscles palsies, headaches, periorbital pain, double vision and to further characterize ocular masses.

Figure 12. A: Longitudinal B-scan. B: Transverse B-scan Figure. C: Axial B-scan
Source: Tak-Man Kimberly Fung OD, 2021

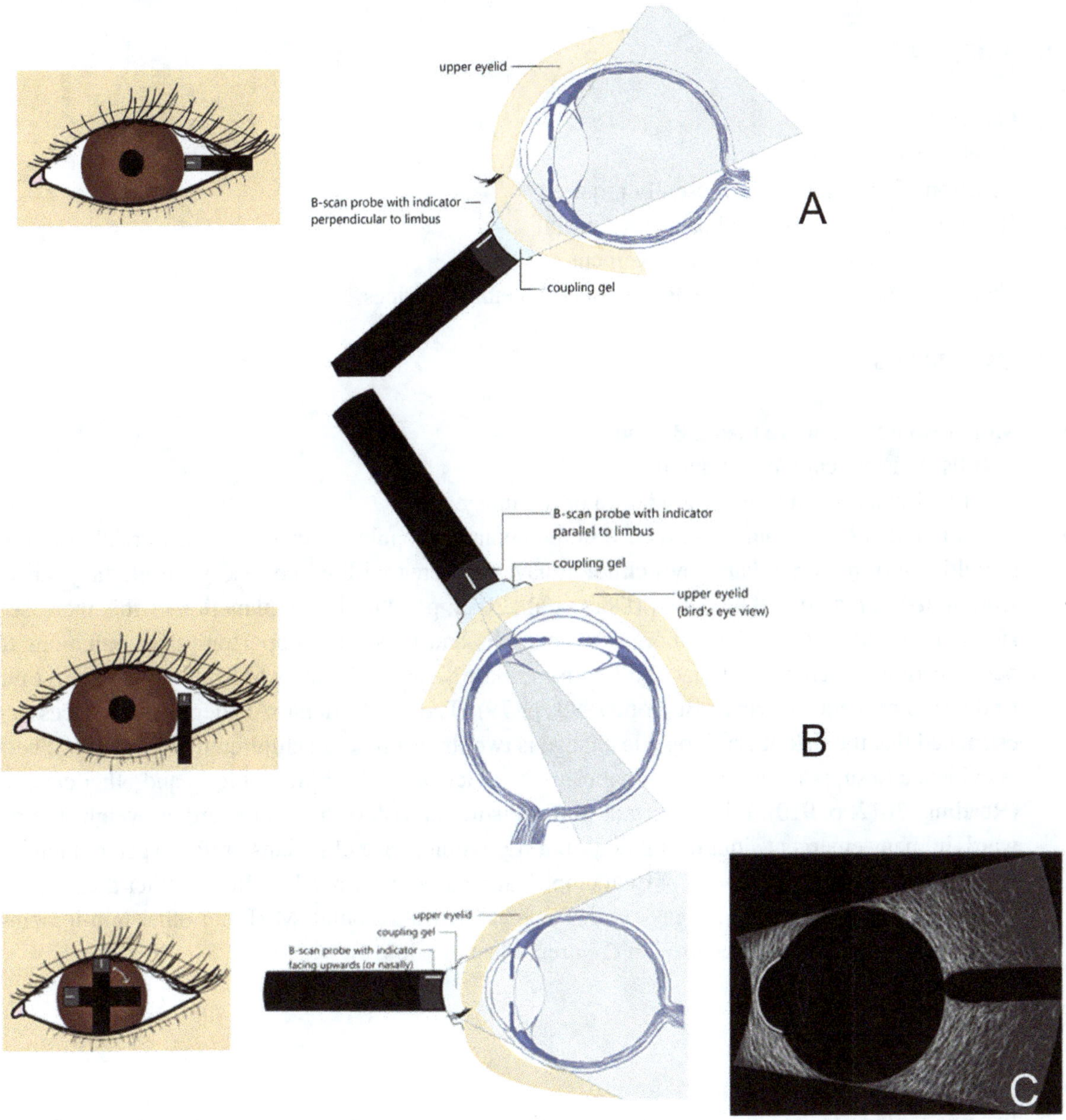

Background

A Commuted Tomography (CT) image is formed from measuring the attenuation of a rotating x-ray beam as it moves around the body. A two-dimensional image is formed by getting multiple x-ray scans from a revolving unit. Bones will appear as white, while soft tissue and fluid-filled spaces will be shades of gray. The scanning technology generally works best for viewing bony structures, although settings can be adjusted to see soft tissue adequately. These scans can be ordered with contrast or without contrast depending on the pathology suspected.

Advantages

- Quick
- Relatively cost effective
- Sedation of the patient is not usually required
- Bony structures are captured particularly well
- Relatively insensitive to patient movement
- Can be performed on patients with implanted metallic devices

Disadvantages

- More resource intensive than a B-scan
- Soft tissue is not captured in detail
- Metallic implants can cause degradation of the image
- Ionizing radiation is required so its use in the pediatric population can be controversial. There is a multitude of research that shows children have an increased lifetime risk of developing cancer from ionizing radiation than adults (Doss et al., 2012, p. 244). The explanation of this increased risk is two-fold: children have more dividing cells and thus more opportunity for mutations to occur leading to cancer, and that children have more years of life ahead of them, thus more time to develop cancers (Slovis & Berdon, 1999, p. 79). The US National Academy of Sciences has estimated that the risk of carcinogenic change is two times higher in children than in adults. There is evidence to support that radiation exposure can increase risk of brain, blood and other cancers (Reading, 2012, p. 910). It is important to make sure the risk of the procedure outweighs the reward. In many emergent situations it does, but if possible, most clinicians prefer to get a Magnetic Resonance Imaging (MRI) scan or treat empirically based on clinical findings, rather than expose a child to ionizing radiation. Many studies suggest that ultrasound, MRI and other non-ionizing imaging modalities should be used in children when possible.

Contrast

- Iodinated contrast dye is standard for use
- In some settings, testing kidney function (see the laboratory studies section) is recommended prior to using contrast in the pediatric and adult population
- The use of contrast is recommended detect areas of inflammation, infection or early ischemia
- Contrast is not generally needed to image bone (e.g., ruling out an orbital fracture)

CT Scans Commonly Ordered for Ocular Examination

- Orbit (Figure 13A)
- Maxillofacial and sinus (Figure 13B)
- Head (Figure 13C)

Scan Orientation Review

- *Sagittal or mid-sagittal plane:* separates the right half of the body from the left half of the body (Nikita, 2017)
- *Coronal plane:* separates the anterior half and the posterior half of the body (i.e. the front of the body from the back of the body) (Nikita, 2017)
- Transverse or axial plane: separates the top of the body from the bottom of the body; this can be measured at different heights. (Nikita, 2017)

Figure 13. A: CT orbits, axial scan without contrast. B: CT maxillofacial sinus, coronal scan, 14-year-old patient. C: CT brain, axial scan, 19-year-old patient

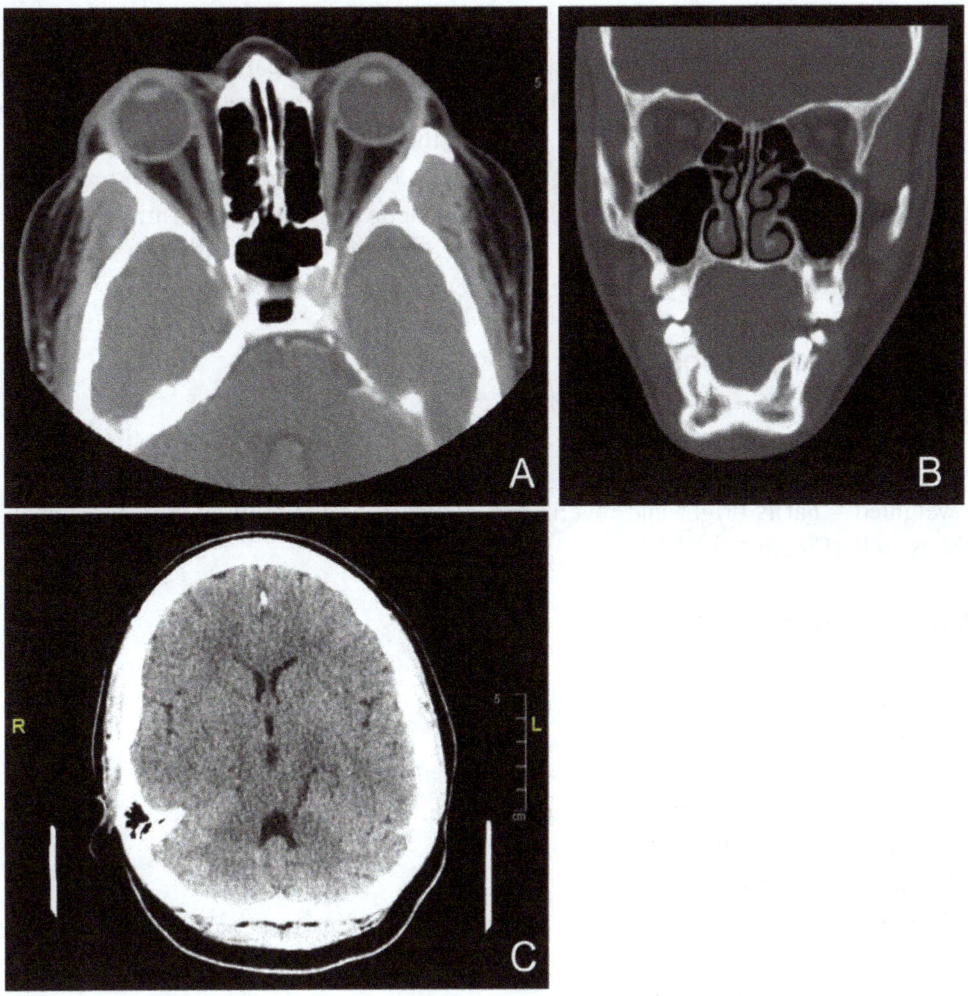

MAGNETIC RESONANCE IMAGING (MRI)

Indications

Magnetic resonance imaging (MRI) is employed when more detailed images of ocular and cranial structures are desired. It can be used to further investigate ocular trauma and rule out orbital fracture and globe rupture. It can be used to characterize proptosis, ptosis and peri-ocular inflammation such as preseptal cellulitis and orbital cellulitis. It can be used to provide more information about extraocular muscle palsies, nystagmus, periorbital pain, double vision, and numbness or weakness. Finally, it can be used to characterize ocular masses, orbital vascular disease, to further investigate unqualified vision loss and optic nerve edema.

Background

Magnetic resonance imaging (MRI), known in some circles as nuclear magnetic resonance imaging (NMR) is a sensitive imaging modality that uses a magnetic field and radiofrequency pulses to view internal structures of the body. The patient is placed in the strong magnetic field and a radiofrequency pulses are applied, which in turn cause protons in tissues to align patterns, which produce an image. The characteristics of the image (light vs dark) is dependent on the type of acquisition sequence applied. This means that different algorithms are used to produce an image. The acquisition sequence is chosen based on where and what pathology the clinician expects to see.

MRI Acquisition Sequences

- T1-weighted – Fat is bright while myelin, glandular tissue and other body tissue is grey, water/liquid is black (Figure 14A)
- T2- weighted – Fat is bright and myelin and glandular is grey although water/aqueous will be bright as well. (Figure 14B)

Other Acquisition Sequences

- T1-weighted with fat suppression
- T2-weighted with fat suppression
    - Fat suppression is used to suppress the signal from adipose tissue for better visualization of pathology, particularly when contrast is being used. It is also used to better characterize tumors (Delfaut et al., 1999)
- Fluid attenuation inversion recovery (FLAIR)
    - This is generally ordered when you suspect demyelinating disease like multiple sclerosis (MS)
- Diffusion weighted imaging (DWI)
    - Ordered to find an acute infarct

Figure 14. A. MRI Brain, T1-weighted image, sagittal scan, 5-year-old patient. B. MRI orbits, T2 weighted, axial scan, 14-year-old patient

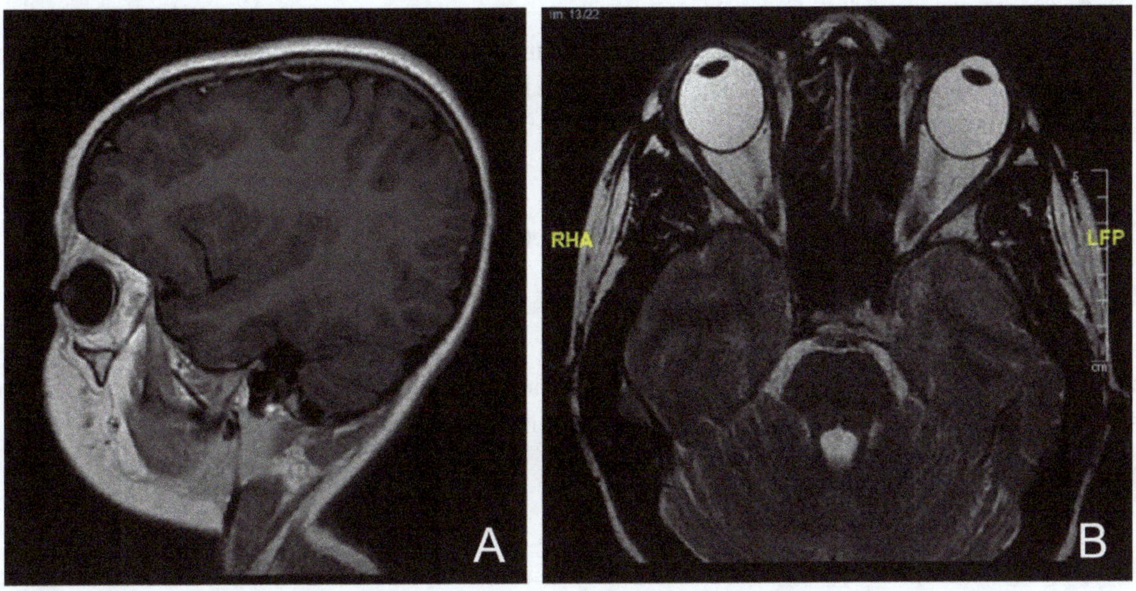

Contrast

- Gadolinium is the contrast dye generally used in MRI imaging
- Rare side effects include renal failure and allergy
- Recommended use when there is a suspicion of inflammation, infection, early ischemia and/or to determine specific characteristics of masses

MRI Scans Commonly Ordered for Ocular Examination

- Orbit
- Maxillofacial and sinus
- Brain

Advantages

- Provides detailed view of soft tissue
- Allows for examination of a greater depth of tissue
- Ionizing radiation is not required, mitigating the risk of carcinogenic exposure. MRIs are generally preferred over CT scans for the pediatric population.

Disadvantages

- Long process
- Sensitive to movement

- The instrument requires a patient to be in a small space, thus people who are claustrophobic may not tolerate it. An open MRI machine is an alternative for patients with claustrophobia.
- Sedation can be required for pediatric patients
- Contraindicated in patients with non-removable metallic implants/prosthesis. There are some implanted devices that are conditionally safe for use in MRI scans. When in doubt contact the device manufacturer

MAGNETIC RESONANCE ANGIOGRAPHY (MRA)

Indications

Indications for this procedure include cases of transient vision loss and amaurosis fugax. It can also be used to characterize arteriovenous malformations, cranial vascular disease and carotid artery fistulas.

Background

This imaging technique employs the same radio waves as with an MRI but is used to look at the arterial blood flow. A low dose of contrast dye gadolinium can be injected and the first pass through the circulatory system is examined. This allows for the evaluation of blood circulation.

Advantages

- Provides detailed view of the circulatory system of the brain
- Can be performed at the same time as an MRI
- Allows for examination of a greater depth of tissue
- Ionizing radiation is not required

Disadvantages

- Long process
- Sensitive to movement
- The instrument requires a patient to be in a small space, thus people who are claustrophobic may not tolerate it. An open MRI machine is an alternative for these patients with claustrophobia
- Sedation can be required for pediatric patients
- Contraindicated in patients with non-removable metallic implants/prosthesis. There are some implanted devices that are conditionally safe for use in MRI scans. When in doubt contact the device manufacturer

MAGNETIC RESONANCE VENOGRAPHY (MRV)

Indications

This technique is generally used to characterize optic nerve edema, cavernous sinus disease and investigate the etiology of headaches.

Background

This imaging technique uses a magnetic field and radio pulses to examine venous blood flow. A low dose of gadolinium can be injected into a vein and the first pass through the venous system is examined. This allows for evaluation of the drainage system of the brain (Figure 15).

Figure 15. MRV brain, 9-year-old patient, sagittal scan

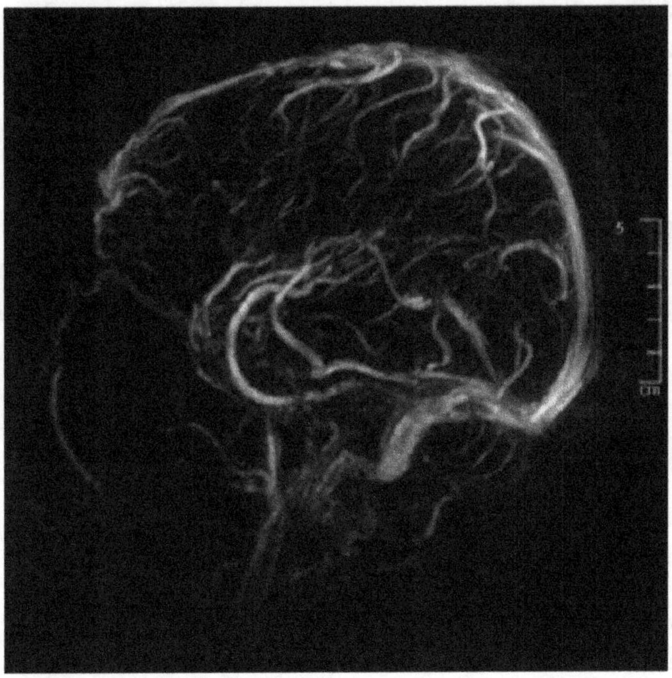

Advantages

- Provides detailed view of the circulatory system of the brain
- Can be performed at the same time as an MRI
- Allows for examination of a greater depth of tissue
- Ionizing radiation is not required

Disadvantages

- Long process
- Sensitive to movement
- The instrument requires a patient to be in a small space, thus people who are claustrophobic may not tolerate it. An open MRI machine is an alternative for these patients with claustrophobia
- Sedation can be required for pediatric patients
- Contraindicated in patients with non-removable metallic implants/prosthesis. There are some implanted devices that are conditionally safe for use in MRI scans, when in doubt, contact the device manufacturer

CONCLUSION

This chapter is intended to aid the clinician examining pediatric patients in an emergency scenario. The different techniques, skills and procedures reviewed are commonly seen in the pediatric population in acute-care bedside and exam lane settings. The authors provide detailed procedures aimed to equip the clinician with the ability to adapt an examination for efficiency and maximal patient comfort, allowing for improved diagnostic and procedural proficiency.

ACKNOWLEDGMENT

The authors would like to thank Tak-Man Kimberly Fung, OD, for her illustration contributions to this chapter.

REFERENCES

Al-Otaibi, A. G. (2012). Non-viral microbial keratitis in children. *Saudi Journal of Ophthalmology, 26*(2), 191–197. doi:10.1016/j.sjopt.2011.10.002 PMID:23960991

Allen, R. C. (2016, December 19). *Placement of a pressure patch*. EyeRounds.Org. https://webeye.ophth.uiowa.edu/eyeforum/atlas-video/placement-of-pressure-patch.htm

American Academy of Ophthalmology. (2020, December 28). Pressure patch. https://www.aao.org/image/pressure-patch

Augeri P. A. (1991). Corneal foreign body removal and treatment. *Optometry Clinics: The Official Publication of the Prentice Society, 1*(4), 59–70.

Bagheri, N. (2017a). *Trauma. In The Wills eye manual: Office and emergency room diagnosis and treatment of eye disease*. Wolters Kluwer.

Bagheri, N. (2017b). *Uveitis. In The Wills eye manual: Office and emergency room diagnosis and treatment of eye disease*. Wolters Kluwer.

Bates, A., & Zanaboni, A. (2020). Ocular burns. *StatPearls.* https://www.ncbi.nlm.nih.gov/books/NBK459221/

Binenbaum, G. (2020, October 8). *Child abuse: Eye findings in children with abusive head trauma (AHT).* UpToDate. https://www.uptodate.com/contents/child-abuse-eye-findings-in-children-with-abusive-head-trauma-aht?search=ocular%20signs%20of%20child%20abuse&source=search_result&selectedTitle=7~150&usage_type=default&display_rank=7

Biousse, V., & Newman, N. J. (2009). *Neuro-Ophthalmology Illustrated* (1st ed.). Thieme.

Bordoni, B., Mankowski, N. L., & Daly, D. T. (2021, February 7). *Neuroanatomy, Cranial Nerve 8 (Vestibulocochlear).* https://www.ncbi.nlm.nih.gov/books/NBK537359/

Brady, C. (2020). How to irrigate the eye and do eyelid eversion - Eye Disorders. In *Merck Manuals Professional Edition.* Merck Manuals. www.merckmanuals.com/professional/eye-disorders/how-to-do-eye-procedures/how-to-irrigate-the-eye-and-do-eyelid-eversion

Breazzano, M. P., Day, H. R. Jr, Tanaka, S., & Tran, U. (2018). Prospective analysis of pediatric ocular chemical burns: Laundry detergent pods. *Journal of American Association for Pediatric Ophthalmology and Strabismus, 22*(6), 426–428. doi:10.1016/j.jaapos.2018.07.349 PMID:30342182

Brown, D. J., Jaffe, J. E., & Henson, J. K. (2007). Advanced Laceration Management. *Emergency Medicine Clinics of North America, 25*(1), 83–99. doi:10.1016/j.emc.2006.11.001 PMID:17400074

Cain, W., & Sinskey, R. M. (1981). Detection of Anterior Chamber Leakage With Seidel's Test. *Archives of Ophthalmology, 99*(11), 2013. doi:10.1001/archopht.1981.03930020889015 PMID:7295152

Child Welfare Information Gateway. (2019). *What Is Child Abuse and Neglect? Recognizing the Signs and Symptoms.* https://www.childwelfare.gov/pubPDFs/whatiscan.pdf

Christian, C. W., & Levin, A. V. (2018). The Eye Examination in the Evaluation of Child Abuse. *Pediatrics, 142*(2), e20181411. Advance online publication. doi:10.1542/peds.2018-1411 PMID:30037976

Chung, I., & Buhr, V. (2000). Topical ophthalmic drugs and the pediatric patient. *Optometry (St. Louis, Mo.), 71*(8), 511–518. PMID:15326908

Cochran, M. L., & Czyz, C. N. (2020, March 31). *Eyelid Laceration.* https://www.ncbi.nlm.nih.gov/books/NBK470367/

COPAN Diagnostics Inc. (2019). *ESwab and Bacterial Keratitis.* www.copanusa.com/eswab-ophthalmology-diagnosing-bacterial-keratitis/

Coulter, R. A. (2004). Pediatric use of topical ophthalmic drugs. *Optometry (St. Louis, Mo.), 75*(7), 419–429. doi:10.1016/S1529-1839(04)70157-8 PMID:15296375

Crosby, N. J., Shepherd, D., & Murray, A. (2013). Mechanical testing of lid speculae and relationship to postoperative ptosis. *Eye (London, England), 27*(9), 1098–1101. doi:10.1038/eye.2013.133 PMID:23788211

Davidson, T. M., & Murphy, C. (1997). Rapid Clinical Evaluation of Anosmia: The Alcohol Sniff Test. *Archives of Otolaryngology—Head & Neck Surgery*, *123*(6), 591–594. doi:10.1001/archotol.1997.01900060033005 PMID:9193218

Delfaut, E. M., Beltran, J., Johnson, G., Rousseau, J., Marchandise, X., & Cotten, A. (1999). Fat Suppression in MR Imaging: Techniques and Pitfalls. *Radiographics*, *19*(2), 373–382. doi:10.1148/radiographics.19.2.g99mr03373 PMID:10194785

Devices@FDA PMA Supplement Bausch & Lomb Purevision (Balafilcon A) Visibility Tinted Contact Lenses-Therapeutic Use. (n.d.). *U.S. Food & Drug Administration*. https://www.accessdata.fda.gov/scripts/cdrh/devicesatfda/index.cfm?db=pma&id=333808

Devices@FDA PMA Supplement Night & Day 30 Night Extended Wear Soft Contact Lens. (n.d.). *U.S. Food & Drug Administration*. https://www.accessdata.fda.gov/scripts/cdrh/devicesatfda/index.cfm?db=pma&id=332525

Devices@FDA PMA Supplement Vistakon (Senofilcon A) Contact Lens Material. (n.d.). *U.S. Food & Drug Administration*. https://www.accessdata.fda.gov/scripts/cdrh/devicesatfda/index.cfm?db=pma&id=336147

Doss, M., Egleston, B. L., & Litwin, S. (2012). Comments on "Studies of the Mortality of Atomic Bomb Survivors, Report 14, 1950–2003: An Overview of Cancer and Noncancer Diseases" (Radiat Res 2012; 177:229–43). *Radiation Research*, *178*(3), 244–245. https://doi.org/10.1667/rr3039.1

Elner, S. G., Elner, V. M., & Arnall, M. (1990). Ocular and Associated Systemic Findings in Suspected Child Abuse. *Archives of Ophthalmology*, *108*(8), 1094. https://doi.org/10.1001/archopht.1990.01070100050033

Epley, K., Tychsen, L., & Lueder, G. T. (2002). The effect of an eyelid speculum on intraocular pressure measurement in children. *American Journal of Ophthalmology*, *134*(6), 926–927. doi:10.10160002-9394(02)01793-2

Gardiner, M. F. (2019). Eyelid lacerations. In T.W. Post, P. Rutgeerts, & S. Grover (Eds.), *UpToDate*. Available from https://www.uptodate.com/contents/eyelid-lacerations?search=eyelid%20laceratin&source=search_result&selectedTitle=1~12&usage_type=default&display_rank=1#H6664674

Guier, C. P., & Thomas, S. J. (2021, February 13). *Cornea foreign body removal*. https://www.ncbi.nlm.nih.gov/books/NBK554478/

Haring, R. S., Sheffield, I. D., Channa, R., Canner, J. K., & Schneider, E. B. (2016). Epidemiologic trends of chemical ocular burns in the United States. *JAMA Ophthalmology*, *134*(10), 1119. doi:10.1001/jamaophthalmol.2016.2645

Howell, A. (2020, November 15). Accident or child abuse? *Optometry Times*. https://www.optometrytimes.com/view/accident-or-child-abuse

Hwang, J. Y., Yoon, H. K., Lee, J. H., Yoon, H. M., Jung, A. Y., Cho, Y. A., Lee, J. S., & Yoon, C. H. (2016). Cranial Nerve Disorders in Children: MR Imaging Findings. *Radiographics*, *36*(4), 1178–1194. https://doi.org/10.1148/rg.2016150163

Kurtz, D., & Carlson, N. B. (2003). *Clinical Procedures for Ocular Examination* (3rd ed.). McGraw-Hill Education / Medical.

Lim, L., & Lim, E. W. L. (2020). Therapeutic Contact Lenses in the Treatment of Corneal and Ocular Surface Diseases - A Review. *Asia-Pacific Journal of Ophthalmology*, *9*(6), 524–532. https://doi.org/10.1097/apo.0000000000000331

Lorch, M., & Teach, S. J. (2010). Facial Nerve Palsy. *Pediatric Emergency Care*, *26*(10), 763–769. https://doi.org/10.1097/pec.0b013e3181f3bd4a

Monaghan, M., Brogan, K., Lockington, D., Rotchford, A. P., & Ramaesh, K. (2019). Variability in measuring pH using litmus paper and the relevance in Ocular Chemical injury. *Eye (London, England)*, *34*(11), 2133–2134. doi:10.103841433-019-0737-z

Nikita, E. (2017). *Osteoarchaeology: A Guide to the Macroscopic Study of Human Skeletal Remains* (1st ed.). Academic Press.

Precision Laboratories. (2020). *How should test strips be stored? | Precision Laboratories Test Strips*. https://www.preclaboratories.com/faq-items/how-should-test-strips-be-stored/

Prentiss, K. A., & Dorfman, D. H. (2008). Pediatric ophthalmology in the emergency department. *Emergency Medicine Clinics of North America*, *26*(1), 181–198. doi:10.1016/j.emc.2007.11.001

Pullen, R. L. (2005). Checking for oculocephalic reflex. *Nursing*, *35*(6), 24. https://doi.org/10.1097/00152193-200506000-00016

Reading, R. (2012). Radiation exposure from CT scans in childhood and subsequent risk of leukaemia and brain tumours: A retrospective cohort study. *Child: Care, Health and Development*, *38*(6), 910. https://doi.org/10.1111/cch.12006_2

Robinson, J., Ellen, J., Hadel, B., & Lighthizer, N. (2016). *Collecting a corneal culture*. https://www.reviewofoptometry.com/article/collecting-a-corneal-culture

Rogan, D. T., & Fang, A. (2020, July 6). *Pediatric Facial Trauma*. https://www.ncbi.nlm.nih.gov/books/NBK558932/

Slovis, T. L., & Berdon, W. E. (1999). Editorial. *Pediatric Radiology*, *29*(2), 79. https://doi.org/10.1007/s002470050544

Syed, Z. (2021). *Hyphema*. Academy of Ophthalmology. EyeWiki. Retrieved from eyewiki.aao.org/Hyphema

Topical Antibiotics. (2009). *Review of Optometry*. https://www.reviewofoptometry.com/article/topical-antibiotics

U.S. Food and Drug Administration. (2019). *Pediatric medical devices*. https://www.fda.gov/medical-devices/products-and-medical-procedures/pediatric-medical-devices

Walker, K. H., Hall, D. W., & Hurst, W. J. (1990). *Clinical Methods: The History, Physical and Laboratory Examinations* (3rd ed.). Butterworth-Heinemann.

ADDITIONAL READING

Suhr, C. L., & DelGiodice, M. (2015, October 1). *Neuroimaging 101 For the Optometrist.* Review of Optometry. https://www.reviewofoptometry.com/article/neuroimaging-101-for-the-optometrist

KEY TERMS AND DEFINITIONS

B-Scan Ultrasound: An ocular imaging apparatus that uses sound waves to create two images of the eye and orbit.

Corneal and Conjunctival Culturing: Sampling and subsequent analysis of causative infectious material of the cornea and conjunctiva.

CT Scan, Imaging, Commuted Tomography: An ocular imaging technique that uses multiple x-ray scans obtained from a revolving unit to form a two-dimensional image.

Magnetic Resonance Angiography: An imaging technique employs the same radio waves as with an MRI but is used to look at the arterial blood flow.

Magnetic Resonance Imaging: A sensitive imaging modality that uses a magnetic field and radio-frequency pulses to view internal structures of the body.

Magnetic Resonance Venography: An imaging technique using a magnetic field and radio pulses to examine venous blood flow. This allows for the evaluation of the drainage system of the brain.

Neurological Testing: Evaluating the function of the cranial nerves.

Ocular Emergency: A serious vision threatening and/or painful occurrence requiring immediate medical attention.

Ocular Imaging: An armamentarium of devices utilized to provide improved understanding of ocular pathology and sequelae of ocular trauma not easily visible during clinical examination.

pH Testing: Measurement of acidity of the ocular surface after exposure to chemical substances.

Seidel Sign: A clinical sign indicating a ruptured globe.

APPENDIX 1

Pediatric Topical Ophthalmic Agents

Introduction

Special consideration should be given to prescribing topical ophthalmic medications for the pediatric population. Prior to the early 2000s, less than 25% of all drugs approved by the Food and Drug Administration (FDA) had indications for pediatric use. The gap in research regarding pediatric drug use was due to a large perceived cost of pediatric clinical trials, ethical dilemmas regarding pediatric clinical trials, and the challenge associated with studying distinct pediatric age groups. Children are physiologically and metabolically different when they are newborns, infants, preschool children, school-aged children, and adolescents. Therefore, when a child enrolls in a multi-year clinical trial, they may advance to the next age-group within the time of the study (Coulter, 2004).

In 1997, the FDA responded to the lack of drugs studied for pediatric use with the "carrot-and-stick" approach. The "carrot," known as the Modernization Act awarded manufacturers patent exclusivity for their participation. The FDA created a "Pediatric Priority List" including drugs that were vulnerable to severe misuse by the pediatric population. (Coulter, 2004).

The "stick," or the Pediatric Rule, enacted by the FDA required that a drug likely to be used by children be tested in the population. Exclusions were granted if the drug was deemed unsafe or ineffective in pediatric patients, if studies were impractical, or if formulation for pediatric administration was unsuccessful. In the early 2000s, the Pediatric Rule was overthrown by the US District Court for the District of Columbia. The ruling found that the FDA could not require drug manufacturers to study drugs in the pediatric population unless the drug was intended for pediatric use (Coulter, 2004). Therefore, at this time, if a drug has not been studied in the pediatric population, it is not necessarily presumed to be unsafe in children.

When classifying drugs for pediatric safety, two terms are often used: *Not established* (NE) and not recommended (NR). *Not established* is a term used for drugs with insufficient evidence to support a specific pediatric indication. If evidence is lacking for the pediatric population or a specific pediatric age group, it will be stated in the "Pediatric use" subsection of the drug label. Drugs that are *not recommended* are associated with adverse drug side effects seen in animal studies and/or anecdotal cases (Chung & Buhr, 2000).

Unfortunately, there is a lack of consistency across sub-specialties when referring to pediatric patients in categorical terms of age groups such as newborn, neonate, preschool, child and adolescent. The FDA defines pediatrics as birth to 21 years of age and further categorizes into a specific breakdown. The FDA recognizes neonates as patients' birth to 28 days. Infants are 29 days to less than 2 years. Children are 2 years old to less than 12 years old. Adolescent patients are 12 years old through 21 years old. The FDA encourages drug manufacturers to analyze data specific to these age groups (U.S. Food and Drug Administration, 2019).

Tables 2 - 6 are intended to help guide the clinician when considering which therapeutic drops can be safely prescribed for a pediatric patient.

Table 2. Topical antibiotic drugs (Topical Antibiotics, 2009)

Brand Name	Generic Name	Manufacturer	Preparation	Pediatric Use	Bottle/Tube
Fluoroquinolones					
Besivance	Besifloxacin 0.6%	Bausch & Lomb	Suspension	^{3}1 yr.	5 mL
Ciloxan	Ciprofloxacin 0.3%	Alcon, generic	Solution/unguent	^{3}1 yr./ ^{3}2 yrs.	2.5 mL, 5 mL, 10 mL/3.5g
Iquix	Levofloxacin 1.5%	Vistakon Pharmacy	Solution	^{3}6 yr.	5 mL
Ocuflox	Ofloxacin 0.3%	Allergan, generic	Solution	^{3}1 yr.	5 mL, 10 mL
Quixin	Levofloxacin 0.5%	Vistakon Pharm.	Solution	^{3} 1 yr.	5 mL
Vigamox	Moxifloxacin 0.5%	Alcon	Solution	^{3} 1 yr.	3 mL
Zymar	Gatifloxacin 0.3%	Allergan	Solution	^{3} 1 yr.	2.5 mL, 5 mL
Aminoglycosides					
Tobrex	Tobramycin 0.3%	Alcon, generic	Solution/unguent	^{3} 2 mos.	5 mL/3.5 g
Genoptic	Gentamicin 0.3%	Allergan, generic	Solution/unguent	NE	1 mL/5 mL
Polymyxin B Combinations					
Polytrim	Polymyxin B/ trimethoprim	Allergan, generic	Solution	^{3} 2 mos.	10 mL
Polysporin	Polymyxin B/ bacitracin	Monarch, generic	Unguent	NE	3.5 g
Neosporin	Polymyxin B/ neomycin/ gramicidin	Monarch, generic	Solution/unguent	^{3} 2 yrs.	10 mL/3.5 g
Other					
AzaSite	Azithromycin 1%	Inspire Pharm.	Solution	^{3} 1 yr.	2.5 mL
Botycin	Erythromycin 0.5%	Dista, generic	Unguent	^{3} 2 mos.	3.5 g
AK-Tracin	Bacitracin 500u/g	Akorn, generic	Unguent	NE	3.5 g/3.75 g

NE= Not established

Table 3. Topical anti-inflammatory drugs

Brand Name	Generic Name	Manufacturer	Preparation	Pediatric Use	Bottle/Tube
		NSAID			
Acular	Ketorolac tromethamine 0.5%	Allergan, generic	Solution	^{3} 2 yrs.	10 mL
Steroids					
Flarex	Fluorometholone acetate 0.1%	Alcon, generic	Suspension	^{3} 2 yrs.	5 mL, 10 mL
Alrex	Loteprednol 0.2%	Bausch & Lomb	Suspension	NE	5 mL, 10 mL
Lotemax	Loteprednol 0.5%	Bausch & Lomb	Suspension/Gel	NE	5 mL, 10 mL, 15 mL
Pred Forte	Prednisolone acetate 1%	Allergan, generic	Suspension	NE	5 mL, 10 mL
Durezol	Difluprednate 0.05%	Novartis	Emulsion	NE	5 mL

NE= Not established

Table 4. Topical steroid-antibiotic combination drugs

Brand Name	Generic Name	Manufacturer	Preparation	Pediatric Use	Bottle/Tube
Tobradex	Tobramycin 0.3% - Dexamethasone 0.1%	Alcon, generic	Suspension	^{3} 2 yrs.	5 mL
Zylet	Loteprednol 0.5% - Tobramycin 0.3%	Bausch & Lomb	Suspension	NE	5 mL, 7.5 mL, 10 mL
Maxitrol	Neomycin 0.35% - Polymyxin B, Dexamethaasone 0.1%	Bausch & Lomb	Suspension/Unguent	^{3} 2 yrs./NE	8 mL/3.5 g

NE= Not established

Table 5. Topical anti-viral drugs

Brand Name	Generic Name	Manufacturer	Preparation	Pediatric Use	Bottle/Tube
Zirgan	Ganciclovir 0.15%	Bausch & Lomb	Gel	^{3} 2 yrs	5g
Viroptic	Trifluoridine 1%	Pfizer	Solution	^{3} 6 yrs	7.5 mL

Table 6. Diagnostic drops

Brand Name	Generic Name	Manufacturer	Preparation	Pediatric Use	Bottle/Tube
Mydriatics					
Phenylephrine	Phenylephrine HCl 2.5% / 10%	Paragon BioTeck, Inc.	Solution	>1 yrs. <1 yr. - 2.5% only	15 mL
Paremyd	Hydroxyamphetamine 1% - Tropicamide 0.25%	Akorn	Solution	NE	15 mL
Tropicamide	Tropicamide 0.5% / 1%	Bausch & Lomb, generic	Solution	All ages	7.5 mL, 15 mL
Cycloplegics					
Cyclopentolate	*Cyclopentolate HCl 0.5% / 1% / 2%	Bausch & Lomb, Akorn, Alcon	Solution	Children: 0.5%, 1% or 2% Small infants: 0.5%	15 mL / 2 mL, 5 mL, 15 mL / 2 mL, 5 mL, 15 mL
Combination drop					
Cyclomydril	*Cyclopentolate HCl 0.2% - Phenylephrine HCl 1%	Alcon	Solution	All ages	2 mL, 5 mL

NE = not established

*The American Academy of Ophthalmology recommends: cyclopentolate 1% for patients 6 months old and Cyclomydril for patients < 6 months old.

APPENDIX 2

Child Abuse and Neglect

There are three categories of child abuse that can be inflicted by a guardian or legally responsible adult. They are physical, emotional/verbal and sexual abuse. Physical abuse is non-accidental physical injury. Emotional/verbal abuse is a non-physical maltreatment that impairs a child's emotional development or sense of self-worth. Sexual abuse occurs when a guardian/legally responsible adult engages or allows someone to engage in sexual acts with a child. A guardian/legally responsible adult can be found guilty of these types of abuse if they allow others to commit abuse to a child in their care. Neglect occurs when a guardian or legally responsible adult harms a child, places a child in imminent danger, and/or does not provide adequate supervision.

Tables 7 – 11 outline signs of the various categories of abuse, as well as ocular specific signs that may be indicative of child abuse.

All healthcare workers are considered mandated reporters, and while acting in their professional capacity must report when there is reasonable cause to suspect the abuse or maltreatment of a child. Each state has specific provisions or procedures for mandated reporters.

Indicators of Maltreatment

Table 7. Indicators of child abuse or neglect

The Child	The Parent or Other Adult Caregiver	The Parent/Other Adult Caregiver & The Child
Has not received help for medical/physical problems that have been brought to the parents' attention	Denies the existence, or blames the child for the child's problems	Rarely look at or touch each other
Is always watchful, preparing for something bad to take place	Shows little concern for the child	Consider their relationship entirely negative
Is overly compliant, passive, or withdrawn	Views the child as entirely bad, burdensome or worthless	State that they do not like each other
Sudden change in behavior and/or school performance	Demands a level of performance (physical or academic) the child cannot achieve	
Learning problems not attributed to physical or psychological causes	Asks other caregivers or teachers to use harsh physical discipline if the child misbehaves	
Comes to school or activities early/stays late/does not want to go home	Looks primarily to the child for attention, care and satisfaction of emotional needs	
Reluctant to be around a particular person		
Discloses maltreatment		
Lacks adult supervision		

(Child Welfare Information Gateway, 2019)

Table 8. Signs of physical abuse

The Child	The Parent or Other Adult Caregiver
Has unexplained physical injuries: bites, burns, bruises, black eyes, broken bones	Offers unconvincing/conflicting or no explanation for child's injury
Has fading bruises/other marks noticeable after an absence from school	Describes the child in a negative way
Frightened of their caregiver and protests or cries when it is time to go home	Uses harsh physical discipline
Shrinks when adults approach	Has a history of abuse as a child
Reports injury by parent/parent/another adult caregiver	

(Child Welfare Information Gateway, 2019)

Table 9. Signs of sexual abuse

The Child	The Parent or Other Adult Caregiver
Has difficulty sitting or walking	Is isolated and secretive
Reports bedwetting or nightmares	Is controlling or jealous with family member
Suddenly refuses to participate in physical activities or change for gym	Severely limits the child's contact with other children, especially those of the opposite sex
Sudden change in appetite	Is unduly protective of the child
Demonstrates sophisticated, bizarre or unusual sexual knowledge/behavior	
Becomes pregnant or contracts a sexually transmitted infection, particularly under the age of 14	
Runs away	
Reports sexual abuse by a parent or other adult caregiver	

(Child Welfare Information Gateway, 2019)

Table 10. Signs of emotional maltreatment

The Child	The Parent or Other Adult Caregiver
Shows extremes in behavior	Constantly berates, blames or belittles the child
Is inappropriately adult or inappropriately infantile	Unconcerned about the child
Delayed in physical or emotional development	Refuses to consider offers of help for the child's problems
Has attempted suicide	Overt rejection of the child
Reports a lack of attachment to the parent or other adult caregiver	

(Child Welfare Information Gateway, 2019)

Table 11. Signs of neglect

The Child	The Parent or Other Adult Caregiver
Frequently absent from school	Appears indifferent towards the child
Steals or begs for food/money	Seems depressed or apathetic
Consistently dirty, has severe body odor	Behaves irrationally or in a bizarre manner
Lacks needed medical/dental/vision care and glasses, immunizations	Is abusing drugs or alcohol
States no one at home provides care	
Abuses alcohol and other drugs	
Lacks sufficient clothing for the weather	

(Child Welfare Information Gateway, 2019)

Table 12. Ophthalmic signs of abusive head trauma

Ophthalmic Finding	Additional notes
Retinal hemorrhages	Too numerous to count Extend to ora serrata Typically, bilateral but can be asymmetric Occur in multiple layers of the retina
Retinal folds	
Retinoschisis	Can be located peripherally or in the macula
Vitreous hemorrhage	
Papilledema	
Optic nerve sheath hemorrhage	
Optic atrophy	

(Binenbaum, 2020)

Table 13. Other ocular signs of abuse. The chart is not all encompassing. Some of the ocular findings can be caused by other etiologies and not only child abuse. It is important to take a detailed history and evaluate the patient's entire clinical picture during examination

Ocular Signs of Physical Abuse	Ocular Signs of Sexual Abuse
Orbital fractures	Phthiriasis palpebrarum of eyelashes
Hyphema	Chlamydial conjunctivitis
Periorbital Ecchymosis	Gonorrheal conjunctivitis
Subconjunctival hemorrhage	Streff Syndrome
Traumatic cataract or subluxated lens	
Iridodialysis	
Iris sphincter tear	
Papilledema	

(Christian, 2018; Elner, 1999; Howell, 2020)

Chapter 16
Myopia Management

Sarah Singh
University of California, Berkeley, USA

ABSTRACT

Myopia is already the most common ocular disorder in the world, and its prevalence continues to increase worldwide. Higher myopic refractive errors are associated with an increased risk of vision-threatening complications, which has led to many investigations into the underlying cause of myopia and the mechanisms of myopia progression in order to prevent or delay the onset of myopia and slow its progression. This chapter briefly reviews ocular development and emmetropization, summarizes the known risk factors for myopia onset and myopia progression, reviews current clinical interventions for controlling myopia, and provides practice management recommendations. Finally, instances of syndromic myopia, which have not been shown to be responsive to myopia control treatments, are reviewed.

INTRODUCTION

Myopia is a visual condition in which light is focused in front of the retina, causing distant objects to appear blurred. It is already the most common ocular disorder in the world and is still increasing in prevalence worldwide (Holden et al., 2016), with the onset of myopia occurring earlier in life (Lin et al., 2004).

Myopia most commonly occurs during school-age years when the eyeball grows too long, as shown in Figure 1.

Historically, myopia has been seen as more of an inconvenience than a disease. However, the anatomical changes associated with myopia, which worsen with higher levels of myopia, are not eliminated with refractive error corrections, and any amount of myopia increases the risk of retinal detachment, myopic maculopathy, glaucoma, and other vision-threatening complications (Flitcroft, 2012). High myopia, defined as refraction greater than -6.00D, is now a leading cause of preventable blindness (Wu et al., 2015).

The myopia epidemic has prompted a renewed interest in efforts to prevent or reduce the progression of myopia, and methods of controlling eye growth are constantly evolving. Current information from the peer-reviewed literature about clinically applicable myopia control is reviewed here along with practical tips for treating children with current effective myopia control options.

DOI: 10.4018/978-1-7998-8044-8.ch016

Figure 1. Compared to the emmetropic eye shown in A, a myopic eye, shown in B, is elongated along the sagittal axis of the globe. This leads to a longer vitreous chamber depth and axial length

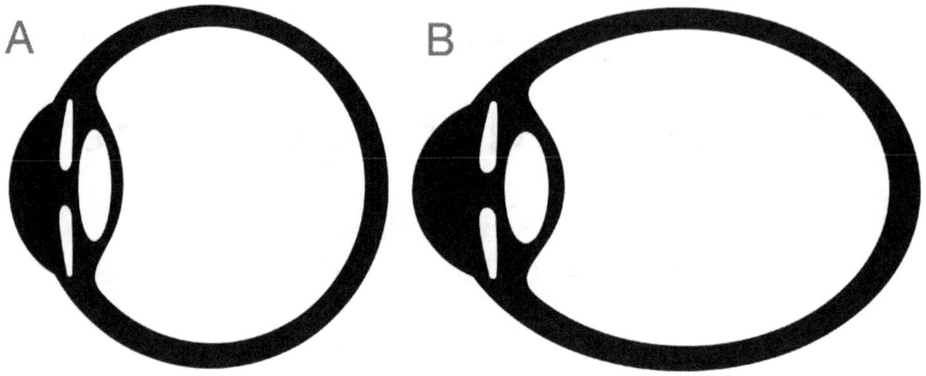

BACKGROUND

Clinical Studies

Risk Factors for Myopia Onset and Progression

The mechanisms and risk factors for myopia onset and progression are important but challenging to study. Myopia is caused by a complex mixture of genetic and environmental risk factors such as less outdoor time and more near work. It is important to be able to identify those at risk of becoming highly myopic to target early interventions. Age of myopia onset was found to be the strongest predictor of high myopia among children in Singapore (Chua et al., 2016), and a large observational cohort study in the United States found that hyperopia lower than expected at a young age was the best predictor of myopia in subsequent years (Zadnik et al., 2015). Therefore, care should be taken to council young children, schoolteachers, nurses, parents, and pediatricians on the consequences of myopia and the importance of early interventions with myopia controlling treatments, which are reviewed in the following sections. The earlier the onset of myopia, the faster the progression (Sankaridurg and Holden, 2014), therefore, the earlier treatment should be initiated.

Clinical Pearl: *The earlier the onset of myopia, the faster myopia progresses. Therefore, the earlier the onset of myopia, the more urgently a myopia-controlling treatment should be initiated.*

Time Outdoors

To date, the most influential and consistent environmental, modifiable factor associated with the onset of myopia is time spent outdoors (French et al., 2013; Xiong et al., 2017). It is unclear whether the benefit is due to increased light exposure, environmental colors and/or textures, viewing distances, the stimulation of retinal dopamine release by brighter light outdoors, or simply that when children are outdoors, they're often doing something other than near work (Hua et al., 2015; Read et al., 2014). However, increasing time outdoors is the most effective method of preventing the onset of myopia (Wu et al., 2018). There is conflicting evidence surrounding the effect of increased outdoor time on the slowing of myopia progression but increased outdoor time can be safely recommended regardless.

Clinical Pearl: *Increased outdoor time in pre-myopic children is the most effective method of delaying the onset of myopia and should be recommended to all children with myopic parents.*

Education and Near Work

Education plays an important role in determining the onset of myopia. In the Singapore Cohort Study of the Risk Factors for Myopia (SCORM), both academic grades and intelligence quotient (IQ) scores were found to be independently associated with myopia in Singaporean children (Saw et al., 2004). In addition, spending more time at school or doing other near work activities is associated with a higher amount of indoor time, and faster myopic progression (Nemeth et al., 2021). Higher socioeconomic status, which is often measured in terms of parental education, also carries a higher likelihood of myopia.

Personal Characteristics

Females tend to show faster progression of myopia than males (Midelfart et al., 2002; Parssinen, 1987; Sun et al., 2012; Zhou et al., 2016), however, this has not been observed in all studies (Gwiazda et al., 2007; Rezvan et al., 2012). Parental history of myopia is a risk factor for myopia. Studies have found that young school children that have two myopic parents have longer axial lengths and less hyperopia than children with one myopic parent or no myopic parents (Mutti et al., 2002; Xiang et al., 2012; Zhang et al., 2015). It is important to note that the effect of parental myopia on their children is likely not entirely due to genetics, but instead of a heritability that includes shared lifestyle, geographic location, education, and socioeconomic status.

Binocular Vision

An increased Accommodative Convergence to Accommodation (AC/A) ratio has been found to be a predictor of myopia onset (Mutti et al., 2017). In addition, there is an association between higher levels of esophoria and accommodative lag at near in myopic children and young adults compared with emmetropes (Allen & O'Leary, 2006; Drobe & de Saint-Andre, 1995; Gwiazda et al., 1995; Nakatsuka et al., 2005). Myopic children also show reduced accommodative facility and elevated AC/A (Gwiazda et al., 1999; Gwiazda et al., 2005; Mutti et al., 2000). Whether this is a cause or a consequence, though, is still debated.

Geographic Location

Children who live in urban environments have higher odds of developing myopia than those from rural environments (Flitcroft et al., 2020; Rudnicka et al., 2016). A group of researchers in Hong Kong found that axial length was significantly longer in children who lived in areas with a higher population density and in a smaller home than children who were living in lower population density areas and larger homes (Choi et al., 2017). Similarly, researchers in China tied a higher prevalence of myopia to living on a higher floor, compared to children who lived in a flat or room on a lower floor, also suggesting that denser urban areas are myopigenic (Wu et al., 2016).

EVIDENCE-BASED CLINICAL MANAGEMENT OF MYOPIA

There are three main categories of targeted approaches for intervening in myopia progression, which include: 1) public health interventions, 2) optical devices including orthokeratology lenses, multifocal soft contact lenses, and novel spectacle lens designs, 3) pharmaceutical treatments which is currently limited to the topical application of atropine, although additional treatments are under active investigation.

Environmental Recommendations

Many studies, including several very well-designed randomized clinical trials, highlight the protective role of increased outdoor time on myopia prevention (He et al., 2015; Jin et al., 2015; Jones et al., 2007; Jones-Jordan et al., 2011; Mutti et al., 2002; Rose et al., 2008; Wu et al., 2018; Wu et al., 2013). The risk of becoming myopic can be reduced by about 30% by increasing outdoor time to 14 hours or more per week (French et al., 2013; Jones et al., 2007). While the mechanism is not understood, there are several theories, such as the brightness of outdoor light, the patterns of defocus and spatial frequency composition that are applied to the retina when outdoors (Flitcroft, 2012; Flitcroft et al., 2020), light-stimulated release of dopamine (French et al., 2013; Jacobsen et al., 2008), and many others. The evidence is strong enough to recommend that all children at risk for developing myopia should be recommended increased outdoor time.

Clinical Pearl: *Children that are at risk for developing myopia should be advised to spend at least 14 hours per week outdoors.*

Clinical Treatment Options

Under-Correction of Myopia

Under-correction of myopia by 0.50 D to 0.75 D does not slow myopia progression (Adler & Millodot, 2006; Chung et al., 2002; Li et al., 2015). In fact, it appears that under-correcting children by even these small amounts may cause myopia to progress *faster (Vasudevan et al., 2014).* A study that compared no correction vs. full correction found that young myopes who went uncorrected exhibited slower myopia progression and axial elongation than fully corrected myopes (Sun et al., 2017).

Clinical Pearl: *Under-correction of myopic refractive error does not slow progression of myopia.*

Clinical Pearl: *Consider prescribing only part-time correction for very low myopes (using glasses only when needed). While part-time correction has not been investigated directly, children who went uncorrected exhibited slower myopia progression than fully corrected myopes, which suggests that part-time correction may be better than full-time correction.*

Bifocal or Multifocal Spectacle Lenses

Many studies have investigated the use of bifocal spectacle lenses for myopia control (Berntsen et al., 2012; Cheng et al., 2014; Fulk et al., 2000; Gwiazda et al., 2003). Bifocal lenses, when used as indicated, can result in myopic defocus applied to part of the visual field therefore slowing the progression of myopia (see Figure 2). Most investigations have found statistically significant slowing of myopia progression with bifocal or multifocal spectacle lenses than single vision lenses, however, few find clinically meaningful results. In the largest randomized clinical trial, the COMET study, the investigators found that children wearing multifocal spectacle lenses progressed 0.20 ± 0.08 D less than children wearing single vision spectacles over 3 years (Gwiazda et al., 2003). The largest treatment effect was found in a 2014 study that prescribed executive bifocal lenses to myopic children (Cheng et al., 2014). This study was unique in that enrollment was limited to subjects who had documented myopia progression in the year prior to entry into the study, which may explain the larger treatment effect that was observed. Until these results can be replicated, multifocal spectacles are not recommended for myopia control.

Figure 2. Light focused anterior to the retina is considered myopic defocus (blue) while light focused posterior to the retina is considered hyperopic defocus (green). Hyperopic defocus stimulates axial elongation, while myopic defocus slows axial elongation of the globe

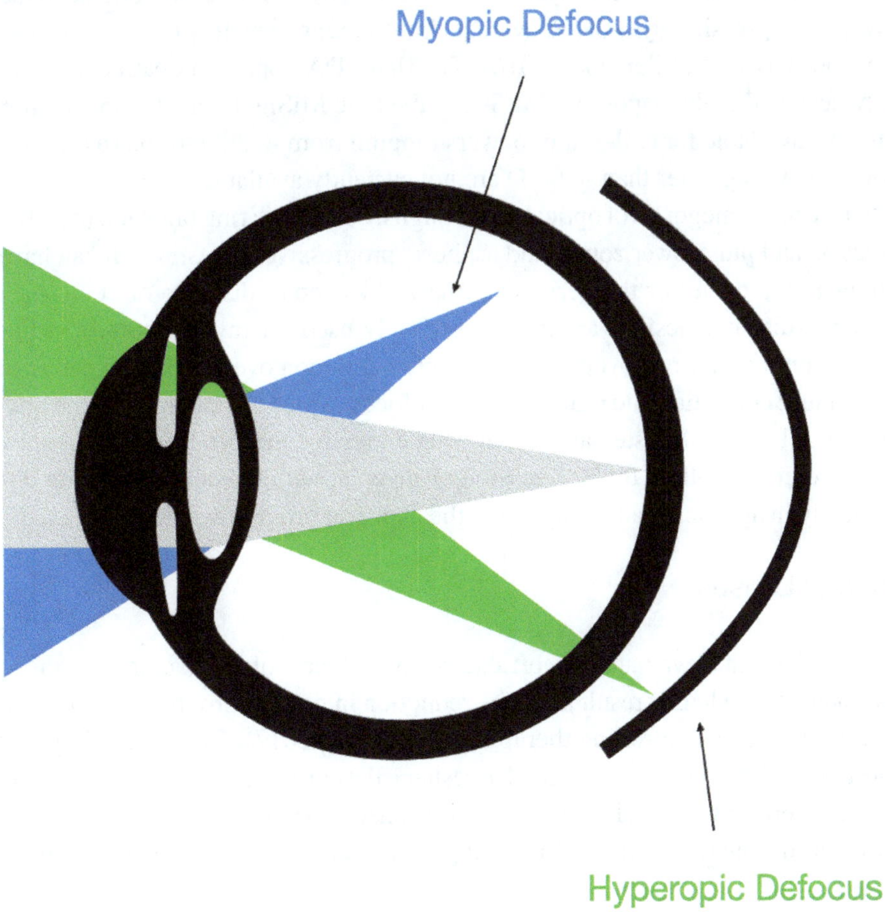

Clinical Pearl: *Multifocal spectacle lenses may provide some myopia control, but not enough to warrant routine prescription for young, progressing myopes.*

Novel Spectacle Lens Designs

There are several novel spectacle lenses that are designed specifically for reducing myopia progression that are being trialed. Research has shown that imposed myopic defocus is a strong inhibitor of myopic eye growth and is the suspected mechanism that underlies the use of orthokeratology and multifocal soft contact lenses for myopia control. One spectacle lens based on this idea, called the Defocus Incorporated Multiple Segments (DIMS) spectacle lens, was developed and trialed in a randomized clinical trial of school-aged children in Hong Kong, and their myopia progression was monitored over the course of 2 years (Lam et al., 2020). Compared to children wearing single-vision lenses, the children wearing DIMS lenses had 59% less myopia progression. These spectacles, among other novel lens designs, show promise as alternative treatment options and are commercially available in Asia, Europe, and Canada, but none are currently available in the United States.

Multifocal Soft Contact Lenses

Multifocal soft contact lenses (MFSCLs) have been used for myopia control since the early 2000's, with a large range of levels of efficacy. A recent systematic review and meta-analysis concluded that they reduce the rate of myopia progression by 38% on average, but the range extends from as low as 25% (Lam et al., 2014) to as much as 72% (Aller et al., 2016). The first FDA-approved treatment for myopia control was a specially designed daily disposable MFSCL called the MiSight lens (CooperVision, Pleasanton, CA), which is now available for children in powers ranging from -0.50D to -6.00D (approved for up to -7.00D, although powers greater than -6.00 D are not currently available).

There are two general categories of optical lens designs: concentric ring bifocal lenses, with alternating distance correction and plus power zones, and aspheric progressive lenses, which can have the distance correction either in the center or the periphery (marked as center-distance or center-near), as shown in Figure 3. Center-distance designs are more commonly used for myopia control, while center-near designs are more common for presbyopia and thus more common overall. Both types of lenses provide simultaneous distance correction and retinal myopic defocus, which is thought to be the underlying cause of the myopia control effect. A systematic review that compared the two lens designs showed that both lenses are effective in controlling the progression of myopia, with the concentric ring design having a slight, but clinically insignificant advantage over the aspheric progressive design.

Orthokeratology Lenses

The same meta-analysis that evaluated the efficacy of multifocal soft contact lenses for myopia control found that orthokeratology lenses result in a 45% reduction in myopia progression compared to children who are not using a myopia controlling therapy (Sankaridurg, 2017). Orthokeratology lenses are rigid gas-permeable contact lenses that are designed to reshape the cornea, temporarily correcting the patient's refractive error. Modern orthokeratology lenses are designed to be worn overnight, providing a temporary reduction of myopia during the daytime, eliminating the need for glasses or contact lenses during the day.

Figure 3. Representative multifocal soft contact lens designs showing a center-distance aspheric lens (A), a center-near aspheric lens (B), and a concentric ring design (C)

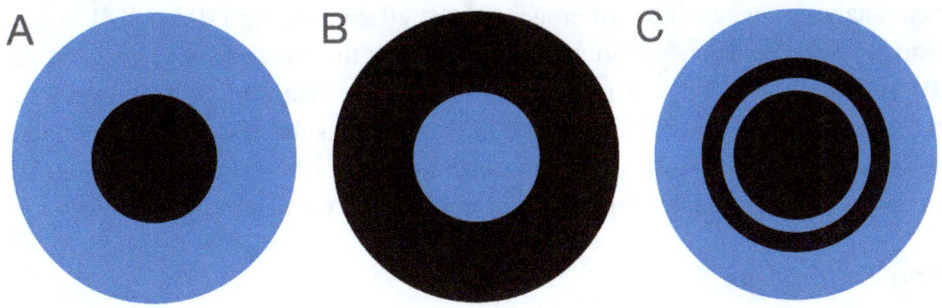

Atropine

The largest and most referenced clinical studies involving atropine are a series of studies referred to as the ATOM studies (Atropine for the Treatment of Childhood Myopia). In the initial ATOM trial, 400 Singaporean children were randomized to be treated either with topical 1% atropine in one eye for two years or with a placebo drop in one eye for two years. Atropine was highly effective in controlling the progression of myopia, resulting in a 77% reduction in the mean progression of myopia compared with the placebo treatment and no change in axial length. However, while no serious adverse events were observed and the monocular treatment was well-tolerated, blurred near vision and light sensitivity prevented this treatment from being widely adopted as a myopia management strategy (Chua et al., 2006).

The same group continued with a new randomized trial to assess the efficacy, safety, and functional impact of three different atropine concentrations for the bilateral treatment of myopia. ATOM 2 was a single-center, double-masked, randomized trial that enrolled 400 children who were randomized to receive bilateral treatment of 0.5%, 0.1%, or 0.01% nightly for two years. Results revealed a dose-dependent response, with 0.5% and 0.1% doses showing a very similar efficacy as the 1% dose in controlling myopia both in terms of refractive error change and axial length change. Interestingly, the 0.01% dose, which was originally intended to be a placebo treatment, showed some efficacy in slowing myopia progression, although there appears to be a difference between the controlling effect on refractive error and the effect on axial length. The axial elongation in the 0.01% group remained significant, leading to uncertainty for the role of very low concentration atropine in myopia control (Chia et al., 2012).

The ATOM studies also found an important effect when atropine treatment was discontinued. Both concentration- and age-related rebound myopia was observed in children followed for a year after termination of atropine treatment (Chia et al., 2014). The pharmacodynamics of atropine would suggest that long-term exposure to a competitive antagonist will cause an upregulation of receptors, resulting in a loss of efficacy to the applied drug over time and exaggerated symptoms when treatment is ended. Younger children and those treated with higher concentrations were shown to have the highest risk of rebound myopia progression in these studies. This leaves an open question about how and when treatment can be safely discontinued.

The ATOM studies as well as those that came before it have shown that as atropine concentration decreases, the number of "nonresponders" (children who continue to experience fast myopia progression despite atropine treatment) increases (Chia et al., 2012; Shih et al., 1999). In addition, although the results of meta-analyses suggest little differences in the efficacy of high (0.5-1.0%), moderate (>0.01 to <0.5%), and low (<0.01%) concentrations, a recent trial of three low atropine concentrations (0.05%, 0.025% and 0.01% doses) found that efficacy increased with concentration, at least over a short-term (2-year) period (Yam et al., 2020), concluding that 0.05% atropine is the best concentration to use in Asian patients. These varied results leave open questions about the relationship between atropine concentration and myopia control efficacy and how optimal dosing might vary on an individual basis.

Combination Treatments

Optical and pharmaceutical treatments are thought to be working via different mechanisms, and therefore, combining pharmaceutical and optical treatments could provide even greater myopia control than either treatment alone. As described above, topical atropine results in a dose-dependent mydriasis and cycloplegia by paralyzing the iris sphincter and the ciliary muscle, respectively. The underlying mechanism for how atropine exerts its anti-myopia effect is unknown. However, the small increase in pupil size or alteration of pupil dynamics may allow for altering the area exposed to additional myopic defocus, potentially improving the efficacy of MFSCLs or orthokeratology lenses.

Another interesting study suggests another possible mechanism for how combination treatments could be more effective than either treatment alone. In a group of children that were using atropine as their myopia control treatment, researchers found that the choroid thickened after the initiation of atropine drops. In addition, the choroid in eyes using atropine no longer thinned in response to hyperopic defocus, suggesting that alterations to choroid thickness may play a key role in eye growth regulation (Chiang et al., 2020).

A few research groups have begun to investigate this possibility. Previously published studies have found that the use of multifocal spectacle lenses in combination with atropine (Shih et al., 2001), and orthokeratology lenses in combination with atropine (Kinoshita et al., 2018; Wan et al., 2018) may provide better myopia control than one treatment alone, although the effect appears more pronounced in children who are younger and have lower myopia. Additionally, there is an ongoing clinical trial in the United States evaluating the use of Biofinity multifocal contact lenses in addition to low-dose atropine treatment, and comparing the result of combination therapy to a historical control, composed of children who previously participated in the BLINK study (Huang et al., 2019). Given the promise that combination therapy holds for fast progressors, it is worthwhile to investigate combination therapy with a contemporary comparison group in a randomized clinical trial.

TREATMENT OPTIONS

The interventions described in the previous section provide several options for managing young children with myopia, providing the necessary background knowledge to translate the risks and benefits of a myopia control treatment to patients and parents. This section attempts to provide best practices for the examination and selection of treatment for young myopic patients.

Orthokeratology

Orthokeratology lenses are reverse-geometry rigid gas permeable contact lenses that are worn overnight and gently reshape the corneal surface so that the cornea maintains the molded contour of the contact lens for many hours after lens wear. Children using this treatment do not need to wear contact lenses or glasses during the day. The central corneal flattening achieved with orthokeratology lenses provides for clear distance vision, and the mid-peripheral steepening and unchanged far periphery of the cornea is thought to provide the myopic defocus and myopia controlling effect.

Clinical Pearl: *Because children are free from glasses and contact lenses during the daytime, this is an excellent treatment option for young children, who may need help with contact lens application, removal, and lens care.*

Clinical Pearl: *Orthokeratology is an ideal treatment option for kids who participate in swimming, other water sports, or sports in dusty environments such as softball or baseball, since they do not need to wear contact lenses during the activity.*

There are many types of orthokeratology lenses available in the US, including Paragon CRT and CRT Dual Axis lenses, iSee lenses, Euclid Emerald and Sapphire lenses, Wave custom orthokeratology lenses, and Abiliti lenses. Eye care practitioners must be certified to fit orthokeratology lenses, and each lens carries its own certificate program. A general approach is provided here:

Equipment

1. Autorefractor/keratometer
2. Corneal topographer
3. Ocular biometer
4. Slit lamp biomicroscope

Patient Selection

1. Refraction: Most lenses treat up to moderate amounts of myopia (myopia ≥ -6.00 D) with low to moderate with-the-rule astigmatism*
   *Check each manufacturer's guidelines for specific FDA-approved criteria
2. Keratometry: In general, it is best not to flatten the cornea to <37.00 D

Example: A patient with -4.00 D of myopia and K's of 45.00 D is a good candidate for orthokeratology (45.00 flat K– 4.00D myopia – 0.50 D Jessen factor = 40.50 D). A patient with -4.00 D of myopia and K's of 39.00 D is not a good candidate for orthokeratology (39.00 D flat K – 4.00 D myopia – 0.50 D Jessen factor = 34.50 D).

3. Pupil size: In ambient room lighting, the ideal candidate's pupil size is smaller than the treated area of the cornea (usually 4-6mm).
4. Corneal topography: Mild or moderate with-the-rule astigmatism is ideal.

Procedure

Step 1: Initial lens selection: There are several options for how to select the initial lens for the patient. Each manufacturer will provide either a digital lens calculator or a consultation service for ordering the lens. At minimum, the following information is required:

Keratometry (flat and steep K)

Manifest refraction (some lenses use only the spherical component; others use sphere and cyl for their lens selector)

Corneal diameter (either white-to-white or horizontal visible iris diameter)

Corneal topography

Step 2: Apply the lens: After carefully inspecting the lens, rinse and massage gas-permeable lens conditioning solution to the front and back surfaces of the lens. Apply one drop of artificial tear to the back surface of the lens just prior to application

Clinical Pearl: *It is not advised to use proparacaine prior to the initial lens fitting. The sensation of discomfort of the contact lens is important for children to experience, so that they can appreciate a normal vs. abnormal level of discomfort when wearing the lenses at home.*

Step 3: Allow the lens to settle for at least 15 minutes

Clinical Pearl: *Initially, we advise patients to keep their eyes closed immediately following lens application because that will be the most comfortable. Once they're able to open their eyes, we recommend having the patient take a walk around for about 10 minutes while waiting for the lenses to settle. This will allow the patient to appreciate the clarity of their vision with the lenses and will take their mind off the initial lens discomfort.*

Figure 4. Representative initial NaFl pattern orthokeratology lens fits for a CRT lens (A) and a Euclid lens (B)

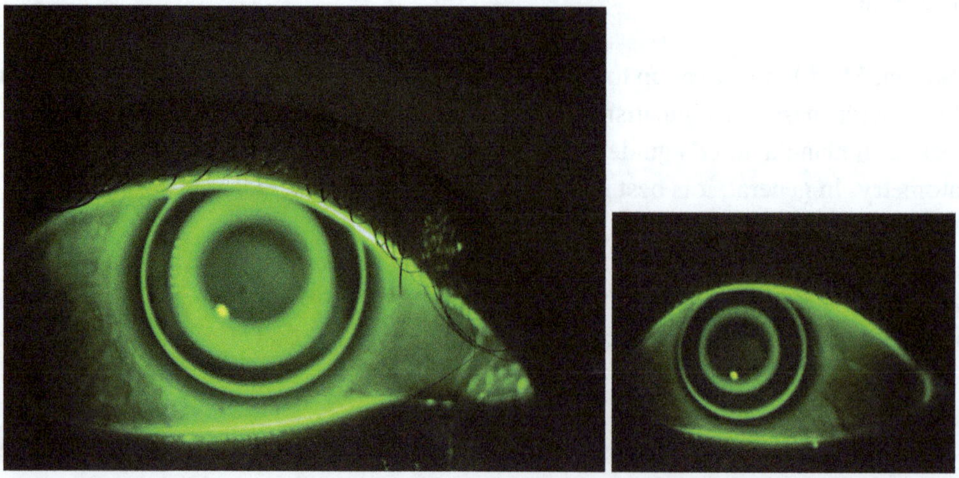

Step 4: Evaluate the lens with sodium fluorescein: The ideal contact lens fit should display a bull's eye pattern as shown in Figure 4
Step 5: Patients should be evaluated in the morning after the first night of lens wear, about 1 week after beginning lens wear, and then again about 1 month after beginning lens wear to ensure appropriate lens fit and vision correction. It is recommended that patients then be followed for myopia control every 3-6 months, depending on their rate of myopia progression and clinician comfort

Multifocal Soft Contact Lenses

MiSight Contact Lenses

The MiSight 1 day lens is currently the only treatment that is approved by the FDA specifically for the indication of correcting myopic refractive error ***and*** for slowing the progression of myopia when initially prescribed for children 8-12 years old. This indication follows the impressive results of a 3-year multicenter, double-masked, randomized clinical trial of MiSight lenses compared to a standard daily disposable soft contact lens, in which children using MiSight lenses were measured to have significantly less myopia progression and axial length change during the trial. After three years, children wearing MiSight lenses had 0.73 D less myopia and 0.32 mm less axial elongation compared to children wearing single-vision lenses (Chamberlain et al., 2019). MiSight contact lenses contain a large center-distance correction area of 3.36 mm surrounded by concentric zones of alternating distance (correction zones) and near (treatment zones) powers. The treatment zones have been shown to contain 2.00 D of plus power, which imposes myopic defocus on the retina.

Equipment

1. Autorefractor/keratometer (recommended)
2. Ocular biometer
3. Slit lamp biomicroscope

Patient Selection

1. Refraction: MiSight lenses are indicated for slowing the progression of myopia in children who have a refraction of -0.75 D to -4.00 D at the initiation of treatment. Lenses are available in powers ranging from -0.5 D to -7.00 D in 0.25 D steps. It is recommended that patients have ≤ 0.75 D of astigmatism.
2. MiSight lenses are indicated for children ages 8-12 years of age.

Procedure

Step 1: Initial lens selection: It is suggested that the initial lens selected match the manifest spherical equivalent refraction, accounting for the vertex distance of the phoropter or the frame if the power is greater than -4.00 D
Step 2: Apply the lens and allow the lenses to settle for at least 5 minutes

Clinical Pearl: *Unlike with orthokeratology lenses, MiSight lenses should be very comfortable upon initial lens application.*

Step 3: Evaluate the lens fit: The lens should be well centered and move with each blink
Step 4: Advise the patient to wear the lenses for at least 10 hours per day for at least 6 days per week. These are daily wear lenses, so the lens should be discarded after each use. Patients should not wear the lenses while sleeping or while showering or swimming
Step 5: Patients should be evaluated 1-2 weeks after beginning lens wear, and then followed for myopia control every 3-6 months, depending on their rate of myopia progression and practitioner comfort

Other Soft Multifocal Contact Lenses

Other than MiSight 1-day lenses, there is one other daily disposable lens that is available in a distance-center design, which is NaturalVue. NaturalVue contact lenses are multifocal lenses with an extended depth-of-focus design, with the myopia correction in the center of the lens and progressively more plus power moving out to the periphery. These lenses are available in a wider range of powers compared to MiSight lenses and are widely used and well-tolerated by young myopic patients, although there have been no clinical trials investigating their use for myopia control and they are used off-label for this purpose.

A handful of commercially available MFSCLs that were originally designed for presbyopia correction have been used off-label as myopia control treatments. All the clinical trials that have been conducted that investigate the use of MFSCLs for the purpose of myopia control use distance-center lens designs, which include the Proclear Multifocal (monthly disposable), the Biofinity Multifocal (monthly disposable), as well as the Biofinity Toric Multifocal (monthly disposable) lenses. MFSCLs provide clear vision by focusing some light on the retina, while simultaneously focusing some light in front of the retina to reduce myopia progression. An important randomized clinical trial called the Bifocal Lenses in Nearsighted Kids (BLINK) study randomly assigned children to wear one of three treatment options for three years: single-vision (non-multifocal) contact lenses, medium add power contact lenses, or high add power contact lenses. This study found that using higher add power lenses, which focus light further in front of the retina compared to medium add power lenses, lead to slower myopia progression, without significant consequences to visual perception (Walline et al., 2020).

Clinical Pearl: *When prescribing multifocal soft contact lenses for myopia control, use the highest add power (usually +2.50 D) that is tolerable to the patient. If necessary, incorporate the spherical over-refraction into the distance power.*

Clinical Pearl: *It is not uncommon for vision to be negatively perceived upon initial trialing of the contact lenses. Discuss this with the patient and their parents. Vision usually improves after 1 week of lens wear.*

Clinical Pearl: *Children need to be confident and independent in their lens care since they will be wearing these lenses during their normal daytime activities. Be encouraging in your application and removal training. There are many YouTube videos that demonstrate proper lens insertion and removal techniques.*

Atropine

Low-dose atropine is commonly used off-label for myopia control. Because atropine is only approved at the 1% concentration in the United States, it needs to be diluted by a compounding pharmacy.

Equipment

1. Autorefractor/keratometer (recommended)
2. Ocular biometer
3. Slit lamp biomicroscope
4. Pupillometer or pupil size ruler
5. Method of measuring near point of accommodation (NPA)
6. Instrument to measure intraocular pressure

Patient Selection

1. Refraction: Atropine can be used with any myopic refractive error.
2. Pupil size: Even the lowest doses of atropine (0.01% atropine sulfate solution) may cause an increase in pupil size (typically about a 1mm increase). It is important to measure the patient's baseline pupil size prior to starting treatment to assess any visual consequences of using atropine.
3. Accommodation: Even the lowest doses of atropine cause a 2-3 D loss of accommodative amplitude. Therefore, this treatment is not recommended for patients with accommodative insufficiency.

Procedure

Step 1: Prior to starting atropine treatment, the following exam procedures should be performed:
Refraction
Slit lamp examination
Measurement of pupil size in bright and dim room illumination
Near point of accommodation
Intraocular pressure
stereopsis (recommended)

Step 2: Release the prescription for the low-dose atropine concentration of choice. For example:
Atropine sulfate solution 0.02%, preserved with BAK
Quantity: 5mL bottle (30-day supply) x 5 refills
Sig: instill one drop in each eye just before bedtime.

Step 3: Patients should be evaluated 1-2 weeks after beginning atropine use, and then followed for myopia control every 3-6 months, depending on their rate of myopia progression and practitioner comfort

Follow-Up Schedules

Follow-up schedules for patients undergoing myopia control treatments are determined by multiple factors, such as the risks of complications, the patient's age, the patient's prior myopia progression history, and the patient's compliance with treatment. Patients should be assessed at least every 6 months to monitor the safety and efficacy of treatment, but general guidelines for each type of treatment are listed in Table 1.

Table 1. Summary of recommended follow-up schedules for the three myopia control treatment options

Multifocal Soft Contact Lenses	Orthokeratology	Low Dose Atropine
• 1-2 weeks after starting lens wear • Every 4-6 months	• The morning after starting lens wear • 1 week after starting lens wear • 1 month after starting lens wear • Every 3-4 months	• 1-2 weeks after starting atropine • Every 4-6 months

CONCLUSION

Eye care practitioners can prevent significant disease risk by employing the treatments described in this chapter. Orthokeratology, multifocal soft contact lenses, and atropine have been shown to be safe and effective methods of slowing myopia progression in children. In addition, environmental modifications, such as increasing outdoor time, can help to prevent or delay the onset of myopia and should be recommended for pre-myopic children.

REFERENCES

Adler, D., & Millodot, M. (2006). The possible effect of undercorrection on myopic progression in children. *Clinical & Experimental Optometry*, *89*(5), 315–321. doi:10.1111/j.1444-0938.2006.00055.x PMID:16907670

Allen, P. M., & O'Leary, D. J. (2006). Accommodation functions: Co-dependency and relationship to refractive error. *Vision Research*, *46*(4), 491–505. doi:10.1016/j.visres.2005.05.007 PMID:16009391

Aller, T. A., Liu, M., & Wildsoet, C. F. (2016). Myopia Control with Bifocal Contact Lenses: A Randomized Clinical Trial. *Optometry and Vision Science*, *93*(4), 344–352. doi:10.1097/OPX.0000000000000808 PMID:26784710

Berntsen, D. A., Sinnott, L. T., Mutti, D. O., & Zadnik, K. (2012). A randomized trial using progressive addition lenses to evaluate theories of myopia progression in children with a high lag of accommodation. *Investigative Ophthalmology & Visual Science*, *53*(2), 640–649. doi:10.1167/iovs.11-7769 PMID:22205604

Chamberlain, P., Peixoto-de-Matos, S. C., Logan, N. S., Ngo, C., Jones, D., & Young, G. (2019). A 3-year Randomized Clinical Trial of MiSight Lenses for Myopia Control. *Optometry and Vision Science*, *96*(8), 556–567. doi:10.1097/OPX.0000000000001410 PMID:31343513

Cheng, D., Woo, G. C., Drobe, B., & Schmid, K. L. (2014). Effect of bifocal and prismatic bifocal spectacles on myopia progression in children: Three-year results of a randomized clinical trial. *JAMA Ophthalmology*, *132*(3), 258–264. doi:10.1001/jamaophthalmol.2013.7623 PMID:24435660

Chia, A., Chua, W. H., Cheung, Y. B., Wong, W. L., Lingham, A., Fong, A., & Tan, D. (2012). Atropine for the treatment of childhood myopia: Safety and efficacy of 0.5%, 0.1%, and 0.01% doses (Atropine for the Treatment of Myopia 2). *Ophthalmology*, *119*(2), 347–354. doi:10.1016/j.ophtha.2011.07.031 PMID:21963266

Chia, A., Chua, W. H., Wen, L., Fong, A., Goon, Y. Y., & Tan, D. (2014). Atropine for the treatment of childhood myopia: Changes after stopping atropine 0.01%, 0.1% and 0.5%. *American Journal of Ophthalmology, 157*(2), 451–457 e451. doi:10.1016/j.ajo.2013.09.020 PMID:24315293

Chiang, S. T., Turnbull, P. R. K., & Phillips, J. R. (2020). Additive effect of atropine eye drops and short-term retinal defocus on choroidal thickness in children with myopia. *Scientific Reports, 10*(1), 18310. doi:10.103841598-020-75342-9 PMID:33110130

Choi, K. Y., Yu, W. Y., Lam, C. H. I., Li, Z. C., Chin, M. P., Lakshmanan, Y., Wong, F. S. Y., Do, C. W., Lee, P. H., & Chan, H. H. L. (2017). Childhood exposure to constricted living space: A possible environmental threat for myopia development. *Ophthalmic & Physiological Optics, 37*(5), 568–575. doi:10.1111/opo.12397 PMID:28643407

Chua, S. Y., Sabanayagam, C., Cheung, Y. B., Chia, A., Valenzuela, R. K., Tan, D., Wong, T. Y., Cheng, C. Y., & Saw, S. M. (2016). Age of onset of myopia predicts risk of high myopia in later childhood in myopic Singapore children. *Ophthalmic & Physiological Optics, 36*(4), 388–394. doi:10.1111/opo.12305 PMID:27350183

Chua, W. H., Balakrishnan, V., Chan, Y. H., Tong, L., Ling, Y., Quah, B. L., & Tan, D. (2006). Atropine for the treatment of childhood myopia. *Ophthalmology, 113*(12), 2285–2291. doi:10.1016/j.ophtha.2006.05.062 PMID:16996612

Chung, K., Mohidin, N., & O'Leary, D. J. (2002). Undercorrection of myopia enhances rather than inhibits myopia progression. *Vision Research, 42*(22), 2555–2559. doi:10.1016/S0042-6989(02)00258-4 PMID:12445849

Drobe, B., & de Saint-Andre, R. (1995). The pre-myopic syndrome. *Ophthalmic & Physiological Optics, 15*(5), 375–378. doi:10.1046/j.1475-1313.1995.9500075o.x PMID:8524558

Flitcroft, D. I. (2012). The complex interactions of retinal, optical and environmental factors in myopia aetiology. *Progress in Retinal and Eye Research, 31*(6), 622–660. doi:10.1016/j.preteyeres.2012.06.004 PMID:22772022

Flitcroft, D. I., Harb, E. N., & Wildsoet, C. F. (2020). The Spatial Frequency Content of Urban and Indoor Environments as a Potential Risk Factor for Myopia Development. *Investigative Ophthalmology & Visual Science, 61*(11), 42. doi:10.1167/iovs.61.11.42 PMID:32986814

French, A. N., Ashby, R. S., Morgan, I. G., & Rose, K. A. (2013). Time outdoors and the prevention of myopia. *Experimental Eye Research, 114*, 58–68. doi:10.1016/j.exer.2013.04.018 PMID:23644222

Fulk, G. W., Cyert, L. A., & Parker, D. E. (2000). A randomized trial of the effect of single-vision vs. bifocal lenses on myopia progression in children with esophoria. *Optometry and Vision Science, 77*(8), 395–401. doi:10.1097/00006324-200008000-00006 PMID:10966065

Gwiazda, J., Bauer, J., Thorn, F., & Held, R. (1995). A dynamic relationship between myopia and blur-driven accommodation in school-aged children. *Vision Research, 35*(9), 1299–1304. doi:10.1016/0042-6989(94)00238-H PMID:7610590

Gwiazda, J., Grice, K., & Thorn, F. (1999). Response AC/A ratios are elevated in myopic children. *Ophthalmic & Physiological Optics, 19*(2), 173–179. doi:10.1046/j.1475-1313.1999.00437.x PMID:10615453

Gwiazda, J., Hyman, L., Dong, L. M., Everett, D., Norton, T., Kurtz, D., Manny, R., Marsh-Tootle, W., Scheiman, M., & Comet, G. (2007). Factors associated with high myopia after 7 years of follow-up in the Correction of Myopia Evaluation Trial (COMET) Cohort. *Ophthalmic Epidemiology, 14*(4), 230–237. doi:10.1080/01658100701486459 PMID:17896302

Gwiazda, J., Hyman, L., Hussein, M., Everett, D., Norton, T. T., Kurtz, D., Leske, M. C., Manny, R., Marsh-Tootle, W., & Scheiman, M. (2003). A randomized clinical trial of progressive addition lenses versus single vision lenses on the progression of myopia in children. *Investigative Ophthalmology & Visual Science, 44*(4), 1492–1500. doi:10.1167/iovs.02-0816 PMID:12657584

Gwiazda, J., Thorn, F., & Held, R. (2005). Accommodation, accommodative convergence, and response AC/A ratios before and at the onset of myopia in children. *Optometry and Vision Science, 82*(4), 273–278. doi:10.1097/01.OPX.0000159363.07082.7D PMID:15829855

He, M., Xiang, F., Zeng, Y., Mai, J., Chen, Q., Zhang, J., Smith, W., Rose, K., & Morgan, I. G. (2015). Effect of Time Spent Outdoors at School on the Development of Myopia Among Children in China: A Randomized Clinical Trial. *Journal of the American Medical Association, 314*(11), 1142–1148. doi:10.1001/jama.2015.10803 PMID:26372583

Holden, B. A., Fricke, T. R., Wilson, D. A., Jong, M., Naidoo, K. S., Sankaridurg, P., Wong, T. Y., Naduvilath, T. J., & Resnikoff, S. (2016). Global Prevalence of Myopia and High Myopia and Temporal Trends from 2000 through 2050. *Ophthalmology, 123*(5), 1036–1042. doi:10.1016/j.ophtha.2016.01.006 PMID:26875007

Hua, W. J., Jin, J. X., Wu, X. Y., Yang, J. W., Jiang, X., Gao, G. P., & Tao, F. B. (2015). Elevated light levels in schools have a protective effect on myopia. *Ophthalmic & Physiological Optics, 35*(3), 252–262. doi:10.1111/opo.12207 PMID:25913873

Huang, J., Mutti, D. O., Jones-Jordan, L. A., & Walline, J. J. (2019). Bifocal & Atropine in Myopia Study: Baseline Data and Methods. *Optometry and Vision Science, 96*(5), 335–344. doi:10.1097/OPX.0000000000001378 PMID:31046016

Jacobsen, N., Jensen, H., & Goldschmidt, E. (2008). Does the level of physical activity in university students influence development and progression of myopia? A 2-year prospective cohort study. *Investigative Ophthalmology & Visual Science, 49*(4), 1322–1327. doi:10.1167/iovs.07-1144 PMID:18385044

Jin, J. X., Hua, W. J., Jiang, X., Wu, X. Y., Yang, J. W., Gao, G. P., Fang, Y., Pei, C. L., Wang, S., Zhang, J. Z., Tao, L. M., & Tao, F. B. (2015). Effect of outdoor activity on myopia onset and progression in school-aged children in northeast China: The Sujiatun Eye Care Study. *BMC Ophthalmology, 15*(1), 73. doi:10.118612886-015-0052-9 PMID:26152123

Jones, L. A., Sinnott, L. T., Mutti, D. O., Mitchell, G. L., Moeschberger, M. L., & Zadnik, K. (2007). Parental history of myopia, sports and outdoor activities, and future myopia. *Investigative Ophthalmology & Visual Science, 48*(8), 3524–3532. doi:10.1167/iovs.06-1118 PMID:17652719

Jones-Jordan, L. A., Mitchell, G. L., Cotter, S. A., Kleinstein, R. N., Manny, R. E., Mutti, D. O., Twelker, J. D., Sims, J. R., Zadnik, K., & Group, C. S. (2011). Visual activity before and after the onset of juvenile myopia. *Investigative Ophthalmology & Visual Science*, *52*(3), 1841–1850. doi:10.1167/iovs.09-4997 PMID:20926821

Kinoshita, N., Konno, Y., Hamada, N., Kanda, Y., Shimmura-Tomita, M., & Kakehashi, A. (2018). Additive effects of orthokeratology and atropine 0.01% ophthalmic solution in slowing axial elongation in children with myopia: First year results. *Japanese Journal of Ophthalmology*, *62*(5), 544–553. doi:10.100710384-018-0608-3 PMID:29974278

Lam, C. S., Tang, W. C., Tse, D. Y., Tang, Y. Y., & To, C. H. (2014). Defocus Incorporated Soft Contact (DISC) lens slows myopia progression in Hong Kong Chinese schoolchildren: A 2-year randomised clinical trial. *The British Journal of Ophthalmology*, *98*(1), 40–45. doi:10.1136/bjophthalmol-2013-303914 PMID:24169657

Lam, C. S. Y., Tang, W. C., Tse, D. Y., Lee, R. P. K., Chun, R. K. M., Hasegawa, K., Qi, H., Hatanaka, T., & To, C. H. (2020). Defocus Incorporated Multiple Segments (DIMS) spectacle lenses slow myopia progression: A 2-year randomised clinical trial. *The British Journal of Ophthalmology*, *104*(3), 363–368. doi:10.1136/bjophthalmol-2018-313739 PMID:31142465

Li, S. Y., Li, S. M., Zhou, Y. H., Liu, L. R., Li, H., Kang, M. T., Zhan, S. Y., Wang, N., & Millodot, M. (2015). Effect of undercorrection on myopia progression in 12-year-old children. *Graefes Archive for Clinical and Experimental Ophthalmology*, *253*(8), 1363–1368. doi:10.100700417-015-3053-8 PMID:26032395

Lin, L. L., Shih, Y. F., Hsiao, C. K., & Chen, C. J. (2004). Prevalence of myopia in Taiwanese schoolchildren: 1983 to 2000. *Annals of the Academy of Medicine, Singapore*, *33*(1), 27–33. https://www.ncbi.nlm.nih.gov/pubmed/15008558 PMID:15008558

Midelfart, A., Kinge, B., Midelfart, S., & Lydersen, S. (2002). Prevalence of refractive errors in young and middle-aged adults in Norway. *Acta Ophthalmologica Scandinavica*, *80*(5), 501–505. doi:10.1034/j.1600-0420.2002.800508.x PMID:12390161

Mutti, D. O., Jones, L. A., Moeschberger, M. L., & Zadnik, K. (2000). AC/A ratio, age, and refractive error in children. *Investigative Ophthalmology & Visual Science*, *41*(9), 2469–2478. https://www.ncbi.nlm.nih.gov/pubmed/10937556 PMID:10937556

Mutti, D. O., Mitchell, G. L., Jones-Jordan, L. A., Cotter, S. A., Kleinstein, R. N., Manny, R. E., Twelker, J. D., Zadnik, K., & Group, C. S. (2017). The Response AC/A Ratio Before and After the Onset of Myopia. *Investigative Ophthalmology & Visual Science*, *58*(3), 1594–1602. doi:10.1167/iovs.16-19093 PMID:28291868

Mutti, D. O., Mitchell, G. L., Moeschberger, M. L., Jones, L. A., & Zadnik, K. (2002). Parental myopia, near work, school achievement, and children's refractive error. *Investigative Ophthalmology & Visual Science*, *43*(12), 3633–3640. https://www.ncbi.nlm.nih.gov/pubmed/12454029 PMID:12454029

Nakatsuka, C., Hasebe, S., Nonaka, F., & Ohtsuki, H. (2005). Accommodative lag under habitual seeing conditions: Comparison between myopic and emmetropic children. *Japanese Journal of Ophthalmology, 49*(3), 189–194. doi:10.100710384-004-0175-7 PMID:15944822

Nemeth, J., Tapaszto, B., Aclimandos, W. A., Kestelyn, P., Jonas, J. B., De Faber, J. H. N., Januleviciene, I., Grzybowski, A., Nagy, Z. Z., Parssinen, O., Guggenheim, J. A., Allen, P. M., Baraas, R. C., Saunders, K. J., Flitcroft, D. I., Gray, L. S., Polling, J. R., Haarman, A. E., Tideman, J. W. L., ... Resnikoff, S. (2021). Update and guidance on management of myopia. European Society of Ophthalmology in cooperation with International Myopia Institute. *European Journal of Ophthalmology, 1120672121998960*(3), 853–883. Advance online publication. doi:10.1177/1120672121998960 PMID:33673740

Parssinen, T. O. (1987). Relation between refraction, education, occupation, and age among 26- and 46-year-old Finns. *American Journal of Optometry and Physiological Optics, 64*(2), 136–143. doi:10.1097/00006324-198702000-00010 PMID:3826288

Read, S. A., Collins, M. J., & Vincent, S. J. (2014). Light exposure and physical activity in myopic and emmetropic children. *Optometry and Vision Science, 91*(3), 330–341. doi:10.1097/OPX.0000000000000160 PMID:24413273

Rezvan, F., Khabazkhoob, M., Fotouhi, A., Hashemi, H., Ostadimoghaddam, H., Heravian, J., Azizi, E., Khorasani, A. A., & Yekta, A. A. (2012). Prevalence of refractive errors among school children in Northeastern Iran. *Ophthalmic & Physiological Optics, 32*(1), 25–30. doi:10.1111/j.1475-1313.2011.00879.x PMID:22023649

Rose, K. A., Morgan, I. G., Ip, J., Kifley, A., Huynh, S., Smith, W., & Mitchell, P. (2008). Outdoor activity reduces the prevalence of myopia in children. *Ophthalmology, 115*(8), 1279–1285. doi:10.1016/j.ophtha.2007.12.019 PMID:18294691

Rudnicka, A. R., Kapetanakis, V. V., Wathern, A. K., Logan, N. S., Gilmartin, B., Whincup, P. H., Cook, D. G., & Owen, C. G. (2016). Global variations and time trends in the prevalence of childhood myopia, a systematic review and quantitative meta-analysis: Implications for aetiology and early prevention. *The British Journal of Ophthalmology, 100*(7), 882–890. doi:10.1136/bjophthalmol-2015-307724 PMID:26802174

Sankaridurg, P. R., & Holden, B. A. (2014). Practical applications to modify and control the development of ametropia. *Eye (London, England), 28*(2), 134–141. doi:10.1038/eye.2013.255 PMID:24310242

Saw, S. M., Tan, S. B., Fung, D., Chia, K. S., Koh, D., Tan, D. T., & Stone, R. A. (2004). IQ and the association with myopia in children. *Investigative Ophthalmology & Visual Science, 45*(9), 2943–2948. doi:10.1167/iovs.03-1296 PMID:15326105

Shih, Y. F., Chen, C. H., Chou, A. C., Ho, T. C., Lin, L. L., & Hung, P. T. (1999). Effects of different concentrations of atropine on controlling myopia in myopic children. *Journal of Ocular Pharmacology and Therapeutics, 15*(1), 85–90. doi:10.1089/jop.1999.15.85 PMID:10048351

Shih, Y. F., Hsiao, C. K., Chen, C. J., Chang, C. W., Hung, P. T., & Lin, L. L. (2001). An intervention trial on efficacy of atropine and multi-focal glasses in controlling myopic progression. *Acta Ophthalmologica Scandinavica, 79*(3), 233–236. doi:10.1034/j.1600-0420.2001.790304.x PMID:11401629

Sun, J., Zhou, J., Zhao, P., Lian, J., Zhu, H., Zhou, Y., Sun, Y., Wang, Y., Zhao, L., Wei, Y., Wang, L., Cun, B., Ge, S., & Fan, X. (2012). High prevalence of myopia and high myopia in 5060 Chinese university students in Shanghai. *Investigative Ophthalmology & Visual Science*, *53*(12), 7504–7509. doi:10.1167/iovs.11-8343 PMID:23060137

Sun, Y. Y., Li, S. M., Li, S. Y., Kang, M. T., Liu, L. R., Meng, B., Zhang, F. J., Millodot, M., & Wang, N. (2017). Effect of uncorrection versus full correction on myopia progression in 12-year-old children. *Graefes Archive for Clinical and Experimental Ophthalmology*, *255*(1), 189–195. doi:10.100700417-016-3529-1 PMID:27796670

Vasudevan, B., Esposito, C., Peterson, C., Coronado, C., & Ciuffreda, K. J. (2014). Under-correction of human myopia—is it myopigenic?: A retrospective analysis of clinical refraction data. *Journal of Optometry*, *7*(3), 147–152. doi:10.1016/j.optom.2013.12.007 PMID:25000870

Walline, J. J., Walker, M. K., Mutti, D. O., Jones-Jordan, L. A., Sinnott, L. T., Giannoni, A. G., Bickle, K. M., Schulle, K. L., Nixon, A., Pierce, G. E., Berntsen, D. A., & Group, B. S. (2020). Effect of High Add Power, Medium Add Power, or Single-Vision Contact Lenses on Myopia Progression in Children: The BLINK Randomized Clinical Trial. *Journal of the American Medical Association*, *324*(6), 571–580. doi:10.1001/jama.2020.10834 PMID:32780139

Wan, L., Wei, C. C., Chen, C. S., Chang, C. Y., Lin, C. J., Chen, J. J., Tien, P. T., & Lin, H. J. (2018). The Synergistic Effects of Orthokeratology and Atropine in Slowing the Progression of Myopia. *Journal of Clinical Medicine*, *7*(9), 259. Advance online publication. doi:10.3390/jcm7090259 PMID:30205439

Wu, L. J., You, Q. S., Duan, J. L., Luo, Y. X., Liu, L. J., Li, X., Gao, Q., Zhu, H. P., He, Y., Xu, L., Jonas, J. B., Wang, W., & Guo, X. H. (2015). Prevalence and associated factors of myopia in high-school students in Beijing. *PLoS One*, *10*(3), e0120764. doi:10.1371/journal.pone.0120764 PMID:25803875

Wu, P. C., Chen, C. T., Lin, K. K., Sun, C. C., Kuo, C. N., Huang, H. M., Poon, Y. C., Yang, M. L., Chen, C. Y., Huang, J. C., Wu, P. C., Yang, I. H., Yu, H. J., Fang, P. C., Tsai, C. L., Chiou, S. T., & Yang, Y. H. (2018). Myopia Prevention and Outdoor Light Intensity in a School-Based Cluster Randomized Trial. *Ophthalmology*, *125*(8), 1239–1250. doi:10.1016/j.ophtha.2017.12.011 PMID:29371008

Wu, P. C., Tsai, C. L., Wu, H. L., Yang, Y. H., & Kuo, H. K. (2013). Outdoor activity during class recess reduces myopia onset and progression in school children. *Ophthalmology*, *120*(5), 1080–1085. doi:10.1016/j.ophtha.2012.11.009 PMID:23462271

Wu, X., Gao, G., Jin, J., Hua, W., Tao, L., Xu, S., & Tao, F. (2016). Housing type and myopia: The mediating role of parental myopia. *BMC Ophthalmology*, *16*(1), 151. doi:10.118612886-016-0324-z PMID:27580859

Xiang, F., He, M., & Morgan, I. G. (2012). The impact of parental myopia on myopia in Chinese children: Population-based evidence. *Optometry and Vision Science*, *89*(10), 1487–1496. doi:10.1097/OPX.0b013e31826912e0 PMID:22922777

Xiong, S., Sankaridurg, P., Naduvilath, T., Zang, J., Zou, H., Zhu, J., Lv, M., He, X., & Xu, X. (2017). Time spent in outdoor activities in relation to myopia prevention and control: A meta-analysis and systematic review. *Acta Ophthalmologica*, *95*(6), 551–566. doi:10.1111/aos.13403 PMID:28251836

Yam, J. C., Li, F. F., Zhang, X., Tang, S. M., Yip, B. H. K., Kam, K. W., Ko, S. T., Young, A. L., Tham, C. C., Chen, L. J., & Pang, C. P. (2020). Two-Year Clinical Trial of the Low-Concentration Atropine for Myopia Progression (LAMP) Study: Phase 2 Report. *Ophthalmology, 127*(7), 910–919. doi:10.1016/j.ophtha.2019.12.011 PMID:32019700

Zadnik, K., Sinnott, L. T., Cotter, S. A., Jones-Jordan, L. A., Kleinstein, R. N., Manny, R. E., Twelker, J. D., & Mutti, D. O. (2015). Prediction of Juvenile-Onset Myopia. *JAMA Ophthalmology, 133*(6), 683–689. doi:10.1001/jamaophthalmol.2015.0471 PMID:25837970

Zhang, X., Qu, X., & Zhou, X. (2015). Association between parental myopia and the risk of myopia in a child. *Experimental and Therapeutic Medicine, 9*(6), 2420–2428. doi:10.3892/etm.2015.2415 PMID:26136998

Zhou, W. J., Zhang, Y. Y., Li, H., Wu, Y. F., Xu, J., Lv, S., Li, G., Liu, S. C., & Song, S. F. (2016). Five-Year Progression of Refractive Errors and Incidence of Myopia in School-Aged Children in Western China. *Journal of Epidemiology, 26*(7), 386–395. doi:10.2188/jea.JE20140258 PMID:26875599

ADDITIONAL READING

American Optometric Association. (2021). *Clinical Report: Myopia Management.* https://aoa.uberflip.com/i/1388672-ebo-myopia-clinical-report-no-spread/0?

International Myopia Institute. (2021). *IMI White Papers & Clinical Summaries: Research Papers & Clinical Summaries.* https://myopiainstitute.org/imi-white-papers/

KEY TERMS AND DEFINITIONS

Emmetropization: The genetic and optical eye growth regulatory process that eliminates most refractive error during early childhood.

Myopia: Also known as nearsightedness, a visual condition in which light is focused in front of the retina, causing distant objects to appear blurred.

Myopia Control: The use of clinical treatments or environmental modifications to delay or slow the progression of myopia in children.

Myopia Progression: The increasing magnitude of refractive error and axial length that is typically observed during school-age years.

Myopia Treatment: The prescription of glasses, contact lenses or atropine for the purpose of myopia control.

Myopigenic: Myopia-inducing, usually referring to a myopia-inducing stimulus.

Orthokeratology: A method of myopia control using reverse-geometry rigid gas permeable contact lenses that are worn overnight and gently reshape the corneal surface and provides for clear distance vision.

Refractive Error: Myopia, hyperopia, or astigmatism resulting from a mismatch between the optical power of the eye and the length of the eye.

Under-Correction: An intentional reduction in the magnitude of myopic correction that is prescribed.

Compilation of References

Adler, D., & Millodot, M. (2006). The possible effect of undercorrection on myopic progression in children. *Clinical & Experimental Optometry*, *89*(5), 315–321. doi:10.1111/j.1444-0938.2006.00055.x PMID:16907670

Adler, P., Scally, A. J., & Barrett, B. T. (2013). Test-retest reproducibility of accommodation measurements gathered in an unselected sample of UK primary school children. *The British Journal of Ophthalmology*, *97*(5), 592–597. doi:10.1136/bjophthalmol-2012-302348 PMID:23426733

Adoh, T. O., & Woodhouse, J. M. (1994). The Cardiff acuity test used for measuring visual acuity development in toddlers. *Vision Research*, *34*(4), 555–560. doi:10.1016/0042-6989(94)90168-6 PMID:8303838

Agrawal, S., Mayer, D. L., Hansen, R. M., & Fulton, A. B. (2009). Visual fields in young children treated with Vigabatrin. *Optometry and Vision Science*, *86*(6), 767–773. doi:10.1097/OPX.0b013e3181a7b3fc PMID:19417698

Agur, A. M., & Dalley, A. F. (2019). *Moore's essential clinical anatomy* (6th ed.). Wolters Kluwer.

Alhammouri, Q., Graf, M., & Lorenz, B. (2011). Bruckner Test Sensitivity to Detect Foveal Dimming. *Journal of Research in Medical Sciences*, *18*, 10–15.

Allen, R. C. (2016, December 19). *Placement of a pressure patch.* EyeRounds.Org. https://webeye.ophth.uiowa.edu/eyeforum/atlas-video/placement-of-pressure-patch.htm

Allen, P. M., & O'Leary, D. J. (2006). Accommodation functions: Co-dependency and relationship to refractive error. *Vision Research*, *46*(4), 491–505. doi:10.1016/j.visres.2005.05.007 PMID:16009391

Aller, T. A., Liu, M., & Wildsoet, C. F. (2016). Myopia Control with Bifocal Contact Lenses: A Randomized Clinical Trial. *Optometry and Vision Science*, *93*(4), 344–352. doi:10.1097/OPX.0000000000000808 PMID:26784710

Al-Otaibi, A. G. (2012). Non-viral microbial keratitis in children. *Saudi Journal of Ophthalmology*, *26*(2), 191–197. doi:10.1016/j.sjopt.2011.10.002 PMID:23960991

American Academy of Ophthalmology. (2020, December 28). Pressure patch. https://www.aao.org/image/pressure-patch

American Academy of Pediatrics, Committee on Fetus and Newborn. (2004). Age Terminology during the Perinatal Period. *Pediatrics*, *114*(5), 1362–1364. doi:10.1542/peds.2004-1915 PMID:15520122

American Academy of Pediatrics. (2006). Committee on Fetus and Newborn, American College of Obstetricians and Gynecologists and Committee on Obstetric Practice. The Apgar Score. *Pediatrics*, *117*(4), 1444–1447. PMID:16585348

American Academy of Pediatrics. (2008). Red Reflex Examination in Neonates, Infants, and Children. *Pediatrics*, *122*(6), 1401–1404. doi:10.1542/peds.2008-2624 PMID:19047263

American Clinical Neurophysiology Society. (2006). Guideline 9B: Guidelines on visual evoked potentials. *Journal of Clinical Neurophysiology*, *23*(2), 138–156. doi:10.1097/00004691-200604000-00011 PubMed

American Optometric Association. (2008). *Optometric Clinical Practice Guideline: Care of the Patient with Learning Related Vision Problems*. https://www.aoa.org/practice/clinical-guidelines/clinical-practice-guidelines?sso=y

American Optometric Association. (2017). *Comprehensive Pediatric Eye and Vision Examination: Evidence-based clinical practice guideline*. https://www.aoa.org/AOA/Documents/Practice%20Management/Clinical%20Guidelines/EBO%20Guidelines/Comprehensive%20Pediatric%20Eye%20and%20Vision%20Exam.pdf

American Optometric Association. (2017). *Evidence-Based Clinical Practice Guideline Comprehensive Pediatric Eye and Vision Examination*. Author.

American Optometric Association. (2017). *Evidence-Based Clinical Practice Guideline: Comprehensive Pediatric Eye and Vision Exam*. https://aoa.uberflip.com/i/807465-cpg-pediatric-eye-and-vision-examination/0?m4=

American Optometric Association. (2021a). *Preschool vision: 2 to 5 years of age*. https://ww1.aoa.org/healthy-eyes/eye-health-for-life/preschool-vision?sso=y

American Optometric Association. (2021b). *School-aged vision: 6 to 18 years of age*. https://www.aoa.org/healthy-eyes/eye-health-for-life/school-aged-vision?sso=y

Amos, J. F. (2001). Chapter 21 Cycloplegic Refraction. In Clinical Ocular Pharmacology (pp. 425-431). Butterworth-Heinemann.

Anderson, A.J., & Johnson, C.A. (2003). Frequency-doubling technology perimetry. *Ophthalmology Clinics of North America, 16*(2), 213-25.

Anderson, D. R. (1987). *Perimetry With and Without Automation* (2nd ed.). CV Mosby Company.

Arora, R., Austin, M., & Bellamy, H. (2014). Applanation tonometry: A comparison of the Perkins handheld and Goldmann slit lamp-mounted methods. *Clinical Ophthalmology*, 605–610. doi:10.2147/OPTH.S53544 PMID:24707165

Augeri P. A. (1991). Corneal foreign body removal and treatment. *Optometry Clinics: The Official Publication of the Prentice Society, 1*(4), 59–70.

Ayton, L. N., Abel, L. A., Fricke, T. R., & McBrien, N. A. (2009). Developmental eye movement test: What is it really measuring? *Optometry and Vision Science*, *86*(6), 722–730. doi:10.1097/OPX.0b013e3181a6a4b3 PMID:19417709

Bagheri, N. (2017a). *Trauma. In The Wills eye manual: Office and emergency room diagnosis and treatment of eye disease*. Wolters Kluwer.

Bagheri, N. (2017b). *Uveitis. In The Wills eye manual: Office and emergency room diagnosis and treatment of eye disease*. Wolters Kluwer.

Balcer, L. J. (2019). Pupillary disorders. In G. T. Liu, G. T. Volpe, & S. L. Galetta (Eds.), *Neuro-ophthalmology diagnosis and management* (3rd ed., pp. 417–421). Elsevier Inc.

Barrett, B. T. (2014). Assessment of binocular vision and accommodation. In D. B. Elliot (Ed.), *Clinical procedures in primary eye care* (4th ed., pp. 147–208). Elsevier Saunders.

Bartolone, A., & Rutner, D. (2020). Quantification of Refractive Error. In P. Schnell, M. Taub, & R. H. Duckman (Eds.), *Visual Development, Diagnosis, and Treatment of the Pediatric Patient* (pp. 300–316). Wolters Kluwer.

Bates, A., & Zanaboni, A. (2020). Ocular burns. *StatPearls*. https://www.ncbi.nlm.nih.gov/books/NBK459221/

Baum, J., Chaturvedi, N., Netland, P. A., & Dreyer, E. B. (1995). Assessment of Intraocular Pressure by Palpation. *American Journal of Ophthalmology, 119*(5), 650–651. doi:10.1016/S0002-9394(14)70227-2 PMID:7733191

Bausch & Lomb. (2019). *Tropicamide ophthalmic solution.* Retrieved on September 28, 2021, from https://www.bausch.com/Portals/77/-/m/BL/United%20States/Files/Package%20Inserts/Pharma/Rx-Generics/Tropicamide-package-insert.pdf?ver=2016-08-26-133847-873

Bausch & Lomb. (2021). *Cyclopentolate hydrochloride.* Retrieved on September 28, 2021, from https://www.bausch.com/Portals/77/-/m/BL/United%20States/Files/Package%20Inserts/Pharma/Rx-Generics/Cyclopentolate-Hydrochloride-Solution.pdf?ver=2016-09-13-101701-047

Bell, R. A., Waggoner, P. M., Boyd, W. M., Akers, R. E., & Yee, C. E. (1993). Clinical grading of relative afferent pupillary defects. *Archives of Ophthalmology, 111*(7), 938–942. doi:10.1001/archopht.1993.01090070056019 PMID:8328935

Benzoni, J. A., & Rosenfield, M. (2012). Clinical amplitude of accommodation in children between 5 and 10 years of age. *Optometry and Vision Development, 43*(3), 109–114.

Berntsen, D. A., Sinnott, L. T., Mutti, D. O., & Zadnik, K. (2012). A randomized trial using progressive addition lenses to evaluate theories of myopia progression in children with a high lag of accommodation. *Investigative Ophthalmology & Visual Science, 53*(2), 640–649. doi:10.1167/iovs.11-7769 PMID:22205604

Bieber, J. (1974). Why nearpoint retinoscopy with children. *The Optometric Weekly, 65*(3), 54–57.

Binenbaum, G. (2020, October 8). *Child abuse: Eye findings in children with abusive head trauma (AHT).* UpToDate. https://www.uptodate.com/contents/child-abuse-eye-findings-in-children-with-abusive-head-trauma-aht?search=ocular%20signs%20of%20child%20abuse&source=search_result&selectedTitle=7~150&usage_type=default&display_rank=7

Biousse, V., & Newman, N. J. (2009). *Neuro-Ophthalmology Illustrated* (1st ed.). Thieme.

Birch, J. (2001). *Diagnosis of defective colour vision* (2nd ed.). Butterworth-Heinemann.

Birnbaum, M. H. (1993). *Optometric management of nearpoint vision disorders.* Butterworth Heinemann.

Blansett, D. K. (2001). Dilation of pupil. In Clinical Ocular Pharmacology (pp. 405-421). Butterworth-Heinemann.

Borchert, M., Wang, Y., Tarczyy-Hornoch, K., Cotter, S., Deneen, J., Azen, S., & Varma, R.The Multi-Ethnic Pediatric Eye Disease Study Group. (2008). Testability of the Retinomax Autorefractor and IOL Master in preschool children. *Ophthalmology, 115*(8), 1422–1425. doi:10.1016/j.ophtha.2007.10.036 PMID:18164067

Bordoni, B., Mankowski, N. L., & Daly, D. T. (2021, February 7). *Neuroanatomy, Cranial Nerve 8 (Vestibulocochlear).* https://www.ncbi.nlm.nih.gov/books/NBK537359/

Boyd, K. (2020, July 8). *Vision development: Newborn to 12 months.* American Academy of Ophthalmology. https://www.aao.org/eye-health/tips-prevention/baby-vision-development-first-year

Brady, C. (2020). How to irrigate the eye and do eyelid eversion - Eye Disorders. In *Merck Manuals Professional Edition.* Merck Manuals. www.merckmanuals.com/professional/eye-disorders/how-to-do-eye-procedures/how-to-irrigate-the-eye-and-do-eyelid-eversion

Breazzano, M. P., Day, H. R. Jr, Tanaka, S., & Tran, U. (2018). Prospective analysis of pediatric ocular chemical burns: Laundry detergent pods. *Journal of American Association for Pediatric Ophthalmology and Strabismus, 22*(6), 426–428. doi:10.1016/j.jaapos.2018.07.349 PMID:30342182

Brown, L. (2011). *Identity-first language.* Autistic Self Advocacy Network. https://autisticadvocacy.org/about-asan/identity-first-language/

Brown, A. M. (1990). Development of visual sensitivity to light and color vision in human infants: A critical review. *Vision Research*, *30*(8), 1159–1188. doi:10.1016/0042-6989(90)90173-I PMID:2205977

Brown, D. J., Jaffe, J. E., & Henson, J. K. (2007). Advanced Laceration Management. *Emergency Medicine Clinics of North America*, *25*(1), 83–99. doi:10.1016/j.emc.2006.11.001 PMID:17400074

Cacho, P., Garcia, A., Lara, F., & Seguí, M. M. (2002). Diagnostic signs of accommodative insufficiency. *Optometry and Vision Science*, *79*(9), 614–620. doi:10.1097/00006324-200209000-00013 PMID:12322932

Cain, W., & Sinskey, R. M. (1981). Detection of Anterior Chamber Leakage With Seidel's Test. *Archives of Ophthalmology*, *99*(11), 2013. doi:10.1001/archopht.1981.03930020889015 PMID:7295152

Caloroso, E. E., & Rouse, M. W. (1993). *Clinical Management of Strabismus* (1st ed.). Butterworth-Heinemann.

Caloroso, E. E., & Rouse, M. W. (1993). *Clinical management of strabismus*. Butterworth-Heinemann.

Carlson, N. B., Kurtz, D., Heath, D., Capone, R. C., & Watanabe, R. K. (2004). Clinical procedures for ocular examination (3rd ed.). McGraw-Hill.

Carlson, N. B., & Kurtz, D. (2016). *Clinical Procedures for Ocular Examination* (4th ed.). McGraw-Hill.

Casser, L., Fingeret, M., & Woodcome, H. T. (1997a). Binocular Indirect Ophthalmoscopy. In *Atlas of Primary Eyecare Procedures* (2nd ed., pp. 226–229). Appleton & Lange.

Casser, L., Fingeret, M., & Woodcome, H. T. (1997b). Scleral Indentation. In *Atlas of Primary Eyecare Procedures* (2nd ed., pp. 234–237). Appleton & Lange.

Centers for Disease Control. (2021a). *CDC's developmental milestones*. https://www.cdc.gov/ncbddd/actearly/milestones/index.html

Centers for Disease Control. (2021b). *Communicating with and about people with disabilities*. https://www.cdc.gov/ncbddd/disabilityandhealth/materials/factsheets/fs-communicating-with-people.html

Cervino, A. (2006). Rebound tonometry: New opportunities and limitations of non-invasive determination of intraocular pressure. *The British Journal of Ophthalmology*, *90*(12), 1444–1446. doi:10.1136/bjo.2006.102970 PMID:17114589

Chamberlain, P., Peixoto-de-Matos, S. C., Logan, N. S., Ngo, C., Jones, D., & Young, G. (2019). A 3-year Randomized Clinical Trial of MiSight Lenses for Myopia Control. *Optometry and Vision Science*, *96*(8), 556–567. doi:10.1097/OPX.0000000000001410 PMID:31343513

Cheng, D., Woo, G. C., Drobe, B., & Schmid, K. L. (2014). Effect of bifocal and prismatic bifocal spectacles on myopia progression in children: Three-year results of a randomized clinical trial. *JAMA Ophthalmology*, *132*(3), 258–264. doi:10.1001/jamaophthalmol.2013.7623 PMID:24435660

Chia, A., Chua, W. H., Cheung, Y. B., Wong, W. L., Lingham, A., Fong, A., & Tan, D. (2012). Atropine for the treatment of childhood myopia: Safety and efficacy of 0.5%, 0.1%, and 0.01% doses (Atropine for the Treatment of Myopia 2). *Ophthalmology*, *119*(2), 347–354. doi:10.1016/j.ophtha.2011.07.031 PMID:21963266

Chia, A., Chua, W. H., Wen, L., Fong, A., Goon, Y. Y., & Tan, D. (2014). Atropine for the treatment of childhood myopia: Changes after stopping atropine 0.01%, 0.1% and 0.5%. *American Journal of Ophthalmology*, *157*(2), 451–457 e451. doi:10.1016/j.ajo.2013.09.020 PMID:24315293

Chiang, S. T., Turnbull, P. R. K., & Phillips, J. R. (2020). Additive effect of atropine eye drops and short-term retinal defocus on choroidal thickness in children with myopia. *Scientific Reports*, *10*(1), 18310. doi:10.103841598-020-75342-9 PMID:33110130

Child Welfare Information Gateway. (2019). *What Is Child Abuse and Neglect? Recognizing the Signs and Symptoms.* https://www.childwelfare.gov/pubPDFs/whatiscan.pdf

Choi, K. Y., Yu, W. Y., Lam, C. H. I., Li, Z. C., Chin, M. P., Lakshmanan, Y., Wong, F. S. Y., Do, C. W., Lee, P. H., & Chan, H. H. L. (2017). Childhood exposure to constricted living space: A possible environmental threat for myopia development. *Ophthalmic & Physiological Optics, 37*(5), 568–575. doi:10.1111/opo.12397 PMID:28643407

Chou, S. Y., & Digre, K. M. (1999). Neuro-ophthalmic complications of raised intracranial pressure, hydrocephalus, and shunt malfunction. *Neurosurgery Clinics of North America, 10*(4), 587–608. doi:10.1016/S1042-3680(18)30160-8 PMID:10529972

Christian, C. W., & Levin, A. V. (2018). The Eye Examination in the Evaluation of Child Abuse. *Pediatrics, 142*(2), e20181411. Advance online publication. doi:10.1542/peds.2018-1411 PMID:30037976

Chrousos, G. A., O'Neill, J. F., Lueth, B. D., & Parks, M. M. (1988). Accommodative deficiency in healthy young individuals. *Journal of Pediatric Ophthalmology and Strabismus, 25*(4), 176–179. doi:10.3928/0191-3913-19880701-07 PMID:3411421

Chua, S. Y., Sabanayagam, C., Cheung, Y. B., Chia, A., Valenzuela, R. K., Tan, D., Wong, T. Y., Cheng, C. Y., & Saw, S. M. (2016). Age of onset of myopia predicts risk of high myopia in later childhood in myopic Singapore children. *Ophthalmic & Physiological Optics, 36*(4), 388–394. doi:10.1111/opo.12305 PMID:27350183

Chua, W. H., Balakrishnan, V., Chan, Y. H., Tong, L., Ling, Y., Quah, B. L., & Tan, D. (2006). Atropine for the treatment of childhood myopia. *Ophthalmology, 113*(12), 2285–2291. doi:10.1016/j.ophtha.2006.05.062 PMID:16996612

Chung, I., & Buhr, V. (2000). Topical ophthalmic drugs and the pediatric patient. *Optometry (St. Louis, Mo.), 71*(8), 511–518. PMID:15326908

Chung, K., Mohidin, N., & O'Leary, D. J. (2002). Undercorrection of myopia enhances rather than inhibits myopia progression. *Vision Research, 42*(22), 2555–2559. doi:10.1016/S0042-6989(02)00258-4 PMID:12445849

Ciuffreda, K. J., & Tannen, B. (1995). *Eye movement basics for the clinician.* Mobsy.

Ciuffreda, M. A., Ciuffreda, K. J., & Santos, D. (2003). Visagraph baseline analysis and procedural guidelines. *Journal of Behavioral Optometry, 14*(3), 60–64.

Cochran, M. L., & Czyz, C. N. (2020, March 31). *Eyelid Laceration.* https://www.ncbi.nlm.nih.gov/books/NBK470367/

Colby, D., Laukkanen, H. R., & Yolton, R. L. (1998). Use of the Taylor Visagraph II system to evaluate eye movements made during reading. *Journal of the American Optometric Association, 69*(1), 22–32. PMID:9479933

Cole, C. H., Wright, K. W., Tarnow-Mordi, W., & Phelps, D. L. (2016). Resolving our uncertainty about oxygen therapy. *Pediatrics, 112*(6), 1415–1419. doi:10.1542/peds.112.6.1415 PMID:14654618

Committee for the Classification of Retinopathy of Prematurity. (1984). An International Classification of Retinopathy of Prematurity. *Archives of Ophthalmology, 102*(8), 1130–1134. doi:10.1001/archopht.1984.01040030908011 PMID:6547831

Committee on Vision. (1980). Recommended standard procedures for the clinical measurement and specification of visual acuity. Report of working group 39. Assembly of Behavioral and Social Sciences, National Research Council, National Academy of Sciences, Washington, D.C. *Advances in Ophthalmology, 41*, 103–148. https://www.ncbi.nlm.nih.gov/pubmed/7001873 PMID:7001873

Cooper, J., & Panariello, G. F. (1988). The pathognomonic pattern of accommodative fatigue in myasthenia gravis. *Binocular Vision & Strabismus Quarterly, 3*(3), 141–148.

COPAN Diagnostics Inc. (2019). *ESwab and Bacterial Keratitis*. www.copanusa.com/eswab-ophthalmology-diagnosing-bacterial-keratitis/

Cordero, I. (2016). Understanding and caring for the direct ophthalmoscope. *Community Eye Health Journal, 29*(93), 17. https://www.cehjournal.org/article/understanding-and-caring-for-the-direct-ophthalmoscope/

Cotter, S. A., Lee, D. Y., & French, A. L. (1999). Evaluation of a new color vision test: "color vision testing made easy. *Optometry and Vision Science*, *76*(9), 631–636. doi:10.1097/00006324-199909000-00020 PMID:10498004

Cotter, S. A., Tarczy-Hornoch, K., Song, E., Lin, J., Borchert, M., Azen, S. P., & Varma, R. (2009). Fixation preference and visual acuity testing in a population-based cohort of preschool children with amblyopia risk factors. *Ophthalmology*, *116*(1), 145–153. doi:10.1016/j.ophtha.2008.08.031 PMID:18962921

Coulter, R. A. (2004). Pediatric use of topical ophthalmic drugs. *Optometry (St. Louis, Mo.)*, *75*(7), 419–429. doi:10.1016/S1529-1839(04)70157-8 PMID:15296375

Coulter, R. A., & Shallo-Hoffman, J. (2000). The presumed influence of attention on accuracy in the Developmental Eye Movement (DEM) Test. *Optometry and Vision Science*, *77*(8), 428–432. doi:10.1097/00006324-200008000-00010 PMID:10966069

Courage, M. L., Adams, R. J., Reyno, S., & Kwa, P. G. (1994). Visual acuity in infants and children with Down syndrome. *Developmental Medicine and Child Neurology*, *36*(7), 586–593. doi:10.1111/j.1469-8749.1994.tb11895.x PMID:8034120

Crosby, N. J., Shepherd, D., & Murray, A. (2013). Mechanical testing of lid speculae and relationship to postoperative ptosis. *Eye (London, England)*, *27*(9), 1098–1101. doi:10.1038/eye.2013.133 PMID:23788211

Cryotherapy for Retinopathy of Prematurity Cooperative Group. (1988). Multicenter trial of cryotherapy for retinopathy of prematurity: Preliminary results. *Archives of Ophthalmology*, *106*(4), 471–479. doi:10.1001/archopht.1988.01060130517027 PMID:2895630

Dang, V. T. (2018, August 1). *Identifying ocular allergy*. Optometric Management. https://www.optometricmanagement.com/issues/2018/august-2018/identifying-ocular-allergy

Daum, K. M. (1983). Accommodative dysfunction. *Documenta Ophthalmologica*, *55*(3), 177–198. doi:10.1007/BF00140808 PMID:6884172

Davidson, T. M., & Murphy, C. (1997). Rapid Clinical Evaluation of Anosmia: The Alcohol Sniff Test. *Archives of Otolaryngology—Head & Neck Surgery*, *123*(6), 591–594. doi:10.1001/archotol.1997.01900060033005 PMID:9193218

Davies, L. N., Bartlett, H., Mallen, E. A. H., & Wolffsohn, J. S. (2006). Clinical evaluation of rebound tonometer. *Acta Ophthalmologica Scandinavica*, *84*(2), 206–209. doi:10.1111/j.1600-0420.2005.00610.x PMID:16637838

Delaney, S. M., Dobson, V., & Mohan, K. M. (2005). Measured visual field extent varies with peripheral stimulus flicker rate in very young children. *Optometry and Vision Science*, *82*(9), 800–886. doi:10.1097/01.opx.0000178059.39998.bd PMID:16189489

Delfaut, E. M., Beltran, J., Johnson, G., Rousseau, J., Marchandise, X., & Cotten, A. (1999). Fat Suppression in MR Imaging: Techniques and Pitfalls. *Radiographics*, *19*(2), 373–382. doi:10.1148/radiographics.19.2.g99mr03373 PMID:10194785

DeRespinis, P. A., Shen, J. J., & Wagner, R. S. (1989). Guillain-Barre syndrome presenting as a paralysis of accommodation. Case report. *Archives of Ophthalmology*, *105*(4), 508–512. doi:10.1001/archopht.1989.01070020352010 PMID:2783058

Devices@FDA PMA Supplement Bausch & Lomb Purevision (Balafilcon A) Visibility Tinted Contact Lenses-Therapeutic Use. (n.d.). *U.S. Food & Drug Administration.* https://www.accessdata.fda.gov/scripts/cdrh/devicesatfda/index.cfm?db=pma&id=333808

Devices@FDA PMA Supplement Night & Day 30 Night Extended Wear Soft Contact Lens. (n.d.). *U.S. Food & Drug Administration.* https://www.accessdata.fda.gov/scripts/cdrh/devicesatfda/index.cfm?db=pma&id=332525

Devices@FDA PMA Supplement Vistakon (Senofilcon A) Contact Lens Material. (n.d.). *U.S. Food & Drug Administration.* https://www.accessdata.fda.gov/scripts/cdrh/devicesatfda/index.cfm?db=pma&id=336147

Dinardo, A., & Walling, P. (2013). The Lost Arts of Optometry, Part One: A Refresher on Scleral Depression. *Review of Optometry.* Retrieved October 2, 2021, from https://www.reviewofoptometry.com/content/c/42459

Dobson, V., Clifford-Donaldson, C. E., Green, T. K., Miller, J. M., & Harvey, E. M. (2009). Normative monocular visual acuity for early treatment diabetic retinopathy study charts in emmetropic children 5 to 12 years of age. *Ophthalmology, 116*(7), 1397–1401. doi:10.1016/j.ophtha.2009.01.019 PMID:19427702

Dobson, V., Quinn, G. E., Tung, B., Palmer, E. A., & Reynolds, J. D. (1995). Comparison of recognition and grating acuities in very-low-birth-weight children with and without retinal residua of retinopathy of prematurity. Cryotherapy for Retinopathy of Prematurity Cooperative Group. *Investigative Ophthalmology & Visual Science, 36*(3), 692–702. PMID:7890499

Dobson, V., & Teller, D. Y. (1978). Visual acuity in human infants: A review and comparison of behavioral and electrophysiological studies. *Vision Research, 18*(11), 1469–1483. doi:10.1016/0042-6989(78)90001-9 PMID:364823

Doss, M., Egleston, B. L., & Litwin, S. (2012). Comments on "Studies of the Mortality of Atomic Bomb Survivors, Report 14, 1950–2003: An Overview of Cancer and Noncancer Diseases" (Radiat Res 2012; 177:229–43). *Radiation Research, 178*(3), 244–245. https://doi.org/10.1667/rr3039.1

Drobe, B., & de Saint-Andre, R. (1995). The pre-myopic syndrome. *Ophthalmic & Physiological Optics, 15*(5), 375–378. doi:10.1046/j.1475-1313.1995.9500075o.x PMID:8524558

Duckman, R. H. (2006). *Visual development, diagnosis, and treatment of the pediatric patient.* Lippincott Williams & Wilkins.

Elliott, D. B. (2007). *Clinical Procedures in Primary Eye Care: Expert Consult: Online and Print* (3rd ed.). Butterworth-Heinemann.

Elner, S. G., Elner, V. M., & Arnall, M. (1990). Ocular and Associated Systemic Findings in Suspected Child Abuse. *Archives of Ophthalmology, 108*(8), 1094. https://doi.org/10.1001/archopht.1990.01070100050033

Epley, K., Tychsen, L., & Lueder, G. T. (2002). The effect of an eyelid speculum on intraocular pressure measurement in children. *American Journal of Ophthalmology, 134*(6), 926–927. doi:10.10160002-9394(02)01793-2

Fantz, R. L. (1963). Pattern Vision in Newborn Infants. *Science, 140*(3564), 296–297. doi:10.1126cience.140.3564.296 PMID:17788054

Feng, C. S., Jin, K. W., Yi, K., & Choi, D. G. (2015). Comparison of Intraocular Pressure Measurements Obtained by Rebound, Noncontact, and Goldmann Applanation Tonometry in Children. *American Journal of Ophthalmology, 160*(5), 937–943.e1. doi:10.1016/j.ajo.2015.07.029 PMID:26210864

Fernandez-Velazquez, F. J., & Fernandez-Fidalgo, M. J. (1995). Do DEM test scores change with respect to the language? Norms for Spanish-speaking population. *Optometry and Vision Science, 72*(12), 902–906. doi:10.1097/00006324-199512000-00009 PMID:8749338

Fern, K. D., & Manny, R. E. (1986). Visual acuity of the preschool child: A review. *American Journal of Optometry and Physiological Optics*, *63*(5), 319–345. doi:10.1097/00006324-198605000-00003 PMID:3717284

Ficarra, A. P., Sorkin, R., & Morrison, C. (2002). Assessment of intraocular pressure in children by digital tension. *Optometry (St. Louis, Mo.)*, *73*(8), 499–506. PMID:12365673

Fierson, W. M. (2018). Screening Examination of Premature Infants for Retinopathy of Prematurity. *Pediatrics*, *142*(6), 1–11. doi:10.1542/peds.2018-3061 PMID:30478242

Flitcroft, D. I. (2012). The complex interactions of retinal, optical and environmental factors in myopia aetiology. *Progress in Retinal and Eye Research*, *31*(6), 622–660. doi:10.1016/j.preteyeres.2012.06.004 PMID:22772022

Flitcroft, D. I., Harb, E. N., & Wildsoet, C. F. (2020). The Spatial Frequency Content of Urban and Indoor Environments as a Potential Risk Factor for Myopia Development. *Investigative Ophthalmology & Visual Science*, *61*(11), 42. doi:10.1167/iovs.61.11.42 PMID:32986814

Frantz, R. L., Ordy, J., & Udelf, M. (1962). Maturation of pattern vision in infants during the first six months. *Journal of Comparative and Physiological Psychology*, *55*(6), 907–917. doi:10.1037/h0044173

Frazier, M., & Jaanus, S. D. (2008). Cycloplegic Refraction. In Clinical Ocular Pharmacology 5th Edition (pp.133). Butterworth Heinmann Elsevier.

French, A. N., Ashby, R. S., Morgan, I. G., & Rose, K. A. (2013). Time outdoors and the prevention of myopia. *Experimental Eye Research*, *114*, 58–68. doi:10.1016/j.exer.2013.04.018 PMID:23644222

Friendly, D. S. (1978). Preschool visual acuity screening tests. *Transactions of the American Ophthalmological Society*, *76*, 383–480. https://www.ncbi.nlm.nih.gov/pubmed/754379 PMID:754379

Friendly, D. S., Jaafar, M. S., & Morillo, D. L. (1990). A comparative study of grating and recognition visual acuity testing in children with anisometropic amblyopia without strabismus. *American Journal of Ophthalmology*, *110*(3), 293–299. doi:10.1016/S0002-9394(14)76347-0 PMID:2396655

Fulk, G. W., Cyert, L. A., & Parker, D. E. (2000). A randomized trial of the effect of single-vision vs. bifocal lenses on myopia progression in children with esophoria. *Optometry and Vision Science*, *77*(8), 395–401. doi:10.1097/00006324-200008000-00006 PMID:10966065

Galetta, K. M., Brandes, L. E., Maki, K., Dziemianowicz, M. S., Laudano, E., Allen, M., Lawler, K., Sennett, B., Wiebe, D., Devick, S., Messner, L., Galetta, S. L., & Balcer, L. J. (2011). The King-Devick test and sports-related concussion: Study of a rapid visual screening tool in a collegiate cohort. *Journal of the Neurological Sciences*, *309*(1-2), 34–39. doi:10.1016/j.jns.2011.07.039 PMID:21849171

Gallaway, M., Scheiman, M., & Mitchell, G. L. (2017). Vision therapy for post-concussion vision disorders. *Optometry and Vision Science*, *94*(1), 68–73. doi:10.1097/OPX.0000000000000935 PMID:27505624

Gandhi, N. G., Jones, S., Prakalapakorn, S. G., & Freedman, S. F. (2011). Icare ONE handheld rebound tonometry versus Goldmann applanation in children with known and suspected glaucoma. *American Journal of Ophthalmology*, *15*(1), 843–849.e1. doi:10.1016/j.ajo.2012.05.003 PMID:22840485

Gardiner, M. F. (2019). Eyelid lacerations. In T.W. Post, P. Rutgeerts, & S. Grover (Eds.), *UpToDate*. Available from https://www.uptodate.com/contents/eyelid-lacerations?search=eyelid%20laceratin&source=search_result&selectedTitle=1~12&usage_type=default&display_rank=1#H6664674

Gilbert, C., Rahi, J. S., & Quinn, G. E. (2003). *The Epidemiology of Eye Disease* (2nd ed.). Arnold.

Goldberg, C. (2018). *Practical guide to clinical medicine.* UCSD School of Medicine and VA Medical Center. https://meded.ucsd.edu/clinicalmed/ros.html

Good-lite. (2021). *Retinoscopy paddles with axis compass.* Retrieved on September 28, 2021, from https://www.good-lite.com/products/506600

Good, W. (2004). Final results of the early treatment for retinopathy of prematurity (ETROP) randomized trial. *Transactions of the American Ophthalmological Society, 102*, 233–250. PMID:15747762

Gorman, J. J., Cogan, D. G., & Gellis, S. S. (1957). An apparatus for grading the visual acuity of infants on the basis of opticokinetic nystagmus. *Pediatrics, 19*(6), 1088–1092. PMID:13441362

Graf, M. H., Becker, R., & Kaufmann, H. (2000). Lea symbols: Visual acuity assessment and detection of amblyopia. *Graefes Archive for Clinical and Experimental Ophthalmology, 238*(1), 53–58. doi:10.1007004170050009 PMID:10664053

Graham, R., Rivara, F. P., Ford, M. A., & Spicer, C. M. (2014). *Sports-related concussions in youth: Improving the science, changing the culture*. The National Academies Press.

Griffin, J. R., & Borsting, E. J. (2010). *Binocular anomalies: theory, testing, and therapy* (5th ed., Vol. 1). Optometric Extension Program Foundation, Inc.

Grigorian, F., Grigorian, A. P., Li, A., Sattar, A., Krishna, R., & Olitsky, S. E. (2015). Comparison of the Icare rebound tonometry with the Goldmann applanation tonometry in a pediatric population. *Journal of American Association for Pediatric Ophthalmology and Strabismus, 19*(6), 572–574. doi:10.1016/j.jaapos.2015.08.009 PMID:26691047

Guier, C. P., & Thomas, S. J. (2021, February 13). *Cornea foreign body removal.* https://www.ncbi.nlm.nih.gov/books/NBK554478/

Gulden Ophthalmics. (2021). *Disposable spray caps (12 pack).* https://guldenophthalmics.com/product/disposable-spray-cap/

Gulden Ophthalmics. (2021). *Disposable spray caps video.* https://guldenophthalmics.com/video/disposable-spray-caps/

Gwiazda, J., Bauer, J., Thorn, F., & Held, R. (1995). A dynamic relationship between myopia and blur-driven accommodation in school-aged children. *Vision Research, 35*(9), 1299–1304. doi:10.1016/0042-6989(94)00238-H PMID:7610590

Gwiazda, J., Grice, K., & Thorn, F. (1999). Response AC/A ratios are elevated in myopic children. *Ophthalmic & Physiological Optics, 19*(2), 173–179. doi:10.1046/j.1475-1313.1999.00437.x PMID:10615453

Gwiazda, J., Hyman, L., Dong, L. M., Everett, D., Norton, T., Kurtz, D., Manny, R., Marsh-Tootle, W., Scheiman, M., & Comet, G. (2007). Factors associated with high myopia after 7 years of follow-up in the Correction of Myopia Evaluation Trial (COMET) Cohort. *Ophthalmic Epidemiology, 14*(4), 230–237. doi:10.1080/01658100701486459 PMID:17896302

Gwiazda, J., Hyman, L., Hussein, M., Everett, D., Norton, T. T., Kurtz, D., Leske, M. C., Manny, R., Marsh-Tootle, W., & Scheiman, M. (2003). A randomized clinical trial of progressive addition lenses versus single vision lenses on the progression of myopia in children. *Investigative Ophthalmology & Visual Science, 44*(4), 1492–1500. doi:10.1167/iovs.02-0816 PMID:12657584

Gwiazda, J., Thorn, F., & Held, R. (2005). Accommodation, accommodative convergence, and response AC/A ratios before and at the onset of myopia in children. *Optometry and Vision Science, 82*(4), 273–278. doi:10.1097/01.OPX.0000159363.07082.7D PMID:15829855

Haag-Strait, U. K. (2020). *Perkins Mk3 Tonometer Brochure.* https://www.haag-streit.com/fileadmin/Haag-Streit_UK/Downloads/CCO_downloads/Perkins_downloads/Perkins_brochure.pdf

Haegerström-Portnoy, G. (1990). Color Vision. In A. A. Rosenbloom & M. W. Morgan (Eds.), *Principles and Practice of Pediatric Optometry* (pp. 449–466). J.B. Lippincott Company.

Haring, R. S., Sheffield, I. D., Channa, R., Canner, J. K., & Schneider, E. B. (2016). Epidemiologic trends of chemical ocular burns in the United States. *JAMA Ophthalmology, 134*(10), 1119. doi:10.1001/jamaophthalmol.2016.2645

Harvey, E. M., Dobson, V., Luna, B., & Scher, M. S. (1997). Grating acuity and visual-field development in children with intraventricular hemorrhage. *Developmental Medicine and Child Neurology, 39*(5), 305–312. doi:10.1111/j.1469-8749.1997.tb07436.x PMID:9236696

Haynes, H. M. (1960). Clinical observations with dynamic retinoscopy. *The Optometric Weekly, 51*, 2243–2246, 2306–2309.

Haynes, H. M. (1985). Clinical approaches to nearpoint lens power determination. *American Journal of Optometry and Physiological Optics, 62*(6), 375–385. doi:10.1097/00006324-198506000-00004 PMID:4014425

Haynes, H. M., White, B. L., & Held, R. (1965). Visual accommodation in human infants. *Science, 148*(3669), 528–530. doi:10.1126cience.148.3669.528 PMID:14263778

Hedin, A., Nyman, K. G., & Derouet, B. (1980). A modified letter matching chart for testing young children's visual acuity. *Journal of Pediatric Ophthalmology and Strabismus, 17*(2), 114–118. doi:10.3928/0191-3913-19800301-13 PMID:7391898

Heijl, A., Lindgren, G., & Olsson, J. (1987). A package for the statistical analysis of computerized visual fields. *Documenta Ophthalmologica, 49*, 153–168. doi:10.1007/978-94-009-3325-5_23

Heijl, A., & Patella, V. M. (2002). *The Field Analyzer Primer: Essential Perimetry* (3rd ed.). Carl Zeiss Meditec.

He, M., Xiang, F., Zeng, Y., Mai, J., Chen, Q., Zhang, J., Smith, W., Rose, K., & Morgan, I. G. (2015). Effect of Time Spent Outdoors at School on the Development of Myopia Among Children in China: A Randomized Clinical Trial. *Journal of the American Medical Association, 314*(11), 1142–1148. doi:10.1001/jama.2015.10803 PMID:26372583

Hennessey, D., Iosue, R. A., & Rouse, M. W. (1984). Relation of symptoms to accommodative infacility in school-aged children. *American Journal of Optometry and Physiological Optics, 61*(3), 177–183. doi:10.1097/00006324-198403000-00005 PMID:6720863

Hokoda, S. C., & Ciuffreda, K. J. (1982). Measurement of accommodative amplitude in amblyopia. *Ophthalmic & Physiological Optics, 2*(3), 205–212. doi:10.1111/j.1475-1313.1982.tb00178.x PMID:7177646

Holden, B. A., Fricke, T. R., Wilson, D. A., Jong, M., Naidoo, K. S., Sankaridurg, P., Wong, T. Y., Naduvilath, T. J., & Resnikoff, S. (2016). Global Prevalence of Myopia and High Myopia and Temporal Trends from 2000 through 2050. *Ophthalmology, 123*(5), 1036–1042. doi:10.1016/j.ophtha.2016.01.006 PMID:26875007

Holmes, J. M., Mutyala, S., Maus, T. L., Grill, R., Hodge, D. O., & Gray, D. T. (1999). Pediatric third, fourth, and sixth nerve palsies: A population-based study. *American Journal of Ophthalmology, 127*(4), 388–392. doi:10.1016/S0002-9394(98)00424-3 PMID:10218690

Home Vision Care. (1994). *Color vision testing made easy*. Terry L. Waggoner.

Howell, A. (2020, November 15). Accident or child abuse? *Optometry Times*. https://www.optometrytimes.com/view/accident-or-child-abuse

Huang, J., Mutti, D. O., Jones-Jordan, L. A., & Walline, J. J. (2019). Bifocal & Atropine in Myopia Study: Baseline Data and Methods. *Optometry and Vision Science, 96*(5), 335–344. doi:10.1097/OPX.0000000000001378 PMID:31046016

Hua, W. J., Jin, J. X., Wu, X. Y., Yang, J. W., Jiang, X., Gao, G. P., & Tao, F. B. (2015). Elevated light levels in schools have a protective effect on myopia. *Ophthalmic & Physiological Optics*, *35*(3), 252–262. doi:10.1111/opo.12207 PMID:25913873

Hwang, J. Y., Yoon, H. K., Lee, J. H., Yoon, H. M., Jung, A. Y., Cho, Y. A., Lee, J. S., & Yoon, C. H. (2016). Cranial Nerve Disorders in Children: MR Imaging Findings. *Radiographics*, *36*(4), 1178–1194. https://doi.org/10.1148/rg.2016150163

Hyvarinen, L., Nasanen, R., & Laurinen, P. (1980). New visual acuity test for pre-school children. *Acta Ophthalmologica*, *58*(4), 507–511. doi:10.1111/j.1755-3768.1980.tb08291.x PMID:7211248

Ismail, E. E., Rouse, M. W., & De Land, P. N. (1994, April). A Comparison of drop instillation and spray application of 1% cyclopentolate hydrochloride. *Optometry and Vision Science*, *71*(4), 235–241. doi:10.1097/00006324-199404000-00001 PMID:8047334

Iuorno, J., Grant, W., & Noel, L. P. (2004). Clinical Comparison of the Welch Allyn SureSight Handheld Autorefractor Versus Cycloplegic Autorefraction and Retinoscopic Refraction. *Journal of AAPOS*, *8*(2), 123–127. doi:10.1016/j.jaapos.2003.10.006 PMID:15088044

Jacobsen, N., Jensen, H., & Goldschmidt, E. (2008). Does the level of physical activity in university students influence development and progression of myopia? A 2-year prospective cohort study. *Investigative Ophthalmology & Visual Science*, *49*(4), 1322–1327. doi:10.1167/iovs.07-1144 PMID:18385044

Jin, J. X., Hua, W. J., Jiang, X., Wu, X. Y., Yang, J. W., Gao, G. P., Fang, Y., Pei, C. L., Wang, S., Zhang, J. Z., Tao, L. M., & Tao, F. B. (2015). Effect of outdoor activity on myopia onset and progression in school-aged children in northeast China: The Sujiatun Eye Care Study. *BMC Ophthalmology*, *15*(1), 73. doi:10.118612886-015-0052-9 PMID:26152123

Jones-Jordan, L. A., Mitchell, G. L., Cotter, S. A., Kleinstein, R. N., Manny, R. E., Mutti, D. O., Twelker, J. D., Sims, J. R., Zadnik, K., & Group, C. S. (2011). Visual activity before and after the onset of juvenile myopia. *Investigative Ophthalmology & Visual Science*, *52*(3), 1841–1850. doi:10.1167/iovs.09-4997 PMID:20926821

Jones, L. A., Sinnott, L. T., Mutti, D. O., Mitchell, G. L., Moeschberger, M. L., & Zadnik, K. (2007). Parental history of myopia, sports and outdoor activities, and future myopia. *Investigative Ophthalmology & Visual Science*, *48*(8), 3524–3532. doi:10.1167/iovs.06-1118 PMID:17652719

Kanehara & Co. Ltd. (1997). The series of plates designed to test for colour-deficiency. Tokyo, Japan: Shinobu Ishihara.

Kanski, J. J., Bowling, B., Nischal, K. K., & Pearson, A. (2011). *Clinical Ophthalmology* (7th ed.). Elsevier Saunders.

Kardon, R. (2008). The pupils and accommodation. In D. M. Albert & J. W. Miller (Eds.), *Albert & Jakobiec's. Principles and practice of ophthalmology* (pp. 4029–4048). Elsevier Inc. doi:10.1016/B978-1-4160-0016-7.50296-4

Kauser, F., Gupta, Y., Amitava, A., Saxena, J., Raza, S., & Masood, A. (2020). Do all children need a cycloplegic refraction? A comparison of Mohindra's versus cycloplegic refraction. *Indian Journal of Ophthalmology*, *68*(11), 2458. doi:10.4103/ijo.IJO_229_20 PMID:33120640

Keifenheim, K. E., Teufel, M., Ip, J., Speiser, N., Leehr, E. J., Zipfel, S., & Herrmann-Werner, A. (2015). Teaching history taking to medical students: A systematic review. *BMC Medical Education*, *15*(1), 159. doi:10.118612909-015-0443-x PMID:26415941

Kelly, K. R., Jost, R. M., De La Cruz, A., & Birch, E. E. (2015). Amblyopic children read more slowly than controls under natural, binocular reading conditions. *Journal of American Association for Pediatric Ophthalmology and Strabismus*, *19*(6), 515–520. doi:10.1016/j.jaapos.2015.09.002 PMID:26610788

Kempf, R., Kurita, Y., Iida, Y., Kaneko, M., Mishima, H. K., Tsukamoto, H., & Sugimoto, E. (2006, August). Understanding eye deformation in non-contact tonometry. In *2006 International Conference of the IEEE Engineering in Medicine and Biology Society*. EMBS Annual International Conference. 10.1109/IEMBS.2006.259905

Kim, S. K., Wang, K. C., Hwang, Y. S., Kim, K. J., Chae, J. H., Kim, I. O., & Cho, B. K. (2008). Epilepsy surgery in children: Outcomes and Complications. *Journal of Neurosurgery. Pediatrics*, *1*(4), 277–283. doi:10.3171/PED/2008/1/4/277 PMID:18377302

Kinoshita, N., Konno, Y., Hamada, N., Kanda, Y., Shimmura-Tomita, M., & Kakehashi, A. (2018). Additive effects of orthokeratology and atropine 0.01% ophthalmic solution in slowing axial elongation in children with myopia: First year results. *Japanese Journal of Ophthalmology*, *62*(5), 544–553. doi:10.100710384-018-0608-3 PMID:29974278

Kirstein, E. M., Lsheikh, A., & Gunvant, P. (2011). Tonometry – Past, Present and Future. In Glaucoma - Current Clinical and Research Aspects (pp. 85–108). Intech. doi:10.5772/37393

Kocabeyoglu, S., Uzum, S., Mocan, M. C., Bozkurt, B., Irkec, M., & Orhan, M. (2013). Comparison of visual field test results obtained through Humphrey Matrix Frequency doubling technology perimetry versus standard automated perimetry in healthy children. *Indian Journal of Ophthalmology*, *61*(10), 276–279. PMID:24145558

Konan Medical. (2021). *objectiveFIELDTM Objective Field Analyzer (OFATM)*. Retrieved October 17, 2021, from https://www.konanmedical.com/objectivefield

Kong, J., Johnson, C., Kran, B., Wright, D., & Mayer, L. (2009). *Assessment of Visual Fields in Deafblind Children* [Poster presentation]. American Academy of Optometry. https://www.aaopt.org/detail/knowledge-base-article/assessment-visual-fields-deafblind-children

Kontiola, A. (1997). A new electromechanical method for measuring intraocular pressure. *Documenta Ophthalmologica*, *93*(3), 265–276. doi:10.1007/BF02569066 PMID:9550354

Kulp, M. T., & Mitchell, G. L. (2005). Randot stereoacuity testing in young children. *Journal of Pediatric Ophthalmology and Strabismus*, *42*(6), 360–364. doi:10.3928/01913913-20051101-05

Kushner, B. J., Lucchese, N. J., & Morton, G. V. (1995). Grating visual acuity with Teller cards compared with Snellen visual acuity in literate patients. *Archives of Ophthalmology*, *113*(4), 485–493. doi:10.1001/archopht.1995.01100040107035 PMID:7710400

Lam, B. L., Thompson, H. S., & Corbett, J. J. (1987). The prevalence of simple anisocoria. *American Journal of Ophthalmology*, *104*(1), 69–73. doi:10.1016/0002-9394(87)90296-0 PMID:3605282

Lam, C. S. Y., Tang, W. C., Tse, D. Y., Lee, R. P. K., Chun, R. K. M., Hasegawa, K., Qi, H., Hatanaka, T., & To, C. H. (2020). Defocus Incorporated Multiple Segments (DIMS) spectacle lenses slow myopia progression: A 2-year randomised clinical trial. *The British Journal of Ophthalmology*, *104*(3), 363–368. doi:10.1136/bjophthalmol-2018-313739 PMID:31142465

Lam, C. S., Tang, W. C., Tse, D. Y., Tang, Y. Y., & To, C. H. (2014). Defocus Incorporated Soft Contact (DISC) lens slows myopia progression in Hong Kong Chinese schoolchildren: A 2-year randomised clinical trial. *The British Journal of Ophthalmology*, *98*(1), 40–45. doi:10.1136/bjophthalmol-2013-303914 PMID:24169657

Lam, S. R., LaRoche, G. R., De Becker, I., & Macpherson, H. (1996). The range and variability of ophthalmological parameters in normal children aged 4 1/2 to 5 1/2 years. *Journal of Pediatric Ophthalmology and Strabismus*, *33*(5), 251–256. doi:10.3928/0191-3913-19960901-10 PMID:8880619

Leat, S. J. (2009). Paediatric Assessment. In Optometry: Science, Techniques and Clinical Management (pp. 451-453). Butterworth Heinemann.

Leat, S. J., Yadav, N. K., & Irving, E. L. (2009). Development of visual acuity and contrast sensitivity in children. *Journal of Optometry*, *2*(1), 19–26. doi:10.3921/joptom.2009.19

Lessell, S., & Kim, J. W. (2008). Clinical examination. In D. M. Albert & J. W. Miller (Eds.), *Albert & Jakobiec's. Principles and practice of ophthalmology* (pp. 3813–3816). Elsevier Inc. doi:10.1016/B978-1-4160-0016-7.50281-2

Lim, L., & Lim, E. W. L. (2020). Therapeutic Contact Lenses in the Treatment of Corneal and Ocular Surface Diseases - A Review. *Asia-Pacific Journal of Ophthalmology*, *9*(6), 524–532. https://doi.org/10.1097/apo.0000000000000331

Lin, L. L., Shih, Y. F., Hsiao, C. K., & Chen, C. J. (2004). Prevalence of myopia in Taiwanese schoolchildren: 1983 to 2000. *Annals of the Academy of Medicine, Singapore*, *33*(1), 27–33. https://www.ncbi.nlm.nih.gov/pubmed/15008558 PMID:15008558

Li, S. Y., Li, S. M., Zhou, Y. H., Liu, L. R., Li, H., Kang, M. T., Zhan, S. Y., Wang, N., & Millodot, M. (2015). Effect of undercorrection on myopia progression in 12-year-old children. *Graefes Archive for Clinical and Experimental Ophthalmology*, *253*(8), 1363–1368. doi:10.100700417-015-3053-8 PMID:26032395

London, R. (2020). Evaluation of ocular motor function. In P. H. Schnell, M. B. Taub, & R. H. Duckman (Eds.), *Visual development, diagnosis, and treatment of the pediatric patient* (2nd ed., pp. 336–353). Wolters Kluwer.

Lorch, M., & Teach, S. J. (2010). Facial Nerve Palsy. *Pediatric Emergency Care*, *26*(10), 763–769. https://doi.org/10.1097/pec.0b013e3181f3bd4a

Maples, W. C. (2017). Oculomotor dysfunctions: Classification of saccadic and pursuit deficiencies. In L. J. Press (Ed.), *Applied concepts in vision therapy* (pp. 262–292). Ridgevue Publishing.

Maples, W. C., Atchley, J., & Ficklin, T. (1992). Northeastern State University College of Optometry's oculomotor norms. *Journal of Behavioral Optometry*, *3*(6), 143–150.

Maples, W. C., & Ficklin, T. W. (1988). Interrater and test-retest reliability of pursuits and saccades. *Journal of the American Optometric Association*, *59*(7), 549–552. PMID:3403903

Master, C. L., Scheiman, M., Gallaway, M., Goodman, A., Robinson, R. L., Master, S. R., & Grady, M. F. (2016). Vision diagnoses are common after concussion in adolescents. *Clinical Pediatrics*, *55*(3), 260–267. doi:10.1177/0009922815594367 PMID:26156977

Mayer, D. L., Beiser, A. S., Warner, A. F., Pratt, E. M., Raye, K. N., & Lang, J. M. (1995). Monocular acuity norms for the Teller Acuity Cards between ages one month and four years. *Investestigative Ophthalmology & Visual Science*, *36*(3), 671-685. https://www.ncbi.nlm.nih.gov/pubmed/7890497

Mayer, D. L. (1986). Acuity of amblyopic children for small field gratings and recognition stimuli. *Investigative Ophthalmology & Visual Science*, *27*(7), 1148–1153. https://www.ncbi.nlm.nih.gov/pubmed/3721793 PMID:3721793

Mayer, D. L., & Fulton, A. B. (2004). *Pediatric Ophthalmology & Strabismus*. Elsevier Science Limited.

Mayer, D. L., Fulton, A. B., & Rodier, D. (1984). Grating and recognition acuities of pediatric patients. *Ophthalmology*, *91*(8), 947–953. doi:10.1016/S0161-6420(84)34209-9 PMID:6493704

McCulloch, D. L., Orbach, H., & Skarf, B. (1999). Maturation of the pattern-reversal VEP in human infants: A theoretical framework. *Vision Research*, *39*(22), 3673–3680. doi:10.1016/S0042-6989(99)00091-7 PMID:10746137

McCulloch, D. L., & Skarf, B. (1991). Development of the human visual system: Monocular and binocular pattern VEP latency. *Investigative Ophthalmology & Visual Science*, *32*(8), 2372–2381. https://www.ncbi.nlm.nih.gov/pubmed/2071348 PMID:2071348

McCullough, S. J., Doyle, L., & Saunders, K. J. (2017). Intra- and inter- examiner repeatability of cycloplegic retinoscopy among young children. *Ophthalmic & Physiological Optics*, *37*(1), 16–23. doi:10.1111/opo.12341 PMID:28030881

McDougal, D. H., & Gamlin, P. D. (2015). Autonomic control of the eye. *Comprehensive Physiology*, *5*(1), 439–473. PMID:25589275

McKee, S. P., Levi, D. M., & Movshon, J. A. (2003). The pattern of visual deficits in amblyopia. *Journal of Vision (Charlottesville, Va.)*, *3*(5), 380–405. doi:10.1167/3.5.5 PMID:12875634

Midelfart, A., Kinge, B., Midelfart, S., & Lydersen, S. (2002). Prevalence of refractive errors in young and middle-aged adults in Norway. *Acta Ophthalmologica Scandinavica*, *80*(5), 501–505. doi:10.1034/j.1600-0420.2002.800508.x PMID:12390161

Miller, N. R., Newman, N. J., Biousse, V., & Kerrison, J. B. (2008). *Walsh and Hoyt's Clinical neuro-ophthalmology: The essentials* (2nd ed.). Wolters Kluwer.

Mohney, B. G., & Holmes, J. M. (2006). An Office-Based Scale for Assessment Control in Intermittent Exotropia. *Strabismus*, *14*(3), 147–150. doi:10.1080/09273970600894716 PMID:16950743

Mohn, G., & Van Hof-van Duin, J. (1986). Development of the binocular and monocular visual fields of human infants during the first year of life. *Clinical Vision Sciences*, *1*, 51–64.

Molia, L., Winterkorn, J. M., & Schneider, S. J. (1996). Hemianopic visual field defects in children with intracranial shunts: Report of two cases. *Neurosurgery*, *39*, 599–603. PMID:8875494

Monaghan, M., Brogan, K., Lockington, D., Rotchford, A. P., & Ramaesh, K. (2019). Variability in measuring pH using litmus paper and the relevance in Ocular Chemical injury. *Eye (London, England)*, *34*(11), 2133–2134. doi:10.103841433-019-0737-z

Moskowitz, A., & Sokol, S. (1983). Developmental changes in the human visual system as reflected by the latency of the pattern reversal VEP. *Electroencephalography and Clinical Neurophysiology*, *56*(1), 1–15. doi:10.1016/0013-4694(83)90002-0 PMID:6190626

Moss, S. E., Klein, K., & Klein, B. E. K. (1987). Accommodative ability in younger-onset diabetics. *Archives of Ophthalmology*, *105*(4), 508–512. doi:10.1001/archopht.1987.01060040078037 PMID:3566603

Mutti, D. O., Jones, L. A., Moeschberger, M. L., & Zadnik, K. (2000). AC/A ratio, age, and refractive error in children. *Investigative Ophthalmology & Visual Science*, *41*(9), 2469–2478. https://www.ncbi.nlm.nih.gov/pubmed/10937556 PMID:10937556

Mutti, D. O., Mitchell, G. L., Jones-Jordan, L. A., Cotter, S. A., Kleinstein, R. N., Manny, R. E., Twelker, J. D., Zadnik, K., & Group, C. S. (2017). The Response AC/A Ratio Before and After the Onset of Myopia. *Investigative Ophthalmology & Visual Science*, *58*(3), 1594–1602. doi:10.1167/iovs.16-19093 PMID:28291868

Mutti, D. O., Mitchell, G. L., Moeschberger, M. L., Jones, L. A., & Zadnik, K. (2002). Parental myopia, near work, school achievement, and children's refractive error. *Investigative Ophthalmology & Visual Science*, *43*(12), 3633–3640. https://www.ncbi.nlm.nih.gov/pubmed/12454029 PMID:12454029

Nakatsuka, C., Hasebe, S., Nonaka, F., & Ohtsuki, H. (2005). Accommodative lag under habitual seeing conditions: Comparison between myopic and emmetropic children. *Japanese Journal of Ophthalmology*, *49*(3), 189–194. doi:10.100710384-004-0175-7 PMID:15944822

National Eye Institute. (2020). *Refractive Error.* Retrieved on September 28, 2021 from https://www.nei.nih.gov/learn-about-eye-health/eye-conditions-and-diseases/refractive-errors

National Research Council (US) Committee on Vision. (1981). *Procedures for Testing Color Vision: Report of Working Group 41.* Washington, DC: National Academies Press (US). Available from: https://www.ncbi.nlm.nih.gov/books/NBK217823/

Nemeth, J., Tapaszto, B., Aclimandos, W. A., Kestelyn, P., Jonas, J. B., De Faber, J. H. N., Januleviciene, I., Grzybowski, A., Nagy, Z. Z., Parssinen, O., Guggenheim, J. A., Allen, P. M., Baraas, R. C., Saunders, K. J., Flitcroft, D. I., Gray, L. S., Polling, J. R., Haarman, A. E., Tideman, J. W. L., ... Resnikoff, S. (2021). Update and guidance on management of myopia. European Society of Ophthalmology in cooperation with International Myopia Institute. *European Journal of Ophthalmology*, *1120672121998960*(3), 853–883. Advance online publication. doi:10.1177/1120672121998960 PMID:33673740

Nikita, E. (2017). *Osteoarchaeology: A Guide to the Macroscopic Study of Human Skeletal Remains* (1st ed.). Academic Press.

Norcia, A. M., & Tyler, C. W. (1985). Spatial frequency sweep VEP: Visual acuity during the first year of life. *Vision Research*, *25*(10), 1399–1408. doi:10.1016/0042-6989(85)90217-2 PMID:4090273

Olleyes. (2020). *Olleyes Virtual Visual Field Products.* Retrieved October 17, 2021, from https://olleyes.com/

Oxford Medical Education. (2016). *History Taking—Overview.* https://www.oxfordmedicaleducation.com/history/medical-general/

Pai, A. S.-I., Rose, K. A., Samarawickrama, C., Fotedar, R., Burlutsky, G., Varma, R., & Mitchell, P. (2012). Testability of refraction, stereopsis, and other ocular measures in preschool children: The Sydney Paediatric Eye Disease Study. *Journal of AAPOS*, *16*(2), 185–192. https://doi.org/10.1016/j.jaapos.2011.09.017

Park, K. A., Oh, S. Y., Min, J. H., Kim, B. J., & Kim, Y. (2019). Acquired onset of third, fourth, and sixth cranial nerve palsies in children and adolescents. *Eye (London, England)*, *33*(6), 965–973. doi:10.103841433-019-0353-y PMID:30760897

Parssinen, T. O. (1987). Relation between refraction, education, occupation, and age among 26- and 46-year-old Finns. *American Journal of Optometry and Physiological Optics*, *64*(2), 136–143. doi:10.1097/00006324-198702000-00010 PMID:3826288

Patel, D. E., Cumberland, P. M., Walters, B. C., Russell-Eggitt, I., & Rahi, J. S.OPTIC Study Group. (2015). Study of Optimal Perimetric Testing in Children (OPTIC): Feasibility, Reliability and Repeatability of Perimetry in Children. *PLoS One*, *10*(6), e0130895. doi:10.1371/journal.pone.0130895 PMID:26091102

Peterson, M. C., Holbrook, J. H., Von Hales, D., Smith, N. L., & Staker, L. V. (1992). Contributions of the history, physical examination, and laboratory investigation in making medical diagnoses. *The Western Journal of Medicine*, *156*(2), 163–165. PMID:1536065

Picken, D., Mann, W., & Rings, M. (2014). *Validation of a computerized color vision test* [Paper presentation]. *Aerospace Medical Conference*, San Diego, CA.

Pola, J. R., & Schnell, P. H. (2020). Eye movements. In P. H. Schnell, M. B. Taub, & R. H. Duckman (Eds.), *Visual development, diagnosis, and treatment of the pediatric patient* (2nd ed., pp. 79–99). Wolters Kluwer.

Precision Laboratories. (2020). *How should test strips be stored? | Precision Laboratories Test Strips*. https://www.preclaboratories.com/faq-items/how-should-test-strips-be-stored/

Prentiss, K. A., & Dorfman, D. H. (2008). Pediatric ophthalmology in the emergency department. *Emergency Medicine Clinics of North America*, *26*(1), 181–198. doi:10.1016/j.emc.2007.11.001

Preston, K. L., McDonald, M., Sebris, S. L., Dobson, V., & Teller, D. Y. (1987). Validation of the acuity card procedure for assessment of infants with ocular disorders. *Ophthalmology*, *94*(6), 644–653. doi:10.1016/S0161-6420(87)33398-6 PMID:3627713

Pullen, R. L. (2005). Checking for oculocephalic reflex. *Nursing*, *35*(6), 24. https://doi.org/10.1097/00152193-200506000-00016

Quinn, G. E., Dobson, V., Hardy, R. J., Tung, B., Palmer, M. D., & Good, W. V. (2011). Visual field extent at 6 years of age in children who had high-risk prethreshold retinopathy of prematurity. *Archives of Ophthalmology*, *129*(2), 127–132. doi:10.1001/archophthalmol.2010.360 PMID:21320954

Quinn, G. E., Dobson, V., Hardy, R. J., Tung, B., Phelps, D. L., & Palmer, M. D. (1996). Visual fields measured with double-arc perimetry in eyes with threshold retinopathy of prematurity from the Cryotherapy for Retinopathy of Prematurity Trial. *Ophthalmology*, *103*(9), 1432–1427. doi:10.1016/S0161-6420(96)30487-9 PMID:8841302

Racette, L., Fischer, M., Bebie, H., Hollo, G., Johnson, C. A., & Matsumoto, C. (2016). *Visual Field Digest: A guide to perimetry and the Octopus perimeter* (6th ed.). Haag-Streit AG.

Rahi, J. S., & Gilbert, C. E. (2005). *Pediatric Ophthalmology and Strabismus* (3rd ed.). Elsevier Saunders.

Reading, R. (2012). Radiation exposure from CT scans in childhood and subsequent risk of leukaemia and brain tumours: A retrospective cohort study. *Child: Care, Health and Development*, *38*(6), 910. https://doi.org/10.1111/cch.12006_2

Read, S. A., Collins, M. J., & Vincent, S. J. (2014). Light exposure and physical activity in myopic and emmetropic children. *Optometry and Vision Science*, *91*(3), 330–341. doi:10.1097/OPX.0000000000000160 PMID:24413273

Retinomax Autorefractor. (n.d.). http://www.righton-oph.com/en/product/objective/

Rezvan, F., Khabazkhoob, M., Fotouhi, A., Hashemi, H., Ostadimoghaddam, H., Heravian, J., Azizi, E., Khorasani, A. A., & Yekta, A. A. (2012). Prevalence of refractive errors among school children in Northeastern Iran. *Ophthalmic & Physiological Optics*, *32*(1), 25–30. doi:10.1111/j.1475-1313.2011.00879.x PMID:22023649

Richmond Products. (2002). *H.R.R. Pseudoisochromatic Plates*. Author.

Ritter, S., & Steiner, A. (2021). *Anomalies of visual sensorimotor function lab manual* (17th ed.). SUNY College of Optometry.

Robinson, J., Ellen, J., Hadel, B., & Lighthizer, N. (2016). *Collecting a corneal culture*. https://www.reviewofoptometry.com/article/collecting-a-corneal-culture

Rogan, D. T., & Fang, A. (2020, July 6). *Pediatric Facial Trauma*. https://www.ncbi.nlm.nih.gov/books/NBK558932/

Rose, K. A., Morgan, I. G., Ip, J., Kifley, A., Huynh, S., Smith, W., & Mitchell, P. (2008). Outdoor activity reduces the prevalence of myopia in children. *Ophthalmology*, *115*(8), 1279–1285. doi:10.1016/j.ophtha.2007.12.019 PMID:18294691

Rosenberg, E. E., Lussier, M. T., & Beaudoin, C. (1997). Lessons for clinicians from physician-patient communication literature. *Archives of Family Medicine*, *6*(3), 279–283. doi:10.1001/archfami.6.3.279 PMID:9161356

Rosenfield, M. (2016). Computer vision syndrome (a.k.a. digital eye strain). *Optometry in Practice*, *17*(1), 1–10.

Rosenfield, M., & Cohen, A. S. (1996). Repeatability of clinical measurements of the amplitude of accommodation. *Ophthalmic & Physiological Optics, 16*(3), 247–249. doi:10.1046/j.1475-1313.1996.95000933.x PMID:8977892

Rouse, M. W. (2006). Optometric assessment: visual efficiency problems. In M. M. Scheiman & M. W. Rouse (Eds.), *Optometric management of learning-related vision problems* (2nd ed., pp. 335–367). Mosby Elsevier.

Rudnicka, A. R., Kapetanakis, V. V., Wathern, A. K., Logan, N. S., Gilmartin, B., Whincup, P. H., Cook, D. G., & Owen, C. G. (2016). Global variations and time trends in the prevalence of childhood myopia, a systematic review and quantitative meta-analysis: Implications for aetiology and early prevention. *The British Journal of Ophthalmology, 100*(7), 882–890. doi:10.1136/bjophthalmol-2015-307724 PMID:26802174

Rydberg, A., Ericson, B., Lennerstrand, G., Jacobson, L., & Lindstedt, E. (1999). Assessment of visual acuity in children aged 1 1/2-6 years, with normal and subnormal vision. *Strabismus, 7*(1), 1–24. doi:10.1076tra.7.1.1.656 PMID:10401500

Sankaridurg, P. R., & Holden, B. A. (2014). Practical applications to modify and control the development of ametropia. *Eye (London, England), 28*(2), 134–141. doi:10.1038/eye.2013.255 PMID:24310242

Saunders, K. J., & Westall, C. A. (1992). Comparison between near retinoscopy and cycloplegic retinoscopy in the refraction of infants and children. *Optometry and Vision Science, 69*(8), 615–622. doi:10.1097/00006324-199208000-00004 PMID:1513557

Saw, S. M., Tan, S. B., Fung, D., Chia, K. S., Koh, D., Tan, D. T., & Stone, R. A. (2004). IQ and the association with myopia in children. *Investigative Ophthalmology & Visual Science, 45*(9), 2943–2948. doi:10.1167/iovs.03-1296 PMID:15326105

Scheiman, M., Cotter, S., Kulp, M.T., Mitchell, G.L., Cooper, J., Gallaway, M., Hopkins, K.B., Bartuccio, M., & Chung, I., the Convergence Insufficiency Treatment Trial Study Group. (2011). Treatment of accommodative dysfunction in children: Results from a random clinical trial. *Optometry and Vision Science: Official Publication of the American Academy of Optometry, 88*(11), 1343-1352. . doi:10.1097/OPX.0b013e31822f4d7c

Scheiman, M., Herzberg, H., Frantz, K., & Margolies, M. (1988). Normative study of accommodative facility in elementary school children. *American Journal of Optometry and Physiological Optics, 65*(2), 127–134. doi:10.1097/00006324-198802000-00009 PMID:3364515

Scheiman, M., & Wick, B. (2019). *Clinical Management of Binocular Vision Heterophoric, Accommodative, and Eye Movement Disorders* (5th ed.). Lippincott Williams & Wilkins.

Scheiman, M., & Wick, B. (Eds.). (2020). *Clinical management of binocular vision: Heterophoric, accommodative, and eye movement disorders* (5th ed.). Wolters Kluwer.

Scher, M. S., Dobson, V., Carpenter, N. A., & Guthrie, R. D. (1989). Visual and neurological outcome of infants with periventricular leukomalacia. *Developmental Medicine and Child Neurology, 31*(3), 353–365. doi:10.1111/j.1469-8749.1989.tb04004.x PMID:2753239

Schlange, D. G., & Maino, D. M. (2001). Clinical behavioral objectives: Assessment techniques for special populations. In D. M. Maino (Ed.), *Diagnosis and management of special populations* (pp. 151–188). Mosby-Year Book, Inc.

Sener, E. C., Mocan, M. C., Gedik, S., Ergin, A., & Sanac, A. S. (2002). The reliability of grading the fixation preference test for the assessment of interocular visual acuity differences in patients with strabismus. [JAAPOS]. *Journal of American Association for Pediatric Ophthalmology and Strabismus, 6*(3), 191–194. doi:10.1067/mpa.2002.122364 PMID:12075297

Shih, Y. F., Chen, C. H., Chou, A. C., Ho, T. C., Lin, L. L., & Hung, P. T. (1999). Effects of different concentrations of atropine on controlling myopia in myopic children. *Journal of Ocular Pharmacology and Therapeutics, 15*(1), 85–90. doi:10.1089/jop.1999.15.85 PMID:10048351

Shih, Y. F., Hsiao, C. K., Chen, C. J., Chang, C. W., Hung, P. T., & Lin, L. L. (2001). An intervention trial on efficacy of atropine and multi-focal glasses in controlling myopic progression. *Acta Ophthalmologica Scandinavica, 79*(3), 233–236. doi:10.1034/j.1600-0420.2001.790304.x PMID:11401629

Skoczenski, A. M., & Norcia, A. M. (1999). Development of VEP Vernier acuity and grating acuity in human infants. *Investigative Ophthalmology & Visual Science, 40*(10), 2411–2417. https://www.ncbi.nlm.nih.gov/pubmed/10476810 PMID:10476810

Slovis, T. L., & Berdon, W. E. (1999). Editorial. *Pediatric Radiology, 29*(2), 79. https://doi.org/10.1007/s002470050544

Spry, P. G. D., Johnson, C. A., Anderson, A. J., Gunvant, P., Fingeret, M., Keltner, J. L., Wall, M., & Werner, J. S. (2008). *A Primer for Frequency Doubling Technology (FDT) Perimetry Using the Humphrey Matrix*. Carl Zeiss Meditec.

Subhi, Y., Schmidt, D. C., Al-Bakri, M., Bach-Holm, D., & Kessel, L. (2021). Diagnostic Test Accuracy of the Red Reflex Test for Ocular Pathology in Infants. *JAMA Ophthalmology, 139*(1), 33–40. doi:10.1001/jamaophthalmol.2020.4854 PMID:33180103

Suharwardy, J., & Elson, J. (1997). The clinical presentation of children with tumours affecting the anterior visual pathways. *Eye (London, England), 11*(6), 838–844. doi:10.1038/eye.1997.215 PMID:9537141

Sun, J., Zhou, J., Zhao, P., Lian, J., Zhu, H., Zhou, Y., Sun, Y., Wang, Y., Zhao, L., Wei, Y., Wang, L., Cun, B., Ge, S., & Fan, X. (2012). High prevalence of myopia and high myopia in 5060 Chinese university students in Shanghai. *Investigative Ophthalmology & Visual Science, 53*(12), 7504–7509. doi:10.1167/iovs.11-8343 PMID:23060137

Sun, Y. Y., Li, S. M., Li, S. Y., Kang, M. T., Liu, L. R., Meng, B., Zhang, F. J., Millodot, M., & Wang, N. (2017). Effect of uncorrection versus full correction on myopia progression in 12-year-old children. *Graefes Archive for Clinical and Experimental Ophthalmology, 255*(1), 189–195. doi:10.100700417-016-3529-1 PMID:27796670

Syed, Z. (2021). *Hyphema*. Academy of Ophthalmology. EyeWiki. Retrieved from eyewiki.aao.org/Hyphema

System Vision. (n.d.). *PlusoptiX A12R & A12C*. Retrieved on September 28, 2021, from http://www.systemvision.eu/plusoptix-a12c-a12r.html

Tannen, B., & Ciuffreda, K. J. (1997). A proposed addition to the standard protocol for the Visagraph II™ eye movement recording system. *Journal of Behavioral Optometry, 18*(6), 143–147.

Tannen, B., Darner, R., Ciuffreda, K. J., Shelley-Tremblay, J., & Rogers, J. (2015). Vision and reading deficits in post-concussion patients: A retrospective analysis. *Vision Development and Rehabilitation, 1*(3), 206–213.

Tarczy-Hornoch, K., Lin, J., Deneen, J., Cotter, S. A., Azen, S. P., Borchert, M. S., Wang, Y., Varma, R., & Multi-Ethnic Pediatric Eye Disease Study Group (2008). Stereoacuity testability in African-American and Hispanic pre-school children. *Optometry and Vision Science: Official Publication of the American Academy of Optometry, 85*(3), 158–163. https://doi.org/ doi:10.1097/OPX.0b013e3181643ea7

Tassinari, J. T., & DeLand, P. (2005). Developmental eye movement test: Reliability and symptomology. *Optometry (St. Louis, Mo.), 76*(7), 387–399. doi:10.1016/j.optm.2005.05.006 PMID:16038866

Taub, M. B. (2012). Comprehensive examination procedures. In M. B. Taub, M. Bartuccio, & D. M. Maino (Eds.), *Vision diagnosis and care of the patient with special needs* (pp. 155–183). Wolters Kluwer Health/Lippincott Williams & Wilkins.

Taub, M. B., & Shallo-Hoffmann, J. (2012). A comparison of three clinical tests of accommodation to Hofstetter's norms to guide diagnosis and treatment. *Optometry and Vision Development*.

Timberlake, G. T., & Kennedy, M. (2005). The Direct Ophthalmoscope How it Works and How to Use It. In *The Direct Ophthalmoscope How it Works and How to Use It* (pp. 1–35). University of Kansas. https://web.media.mit.edu/~raskar/Eye/TheDirectOphthalmoscope.pdf

Tjark, B. J., Dorman, J. C., Valentine, V. D., Munce, T. A., Thompson, P. A., Kindt, S. L., & Bergeron, M. F. (2013). Comparison and utility of King Devick and ImPACT® composite scores in adolescent concussion patients. *Journal of the Neurological Sciences*, *334*(1-2), 148–153. doi:10.1016/j.jns.2013.08.015 PMID:24007870

Topical Antibiotics. (2009). *Review of Optometry.* https://www.reviewofoptometry.com/article/topical-antibiotics

Turbert, D. (2020). Vision Development: Childhood. *American Academy of Ophthalmology.* https://www.aao.org/eye-health/tips-prevention/children-vision-development

U.S. Food and Drug Administration. (2019). *Pediatric medical devices.* https://www.fda.gov/medical-devices/products-and-medical-procedures/pediatric-medical-devices

US Preventive Services Task Force. (2011). Vision screening for children 1 to 5 years of age: US Preventive Services Task Force Recommendation Statement. American Academy of Pediatrics, 127(2), 340–346. doi:10.1542/peds.2010-3177

Van den Broek, E. G. C., Janssen, C. G. C., Van Ramshorst, T., & Deen, L. (2006). Visual impairments in people with severe and profound multiple disabilities; an inventory of visual functioning. *Journal of Intellectual Disability Research*, *50*(6), 470–475. doi:10.1111/j.1365-2788.2006.00804.x PMID:16672040

Van Herick, W., Shaffer, R. N., & Schwartz, A. (1969). Estimation of width of angle of anterior chamber. Incidence and significance of the narrow angle. *American Journal of Ophthalmology*, *68*(4), 626–629. doi:10.1016/0002-9394(69)91241-0 PMID:5344324

Van Hof-van Duin, J., Cioni, G., Bertuccelli, B., Fazzi, B., Romano, C., & Boldrini, A. (1998). Visual outcome at 5 years of newborn infants at risk of cerebral visual impairment. *Developmental Medicine and Child Neurology*, *40*, 302–309. PMID:9630257

Van Staden, D., Noor Mahomed, F., Govender, S., Lengisi, L., Singh, B., & Aboobaker, O. (2018). Comparing the validity of an online Ishihara colour vision test to the traditional Ishihara handbook in a South African university population. African Vision and Eye Health, 77(1). doi:10.4102/aveh.v77i1.370

Vasudevan, B., Esposito, C., Peterson, C., Coronado, C., & Ciuffreda, K. J. (2014). Under-correction of human myopia—is it myopigenic?: A retrospective analysis of clinical refraction data. *Journal of Optometry*, *7*(3), 147–152. doi:10.1016/j.optom.2013.12.007 PMID:25000870

Vision in Preschoolers Study. (2005). Preschool vision screening tests administered by nurse screeners compared with lay screeners in the vision in preschoolers study. *Investigative Ophthalmology & Visual Science, 46*(8), 2639-2648. doi:10.1167/iovs.05-0141

Volk Optical. (2021a). *90D.* https://www.volk.com/collections/slit-lamp-lens/products/slit-lamp-lens-non-contact-90d

Volk Optical. (2021b). *78D.* https://www.volk.com/collections/slit-lamp-lens/products/slit-lamp-non-contact-78d

von Noorden, G. K., & Campos, E. C. (2002). *Binocular Vision and Ocular Motility: Theory and Management of Strabismus* (6th ed.). Mosby, Inc.

Walker, K. H., Hall, D. W., & Hurst, W. J. (1990). *Clinical Methods: The History, Physical and Laboratory Examinations* (3rd ed.). Butterworth-Heinemann.

Wallace, D. K. (2005). Tests of fixation preference for amblyopia. *The American Orthoptic Journal, 55*(1), 76–81. doi:10.3368/aoj.55.1.76 PMID:21149113

Walline, J. J., Walker, M. K., Mutti, D. O., Jones-Jordan, L. A., Sinnott, L. T., Giannoni, A. G., Bickle, K. M., Schulle, K. L., Nixon, A., Pierce, G. E., Berntsen, D. A., & Group, B. S. (2020). Effect of High Add Power, Medium Add Power, or Single-Vision Contact Lenses on Myopia Progression in Children: The BLINK Randomized Clinical Trial. *Journal of the American Medical Association, 324*(6), 571–580. doi:10.1001/jama.2020.10834 PMID:32780139

Wan, L., Wei, C. C., Chen, C. S., Chang, C. Y., Lin, C. J., Chen, J. J., Tien, P. T., & Lin, H. J. (2018). The Synergistic Effects of Orthokeratology and Atropine in Slowing the Progression of Myopia. *Journal of Clinical Medicine, 7*(9), 259. Advance online publication. doi:10.3390/jcm7090259 PMID:30205439

Warburg, M. (1994). Visual impairment among people with developmental delay. *Journal of Intellectual Disability Research, 38*(4), 423–432. doi:10.1111/j.1365-2788.1994.tb00421.x PMID:7949793

Weakley, D. R. Jr. (2001). The association between nonstrabismic anisometropia, amblyopia, and subnormal binocularity. *Ophthalmology, 108*(1), 163–171. doi:10.1016/S0161-6420(00)00425-5 PMID:11150283

Webber, A. L., & Wood, J. (2005). Amblyopia: Prevalence, natural history, functional effects and treatment. *Clinical & Experimental Optometry, 88*(6), 365–375. doi:10.1111/j.1444-0938.2005.tb05102.x PMID:16329744

Weinstein, J. M., Zweifel, T. J., & Thompson, H. S. (1980). Congenital Horner's syndrome. *Archives of Ophthalmology, 98*(6), 1074–1078. doi:10.1001/archopht.1980.01020031064011 PMID:7387512

Welch Allyn. (2013). *PanOptic Ophthalmoscope Brochure.* Retrieved September 27, 2021, from https://www.canmed-healthcare.com/parent/WelchAllyn_PanOptic_Ophthalmoscope.pdf

Welch Allyn. (2018). *Spot® Vision Screener-Autorefractor.* Retrieved on September 28, 2021, from https://www.hillrom.com/en/products/spot-vision-screener-autorefractor/

Wickum, S. M., & Amos, J. F. (2008). Cycloplegic Refraction. In Clinical Ocular Pharmacology 5th Edition (pp.344-346). Butterworth Heinmann Elsevier. doi:10.1016/B978-0-7506-7576-5.50026-4

Wild, J. M., Ahn, H. S., Baulac, M., Bursztyn, J., Chiron, C., Gandolfo, E., Safran, A. B., Schiefer, U., & Perucca, E. (2007). Vigabatrin and epilepsy: Lessons learned. *Epilepsia, 48*(7), 1318–1327. doi:10.1111/j.1528-1167.2007.01133.x PMID:17635558

Wong, A. M. (2007). *Eye movement disorders.* Oxford University Press.

World Health Organization. (2021). *Adolescent Health.* https://www.who.int/health-topics/adolescent-health#tab=tab_1

Wright, K. W., Sami, D., Thompson, L., Ramanathan, R., Joseph, R., & Farzavandi, S. (2006). A Physiologic reduced oxygen protocol decreases the incidence of threshold retinopathy of prematurity. *Transactions of the American Ophthalmological Society, 104*, 78–84. PMID:17471328

Wright, K. W., Walonker, F., & Edelman, P. (1981). 10-Diopter fixation test for amblyopia. *Archives of Ophthalmology, 99*(7), 1242–1246. doi:10.1001/archopht.1981.03930020116012 PMID:7259597

Wu, L. J., You, Q. S., Duan, J. L., Luo, Y. X., Liu, L. J., Li, X., Gao, Q., Zhu, H. P., He, Y., Xu, L., Jonas, J. B., Wang, W., & Guo, X. H. (2015). Prevalence and associated factors of myopia in high-school students in Beijing. *PLoS One, 10*(3), e0120764. doi:10.1371/journal.pone.0120764 PMID:25803875

Wu, P. C., Chen, C. T., Lin, K. K., Sun, C. C., Kuo, C. N., Huang, H. M., Poon, Y. C., Yang, M. L., Chen, C. Y., Huang, J. C., Wu, P. C., Yang, I. H., Yu, H. J., Fang, P. C., Tsai, C. L., Chiou, S. T., & Yang, Y. H. (2018). Myopia Prevention and Outdoor Light Intensity in a School-Based Cluster Randomized Trial. *Ophthalmology, 125*(8), 1239–1250. doi:10.1016/j.ophtha.2017.12.011 PMID:29371008

Wu, P. C., Tsai, C. L., Wu, H. L., Yang, Y. H., & Kuo, H. K. (2013). Outdoor activity during class recess reduces myopia onset and progression in school children. *Ophthalmology, 120*(5), 1080–1085. doi:10.1016/j.ophtha.2012.11.009 PMID:23462271

Wu, X., Gao, G., Jin, J., Hua, W., Tao, L., Xu, S., & Tao, F. (2016). Housing type and myopia: The mediating role of parental myopia. *BMC Ophthalmology, 16*(1), 151. doi:10.118612886-016-0324-z PMID:27580859

Xiang, F., He, M., & Morgan, I. G. (2012). The impact of parental myopia on myopia in Chinese children: Population-based evidence. *Optometry and Vision Science, 89*(10), 1487–1496. doi:10.1097/OPX.0b013e31826912e0 PMID:22922777

Xiong, S., Sankaridurg, P., Naduvilath, T., Zang, J., Zou, H., Zhu, J., Lv, M., He, X., & Xu, X. (2017). Time spent in outdoor activities in relation to myopia prevention and control: A meta-analysis and systematic review. *Acta Ophthalmologica, 95*(6), 551–566. doi:10.1111/aos.13403 PMID:28251836

Yam, J. C., Li, F. F., Zhang, X., Tang, S. M., Yip, B. H. K., Kam, K. W., Ko, S. T., Young, A. L., Tham, C. C., Chen, L. J., & Pang, C. P. (2020). Two-Year Clinical Trial of the Low-Concentration Atropine for Myopia Progression (LAMP) Study: Phase 2 Report. *Ophthalmology, 127*(7), 910–919. doi:10.1016/j.ophtha.2019.12.011 PMID:32019700

Zadnik, K., Sinnott, L. T., Cotter, S. A., Jones-Jordan, L. A., Kleinstein, R. N., Manny, R. E., Twelker, J. D., & Mutti, D. O. (2015). Prediction of Juvenile-Onset Myopia. *JAMA Ophthalmology, 133*(6), 683–689. doi:10.1001/jamaophthalmol.2015.0471 PMID:25837970

Zellers, J. A., Alpert, T. L., & Rouse, M. W. (1984). A review of the literature and a normative study of accommodative facility. *Journal of the American Optometric Association, 55*(1), 31–37. PMID:6699343

Zeppieri, M., & Johnson, C. A. (2008). *Frequency Doubling Technology (FDT) Perimetry.* Imaging and Perimetry Society. Retrieved October 17, 2021, from http://webeye.ophth.uiowa.edu/ips/perimetryhistory/FDP/

Zhang, X., Qu, X., & Zhou, X. (2015). Association between parental myopia and the risk of myopia in a child. *Experimental and Therapeutic Medicine, 9*(6), 2420–2428. doi:10.3892/etm.2015.2415 PMID:26136998

Zhou, W. J., Zhang, Y. Y., Li, H., Wu, Y. F., Xu, J., Lv, S., Li, G., Liu, S. C., & Song, S. F. (2016). Five-Year Progression of Refractive Errors and Incidence of Myopia in School-Aged Children in Western China. *Journal of Epidemiology, 26*(7), 386–395. doi:10.2188/jea.JE20140258 PMID:26875599

About the Contributors

Lily Zhu-Tam graduated from SUNY College of Optometry and completed her residency program at Salus University in pediatric and binocular vision. Thereafter, she joined the faculty at SUNY College of Optometry as an Assistant Clinical Professor. She was then promoted to Director of the Optometry Residency Program at the Bronx Care Health System. Where she was the co-founder of the Primary Care and Ocular Disease Residency Program for advance clinical training at the hospital and the creator of the on-call program for optometry residents in the hospital's emergency department. Later she created the first Pediatric Optometry Clinic for Mt. Sinai at Queens General Hospital. She has published clinical articles, lectured at CE classes and was an active research examiner in the Convergence Insufficiency Treatment Trial, a national randomized multi-center trial sponsored by the National Eye Institute. Along with her decade of academic experience, she also has experience working as the medical director of a multi-office private practice. Given her academic and clinical experiences combined with her passion for pediatrics, it has led her to become the founder of Citywide Eye Care.

Ida Chung is the Associate Dean of Academic Affairs and associate professor of optometry at Western University of Health Sciences in Pomona, CA. She received her Bachelor of Science in Biology from Cornell University in 1989, her Doctor of Optometry from the SUNY College of Optometry in 1993 and completed a residency in pediatrics and binocular vision at the Pennsylvania College of Optometry in 1994. Dr. Chung obtained her fellowship in developmental vision and vision therapy from the College of Optometrists in Vision Development (COVD) in 1996 and became a fellow of the American Academy of Optometry in 2001. She taught for 19 years at the SUNY College of Optometry where she served as Chief of Pediatrics at the Eye Care Institute and a vision consultant for various community agencies. Dr. Chung is currently serving as the President of the California Optometric Association, is past president of COVD, and served on the executive board of the New York State Optometric Association. She is a principal investigator for the Pediatric Eye Disease Investigator Group with research interest in the areas of pediatric vision care. Dr. Chung has published extensively and is a frequent invited lecturer to practicing optometrists both domestically and internationally.

* * *

Surbhi Bansal graduated from The New England College of Optometry in 2012 and completed the Dr. Irwin B. Suchoff Residency in Vision Therapy and Rehabilitation at the SUNY College of Optometry in New York in 2013. Dr. Bansal provides neuro-optometric rehabilitation services to patients post-traumatic brain injury and specialty contact lenses for infants, toddlers, and pediatric patients at the Byers Eye Institute at Stanford University. Dr. Bansal participates in clinical research in the areas of traumatic brain injury, vision development, and is a clinical investigator for the Pediatric Eye Disease Investigative Group (PEDIG). She previously held positions as an Assistant Clinical Professor at UC Berkeley School of Optometry and Nova Southeastern College of Optometry. She has residency training in pediatrics, binocular vision, and vision therapy/rehabilitation.

Olivia Bass was born and raised in Miami, FL. She attended Florida State University where she graduated cum laude with a Bachelor of Science in Chemical Science and a minor in Environmental Science. She then graduated as salutatorian from the New England College of Optometry in Boston, MA after completing clinical training at Veterans Affairs Hudson Valley Health Care System, Open Cities Health Center in St. Paul, MN, Eye Centers of South Florida, and Yukon-Kuskokwim Health Corporation in Bethel, AK. She was an active member of the Public Health Club and conducted research regarding eye care for the homeless population of Boston. She completed a residency in Pediatric Optometry/ Ocular Disease residency at BronxCare Health System in the Bronx, NY. She is currently an attending optometrist at Fromer Eye Centers, USA. Dr. Bass' interests include fitting pediatric specialty contact lenses, the treatment of strabismic, refractive and deprivational amblyopia, refractive and non-refractive forms of strabismus, binocular vision disorders, and pediatric and adult ocular- and neuro-pathology.

M. H. Esther Han specializes in neuro-optometric rehabilitation. She is a full-time Associate Clinical Professor at the SUNY College of Optometry and the Residency Program Supervisor for the Neuro-Optometric Rehabilitation Residency. Dr. Han received her Bachelor of Arts in Neurobiology and Behavior from Cornell University in 1995. She earned her Doctor of Optometry degree from the SUNY College of Optometry in 2001 and subsequently completed a Residency in Vision Therapy and Rehabilitation at the SUNY College of Optometry in 2002. Dr. Han was a member of the COVD International Exam and Certification Board (IECB) from 2014-2021 and a board member for the Eastern States Optometric Congress (ESOC) from 2013-2021. Dr. Han is well-published in the areas of vision therapy and neuro-optometric rehabilitation. She has lectured domestically and internationally in the areas of neuro-optometric rehabilitation, optometric vision therapy, and Visual Snow Syndrome management.

Joy Harewood is a graduate of University of Toronto, Trinity College, and of the UC Berkeley School of Optometry. She completed a residency in ocular disease at the State University of New York (SUNY) College of Optometry, achieved Fellowship of the American Academy of Optometry and is a Diplomate in the American Board of Optometry. She has extensive experience in hospital-based eye care and was the first fulltime optometrist performing inpatient consults at Northwell Health's Staten Island University Hospital. Dr. Harewood then worked as a faculty member in the Department of Ophthalmology at BronxCare Health System. There, she taught optometry and ophthalmology residents in a clinical and didactic setting, and provided direct patient care. She was a panelist in the highly regarded "Race in Optometry' series in the summer of 2020 and currently serves on the UC Berkeley Optometry Council for Diversity, Equity, Inclusion and Belonging (DEIB). She is currently the inaugural Director for Diversity, Equity, Inclusion and Belonging at SUNY College of Optometry, and an Associate Clinical Professor.

Brandon Johnson is a board-certified ophthalmologist, member of the American Society of Retina Specialists, and member of the American Academy of Ophthalmology. He graduated from Haverford College Magna Cum Laude, where he double majored in Biology and Music. He then received his Doctor of Medicine from the Perelman School of Medicine at the University of Pennsylvania, a top three medical school, where he was awarded for outstanding research. After a one-year internship in general surgery at the Hospital of the University of Pennsylvania, Dr. Johnson completed an ophthalmology residency at the Wills Eye Institute in Philadelphia, which has been ranked the best ophthalmology residency program in the United States. He then completed a fellowship in vitroretinal surgery at the prestigious Emory University in Atlanta, Georgia. Dr. Johnson's outside passions include music. He is a classically trained pianist and a member of the New York Choral Society.

Kristen Kerber is an Associate Professor at the New England College of Optometry (NECO). She graduated from NECO in 2016 with both her Doctorate of Optometry and Master of Science in Vision Science. She then went on to complete her residency in Pediatric Optometry at NECO for which she earned the Terrance N. Ingraham Pediatric Optometry Residency Award. Dr. Kerber joined faculty in the Specialty and Advanced Care department at NECO in 2017 where she teaches and conducts research. She is the attending pediatric optometrist at the Dimock Community Health Center where she precepts 2nd, 3rd and 4th year optometry students as well as the community health optometry resident. She is a fellow of the American Academy of Optometry. Dr. Kerber's research interests include myopia control, refractive error development and pediatric vision screening.

Alanna Khattar is a graduate of Southern College of Optometry. She completed her Primary Eye Care/Ocular Disease residency at Bronx-Lebanon Hospital Center and has been practicing hospital based optometry since the completion of her residency. She joined BronxCare Health System (formerly Bronx-Lebanon Hospital Center) as a faculty member after her residency, and is now Co-Supervisor of the Ocular Disease/Primary Care Optometry Residency Program. Dr. Khattar is also an attending for the Pediatric/Ocular Disease Residency Program at BronxCare Health System. She provides comprehensive eye care with a concentration in ocular disease in a multidisciplinary setting. Dr. Khattar holds an appointment as an Adjunct Assistant Clinical Professor at SUNY College of Optometry. She is a Fellow of the American Academy of Optometry, a Diplomate of the American Board of Optometry and a member of the American Optometric Association and the New York State Optometric Association.

Jacky Kong is a pediatric optometrist and holds a faculty position at the New England College of Optometry. Dr. Kong is a fellow of the American Academy of Optometry. His research and clinical interests include amblyopia, strabismus, binocular vision, visual field assessment in children, and functional vision assessment in children with special needs. During Dr. Kong's research on visual fields in children, he developed an LED based device which uses variable flicker frequencies and illumination to capture and map out gross fields of vision in children with special needs. These devices have been donated to and is currently being used at the Perkins School for the Blind in Watertown, MA. Dr. Kong is the founder of the New England College of Optometry Lions Club chapter and actively participates in community-based vision screening with Boston Chinatown Lions Club. Under sponsorship of FADCANIC and Williams College, Dr. Kong had an opportunity to spend time doing humanitarian work in Nicaragua, including the Rama Cay island where he gave eye exams and dispensed donated glasses to the people in need. Dr. Kong has also spent time in Bogotá, Columbia doing humanitarian work for VOSH.

Danielle Ledoux is a board-certified ophthalmologist, member of the American Association of Pediatric Ophthalmology and Strabismus, and a member of the American Academy of Ophthalmology. She graduated from Cornell University with Distinction in All Subjects, with a major in Biology in Society with a focus on Women's Health. She received her Doctor of Medicine from Emory University and completed a medical internship at the University of Massachusetts. She completed an ophthalmology residency at New York University/Manhattan Eye Ear and Throat Hospital and a pediatric ophthalmology fellowship at the Medical University of South Carolina. She has an appointment at Harvard University as a clinical instructor and works part-time at Boston Children's Hospital. She also founded a private practice in Massachusetts, Specialized Pediatric Eye Care, that provides comprehensive eye care (medical and surgical) to the pediatric population of New England as well as adults with developmental delays and adults who suffer from strabismus and double vision.

Iason Mantagos graduated from the Boston University School of Medicine. He completed a residency in Ophthalmology at Boston Medical Center - Boston University prior to completing a fellowship in Pediatric Ophthalmology and Adult Strabismus at Boston Children's Hospital - Harvard Medical School. He completed his PhD at the University of Patras in Greece, with a thesis on the ophthalmologic manifestations of Progeria. Dr. Mantagos is an Assistant Professor of Ophthalmology at Harvard Medical School and the Fellowship Director for Pediatric Ophthalmology and Adult Strabismus at Boston Children's Hospital. His clinical expertise is pediatric cataract surgery, adult and pediatric strabismus, retinopathy of prematurity and Stevens-Johnson syndrome. Dr. Mantagos has more than 30 peer-reviewed publications and has received multiple awards for his teaching and research.

Siva Meiyeppen graduated from the University of British Columbia and received her Doctor of Optometry from the Illinois College of Optometry. She completed a residency at Salus University in Pediatrics and Binocular vision. She is currently an assistant professor in the Pediatrics and Binocular Vision Service at Salus University. She teaches clinically as well as in Binocular Vision, Acquired Brain Injury, and Advanced Studies courses. She has lectured nationally and internationally on strabismus and pediatric optometry. She has a special interest in binocular vision, concussion, and vision therapy.

Issac Moradi graduated from the SUNY Downstate Medical Center College of Medicine in 1995. Dr. Moradi completed his residency at Stony Brook University Hospital and his fellowship in vitreoretinal disease and surgery in 2001. He is a surgical retinal specialist who is affiliated with Bronx Lebanon Hospital Center, Brookdale University Hospital Medical Center, Montefiore Medical Center, Montefiore Medical Center Einstein Campus, Montefiore Wakefield Campus and New York Eye & Ear Infirmary of Mount Sinai.

Amy Moy is the Director of the New England College of Optometry's Health Center Network and Chief Clinical Compliance Officer. She has been a laboratory instructor and lectures nationally on Infection Control for Optometry. Dr. Moy was the Director of Optometry for 15 years at the Martha Eliot Health Center, a multi-disciplinary health center affiliated with Boston Children's Hospital, where she continues to clinically precept optometry students and provides comprehensive eye care to patients of all ages. Dr. Moy is a Fellow of the American Academy of Optometry and is a member of the American Optometric Association and the Massachusetts Society of Optometrists. She earned her OD degree from The New England College of Optometry in 2003 and completed a residency at the Bedford VA Medical Center in primary eye care and geriatric optometry with an emphasis on ocular disease. Dr. Moy's clinical specialty area is ocular disease and community health. She has been the principal investigator in the "Boston Latino Eye Study", a collaborative project between Martha Eliot Health Center and Dimock Community Health Center. She is also passionate about providing vision care access to those with disabilities. She has been involved in developing eye care social stories for children with disabilities as part of the Resources, Education, Access for Children with Disabilities (READ) grant.

Ruth Shoge received her Doctor of Optometry degree from the Pennsylvania College of Optometry, where she also completed a residency in Pediatrics and Vision Therapy. She is currently the Director of Diversity, Equity, Inclusion, and Belonging (DEIB) at the University of California Berkeley Herbert Wertheim School of Optometry and Vision Science. She received her Master of Public Health from Temple University with a concentration in Social and Behavioral Science. During that time, she developed a special interest in better understanding how to reduce health disparities and improve health outcomes in minority populations. Dr. Shoge has been involved in several DEIB initiatives, including bias awareness and cultural competency training, recruitment and retention strategies, and curriculum reform. She also started her own consulting company, RYS Consultants, to create strategic plans and workshops for academic and corporate settings, practitioners, and student members of the optometric community. Dr. Shoge's clinical interests include pediatric primary care, binocular vision disorders, vision disorders related to traumatic brain injury, and vision therapy. In the clinical setting, Dr. Shoge aims to provide and model clinical competence and cultural humility to her students as they care for their patients. She has served as an investigator in several federally funded research studies and has had the opportunity to present nationally and internationally about binocular vision, vision therapy, the management of concussion-related vision disorders, clinical cultural competency, and humility training.

Sarah Singh is an Assistant Clinical Professor at the School of Optometry at the University of California at Berkeley. She is a "Berkeley Lifer," having received her Bachelor's Degree in Molecular and Cell Biology, her Doctorate of Optometry, her Pediatrics & Primary Care Residency Certificate, and her PhD all from UC Berkeley. Her time as an instructor is divided into teaching the first-year ocular anatomy course as well as clinical instruction in the myopia control and pediatrics clinics, and conducting research in myopia and refractive error. She loves living in the Bay Area and exploring all it has to offer with her husband and two dogs.

Gayathri Srinivasan is an Associate Professor of Optometry in the Specialty and Advanced Care Department at the New England College of Optometry (NECO). She is the Instructor of Record for the Binocular Vision and Accommodative Anomalies course and is the Director of the Pediatric Special Programs. She is the attending pediatric optometrist at the Codman Square Health Center and NECO Center for Eye Care at Commonwealth. Dr. Srinivasan earned a Bachelor of Science degree in optometry from Elite School of Optometry (India) in 2005. After practicing for a brief period in India, she received a Master's of Science in Physiological Optics from the University of Missouri-St. Louis College of Optometry in 2009, followed by receiving her Doctor of Optometry from NECO in 2011, and completing a residency in pediatric optometry in 2012.

Marilyn Vricella is an Associate Clinical Professor at the State University of New York (SUNY) College of Optometry. She received her Doctor of Optometry from SUNY College of Optometry. Dr. Vricella completed her residency in Pediatrics and Infant Vision at SUNY College of Optometry before joining the College as a faculty member and received her fellowship from the College of Optometrists in Vision Development. Dr. Vricella is the pediatric optometry residency supervisor and she is an attending pediatric optometrist in the Barbara Saltzman Center for Pediatric Eye Care in the University Eye Center. Some of her other roles include being the Principal Investigator for the Pediatric Eye Disease Investigator Group, and serving as the liaison for the American Optometric Association Faculty and Student Membership. She has lectured both nationally and internationally in the areas of pediatrics and binocular vision and has numerous professional publications.

Index

D

E

F

G

H

I

J

K

L

M

N

O

P

R

S

www.ingramcontent.com/pod-product-compliance
Lightning Source LLC
LaVergne TN
LVHW060300011026
849161LV00011B/2742